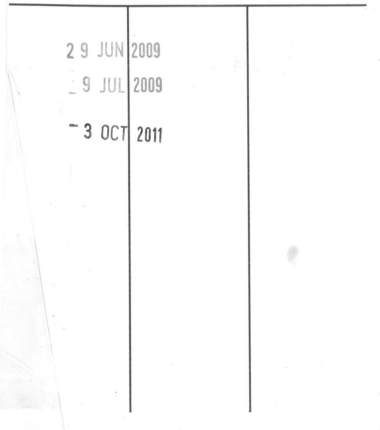

CHURCHILL'S POCKETBOOK OF
Psychiatry

Dedicated to
My late father and mother who both died young and
my little Haris

R.Z.

Commissioning Editor: Michael Parkinson
Project Development Manager: Siân Jarman
Design Direction: Erik Bigland
Project Manager: Frances Affleck

CHURCHILL'S POCKETBOOK OF
Psychiatry

Rashid Zaman

BSc (Hons) MBBChir (Cantab) DGM MRCGP MRCPsych
Lecturer and Honorary Specialist Registrar
Division of Neuroscience and Psychological Medicine
Imperial College School of Medicine
London

Akmal Makhdum

MBBS CavMed DPM MRCPsych
Consultant Psychiatrist
Lead Consultant and Chairman, Division of Psychiatry (East Suffolk)
Local Health Partnership NHS Trust
Ipswich

CHURCHILL LIVINGSTONE

EDINBURGH LONDON NEW YORK OXFORD PHILADELPHIA
ST LOUIS SYDNEY TORONTO 2000

CHURCHILL LIVINGSTONE
An imprint of Elsevier Limited

First published 2000
    Reprinted 2004, 2006, 2007

ISBN 978 0 443 05979 7

British Library Cataloguing in Publication Data
A catalogue record for this book is available from the British Library

Library of Congress Cataloguing in Publication Data
A catalogue record for this book is available from the Library of Congress

Note
Medical knowledge is constantly changing. As new information becomes
available, changes in treatment, procedures, equipment and the use of drugs
become necessary. The author, contributor and the publishers have, as far as
it is possible, taken care to ensure that the information given in this text is
accurate and up to date. However, readers are strongly advised to confirm
that the information, especially with regard to drug usage, complies with the
latest legislation and standards of practice.

ELSEVIER   your source for books,
           journals and multimedia
           in the health sciences
www.elsevierhealth.com

Working together to grow
libraries in developing countries

www.elsevier.com | www.bookaid.org | www.sabre.org

ELSEVIER   BOOK AID
           International   Sabre Foundation

The
publisher's
policy is to use
**paper manufactured
from sustainable forests**

Printed in China

Preface

As a new trainee in psychiatry you may arrive with preconceived ideas, some apprehension and you may even be somewhat mystified with what the practice of this speciality is about, despite exposure during undergraduate training. Practice of psychiatry is not a soft option, nor is it totally unscientific and requiring no organization of thinking by the practitioner. On the contrary, it is an established discipline within the field of medicine and continues to build upon its scientific foundations. It remains challenging both intellectually and emotionally.

The aim of this book is to provide practical guidance, reduce the excessive amount of anxiety (you will still need some for optimal performance; remember the Yerkes–Dodson law) and bewilderment and the tendency to continually turn to one's seniors for answers (though we do not wish to totally discourage this either). It is mainly aimed at new trainees in psychiatry, whether they wish to specialize in the discipline or gain short experience. Those involved in teaching will also find it useful, as will general practitioners, casualty officers, medical students and practitioners of other specialities.

The information in this book is as up-to-date and accurate as possible; however, psychiatric practice continues to change and evolve and this is especially true for drug treatments. If you are in doubt, you are advised to consult your senior colleagues or consultant and a recent reference source.

In addition, we have tried to be as clear and concise as possible. However, like practice of medicine, psychiatry is a science as well as an art. Therefore, do not be surprised by the differences you may encounter in the practice of psychiatry. Your aim should be to enjoy, learn and gain sufficient experience in the practice of psychiatry, which should not only be conventional and effective but also safe. We wish you the best in your endeavour, whether it is to gain short-term experience in psychiatry or to go on to complete full training, and eventually practice as a specialist. Hopefully the gains will far outweigh the pains!

We wish to thank our patients, past teachers, colleagues and students who have given us inspiration and ideas for this book. Amongst those we wish to thank for the support and advice include, N. Arzenton, G. Barroso, V. Excell (secretarial work), M. Mahoney (secretarial work), A. Malaspina, K. Murray, B.B. Pedersen, B.K. Puri, I.H. Treasaden and S.H. Zaman. Finally we would like to thank the publishing staff involved in the production of this book, especially S. Jarman and M. Parkinson for their support and enduring patience.

September 2000   R.Z.
                                                                   A.M.

Contents

1. Training and the job   *1*
The training and career in
   psychiatry   *2*
The job   *7*
Multidisciplinary team   *18*
Planning for discharge   *28*

2. Psychiatric assessment   *31*
History taking   *32*
The Mental State Examination
   (MSE)   *43*
Mini Mental State Examination
   (MMSE)   *51*
Physical examination   *54*

3. Specific psychiatric disorders   *71*
Anorexia and bulimia nervosa   *72*
Anxiety disorders   *76*
Bipolar affective disorder   *83*
Depressive disorders   *87*
Personality disorders   *91*
Schizophrenia   *99*

**4. Pharmacotherapy and other
   treatments**   *105*
Pharmacotherapy   *106*
Pharmacology   *118*
Specific psychiatric disorders:
   drug treatments and
   some management issues   *121*
Other physical treatments   *191*
Future treatment methods in
   psychiatry   *199*

5. Psychological treatments   *201*
Assessment for psychotherapy   *202*

Counselling   *203*
The holistic view   *204*
Cognitive therapy   *205*
Behavioural psychotherapy   *206*
Other therapies   *208*
Psychological treatments for
   alcohol-related addiction/
   dependence disorders   *211*

**6. Psychiatric emergencies
   and their management**   *213*
Emergency assessment and
   admission   *216*
Dealing with psychiatric
   emergencies   *217*
Specific psychiatric
   emergencies   *220*
Drugs-related (including
   alcohol) psychiatric
   emergencies   *249*
Substance withdrawal   *259*
Lithium toxicity   *262*
Serotonin syndrome   *264*
Hypertensive crisis due to
   MAOIs   *264*
Antidopaminergics:
   acute side effects   *265*
Neuroleptic malignant
   syndrome   *267*
Other possible medical
   problems on psychiatric
   wards   *270*

**7. Legal issues and the Mental
   Health Act**   *271*
Nominated deputies   *272*

Definitions in the Mental
  Health Act 1983   272
Civil sections   273
Assessment of patients   277
Forensic sections   278
Hospital orders (Section 37)   281
Mental Health Act
  Commission   282
Mental Health Review
  Tribunal   282
Other legal issues   284
Writing a psychiatric report   287
Mental health legislation in
  Scotland   293
Mental health legislation in
  Northern Ireland   294

Mental health legislation in
  Eire   295
Legislation in the USA,
  Canada, Australia and
  New Zealand   296

Appendices   299
  Descriptive psychopathology   300
  Classification in psychiatric
    practice: ICD-10 and
    DSM-IV   311

Glossary   317

Useful addresses   325

Index   329

CHAPTER 1

TRAINING AND THE JOB

The training and career in psychiatry 2

The job 7

Multidisciplinary team 18

Planning for discharge 28

THE TRAINING AND CAREER IN PSYCHIATRY

The training for specialization in psychiatry in the UK is reasonably well structured and fairly tightly regulated.

During the basic specialist training the psychiatric trainee is advised to achieve the following:

- Gain supervised clinical experience from recommended clinical psychiatric specialties. This should include sufficient experience at managing a variety of psychiatric patients, presenting at ward rounds and carrying out on-call emergency work
- Receive regular one-to-one supervision from his or her consultant/ supervisor
- Attend recommended courses such as those held for MRCPsych examinations
- Pass Parts I and II of MRCPsych examinations
- Carry out psychotherapy under supervision (at least with one patient)
- Take part in research, and publish if at all possible.

In general the specialist training in psychiatry in the UK is divided into *basic* and *higher*.

BASIC SPECIALIST TRAINING

The basic specialist training consists of a number of senior house officer posts (in some cases it will still include pre-Calman registrars who may have passed Part I of the MRCPsych examination). These posts usually include general adult psychiatry, psychiatry of old age, and a number of other subspecialist posts, such as liaison psychiatry, learning disability, forensic psychiatry, child psychiatry, etc. Usually if the trainee is part of one specific training scheme they are likely to change posts every 6–9 months. Changing may also involve moving from one hospital/NHS Mental Health Trust to another which is participating in that training scheme. Some training schemes (such as The Maudsley Hospital training scheme, London) include pure research posts and even the participation of private hospitals, with occasional periods in other training schemes offering more specialized jobs.

The usual period for a basic training scheme is around 3 years, during which it is expected that the trainee will pass Parts I and II of the MRCPsych (Membership of the Royal College of Psychiatrists). It is then usual for the trainee to apply for a specialist registrar (SpR) post (previously known as Senior Registrars).

HIGHER SPECIALIST PSYCHIATRIC TRAINING/SPECIALIST REGISTRAR (SpR) TRAINING

The period of SpR (previously known as senior registrar) training, also known as higher specialist training in psychiatry, usually lasts 3 years. If individuals wish to pursue an academic higher training they may apply for a lecturers' post in an academic department, in such case the higher training lasts 4 years and the lecturer 'trainee' usually holds an honorary contract (Hon. SpR) with a specific Mental Health NHS Trust/hospital.

Currently, a typical SpR's weekly time-table is divided into six clinical sessions, two sessions for special interest and two for research (note each session represents a half day) whilst a lecturer/Hon SpR's time-table differs by having two clinical sessions replaced by two extra sessions for research.

The academic responsibility usually means organizing/teaching of medical students and postgraduate trainees (pre-membership trainees), or helping their professors or senior lecturers. Many lecturers register for a higher degree such as MD or PhD especially, if they have the opportunity to do in-depth original research. Yet another route into higher training is as a research fellow, where the trainee is likely to be carrying out a specific research project. Again this may be registered as a higher degree, such as MD or PhD. Furthermore, if there is sufficient time the higher trainee may continue various honorary clinical posts made up of 1–4 sessions. The length of clinical training may last 4–6 years, depending on the number of clinical sessions carried out.

The SpR trainee may choose to train in either a single or a dual speciality, e.g. adult and old age. Training for the latter lasts 4 years. Training may also be in one of a number of subspecialties, e.g. old age, child psychiatry, psychotherapy, learning disabilities, forensic psychiatry, etc.

At the end of a satisfactory higher specialist training, a certificate in completion (CCST) is issued to the higher trainee, which enables them to register and work as a specialist/consultant in Britain.

Some common subspecialties in psychiatry

Child psychiatry
Community psychiatry
Old-age psychiatry (psychogeriatrics)
Forensic psychiatry
Liaison psychiatry
Substance misuse psychiatry
Learning disability

RESPONSIBLE MEDICAL OFFICER (RMO)/CONSULTANT

The patients cared for by the trainee psychiatrist will have a responsible medical officer (RMO), who will usually be a consultant psychiatrist in overall charge of provision of psychiatric care. The RMO is also likely to be responsible for your supervision and training.

The RMO's clinical duties include:

- Being in charge of the provision of psychiatric care for specific patients (inpatient, outpatient), leading ward rounds, carrying out outpatient clinics
- Dealing with the legal issues affecting the patient being treated involuntarily, such as recommending for or discharging from a section, recommending leave (e.g. signing leave papers), guiding junior psychiatrists in clinical matters
- Attending meetings relating to clinical matters.

SUPERVISION OF PSYCHIATRIC TRAINING

A number of senior psychiatrists are likely to be involved in the supervision of your training: it is essential that you keep regular contact with them and turn to them for advice regarding your training.

TRAINER/CONSULTANT

This is your immediate boss during the period of your particular psychiatric post. It is essential that you receive weekly 1-hour, one-to-one supervision sessions, which should be used to discuss various issues such as your performance and any difficulties that you may have encountered. Clinical issues of educational value may also be discussed; other matters that may also be brought up include your professional development, examinations and career issues.

TUTOR FOR THE TRAINING SCHEME

The training scheme tutor usually meets each trainee during certain periods of the training (e.g. before changing posts), discussing overall performance and moves to specific posts within the training scheme. The tutor may also be responsible for approving attendance at courses.

GENERAL PRACTICE (GP) TRAINEES

In the UK the general practice training scheme (also known as vocational training) usually consists of 2 years of a number of suitable hospital posts and a year spent in a general practice as a GP registrar.

The 2 years of hospital work consist mainly of four 6-monthly posts, such as accident and emergency, paediatrics, elderly medicine, psychiatry, obstetrics and gynaecology, or another relevant specialty post.

Many training schemes include psychiatry as a 6-month post, but those making up their own training scheme may also opt for psychiatry as one of the 6-monthly posts. During the psychiatry post the GP trainee usually works alongside the career trainees and essentially does the same work during the placement. However, a different emphasis is usually placed upon the structure of the training: while the career trainee concentrates on longer-term specialist training needs, such as passing the MRCPsych examinations and research, the GP trainee is best advised to learn about those aspects of psychiatry that will allow him or her to deal with psychiatric issues in a GP setting more effectively, aiming to broaden his or her experience and learning to differentiate between the psychiatric illnesses that could effectively be managed in the GP setting from those that need specialist treatment/management.

In addition, the GP trainee should consider the following issues during their psychiatry post:

- Learn about common psychiatric illnesses and basic psychopathology
- Gain experience regarding drugs commonly used in psychiatry
- Gaining and improving upon interviewing and history-taking skills
- How to deal with difficult patients
- Gain experience about common psychiatric emergencies, e.g. threats of suicide
- When to refer to a specialist psychiatric service, and when not to
- The appropriate and useful information that should accompany an outpatient referral to the psychiatrist and other members of the multidisciplinary team (MDT)
- How to make the best use of other members of the multidisciplinary team (CPNs, social workers, psychologists, etc.)
- How to look after psychiatric patients in collaboration with hospital specialists
- What services are available for people with psychiatric illness, and how to access them.

OVERSEAS TRAINEES/DOCTORS

Doctors who trained outside the UK and EU face certain restrictions with regard to work and training in the UK.

Many overseas doctors come to Britain to take up SHO/registrar posts: some, if they are appropriately qualified and satisfy certain criteria, may be appointed to permanent posts such as staff grade and consultant. However, most return to their respective home countries to carry on their psychiatric work. There are also specific posts which are under the aegis of the overseas doctors training scheme (ODTS) of the Royal College of Psychiatrists.

After the Calman reforms training was divided into types I and II: type I is for British and EU trainees who are accorded the certificate of completion of specialist training, the CCST, after successful completion of approved training. For type II training approved posts are specifically allocated to overseas trainees, who are either brought under the ODTS or through consultant sponsorship through the Royal College of Psychiatrists. These trainees are not automatically granted the CCST but are expected to return to their respective countries. There are moves to change this because the CCST is considered a relevant document in the home countries, certifying the quality of the trainees' education.

The MRCPsych is recognized in many countries, especially in New Zealand, Australia, Canada, most of the Asian countries and in Africa. There is reciprocal recognition of training between the USA and the UK from year to year, but UK trainees have to take the evaluation examinations of the USA or Canada.

The Royal College of Psychiatrists runs various workshops and induction courses for overseas trainees, specifically for those who have come to the UK through the ODTS.

The ODTS is for those doctors who have completed approximately 5 years of psychiatric training in their own countries many of whom will have acquired diplomas and postgraduate degrees. They are sponsored by one of their consultants, who should be a member or a fellow of the Royal College of Psychiatrists. The Royal College processes their application, and the GMC then evaluates their experience with a view to granting limited registration. Once their application is approved they are slotted, first come first served, into various posts made available to the ODTS.

ODTS has matured as a scheme and the problems encountered by the earlier trainees seldom occur: most of them are now dealt with by the employing NHS Trusts, with the help of the ODTS department of the Royal College of Psychiatrists.

OTHER TRAINEES

Occasionally there are doctors from other specialties (e.g. neurology) who may wish to gain experience in psychiatry; in UK this is certainly possible with some training schemes. Opportunities also exist for doctors to take part in specifically designed part-time training schemes, which of course last considerably longer.

THE JOB

The first psychiatric post for a junior doctor cannot be described as an easy option. Most of you should have been through the house officers' posts and will know that, although physically demanding and arduous, these jobs are usually well supervised. Yet at the start of your first psychiatric post not only are you required to deal with different and sometimes bewildering psychiatric problems, you are also expected to advise others.

Although in theory you are supervised the reality may be that the supervision takes the form of a telephone consultation, or at a later stage, during ward rounds or formal supervision sessions. If you are lucky the seniors will be proactive in teaching and supervision, but more often than not it is you who will have to seek it out. Variations of course do occur. However, fortunately the requirements for both trainees and trainers are reasonably formalized and regularly assessed by the Royal College of Psychiatrists for accreditation purposes. Another difficult aspect of a psychiatric post is the extra emotional pressure you may face. This too will need to be addressed, and many training schemes encourage trainees to deal with these issues with the help of a named supervisor, who may be a local psychotherapist or the trainee's supervisor/trainer.

Adaptation into psychiatric training may be less painful for a relatively newly qualified doctor but may prove far more difficult for those who come armed with experience, and even qualifications, from other branches of medicine.

Some of the difficult aspects that the new trainees in psychiatry must adapt to include:

- The ability to work in a multidisciplinary setting where sometimes hierarchy and responsibilities become rather blurred
- Ward rounds which may seem to go on for ever and appear to be a lot less structured
- The patients coming to the ward rounds, instead of the doctor going to them
- Having to deal with a seemingly bewildering number of professionals involved in the care of the patient
- The apparently slow pace at which assessments seem to take place
- The blurring of diagnostic categories
- Changes in diagnostic labels for a particular patient with the progression of time (see Box).

Remember that a number of major revisions of diagnostic categories have taken place over the years. Although the **specificity** of psychiatric diagnoses has improved, little progress has been made with regard to their **validity**.

Psychiatric disorders/syndromes generally consist of groups of abnormal symptoms and behaviours that deviate significantly from the norm.

In psychiatry a diagnosis is mainly based on an accurate history (which sometimes has to be obtained over a longer period) and currently there are no laboratory tests available to confirm most psychiatric diagnoses. Often, a psychiatrist has to build a case using factors for and against a certain preferred diagnostic category.

Many patients will have more than one diagnosis, and it has become fashionable to use terms such as **dual diagnosis** (in cases of drugs and alcohol abuse) and **comorbidity** (e.g. with personality disorders).

- Unavailability of (or difficulty in obtaining) some physical investigation that is commonly used in non-psychiatric branches of medicine
- Too often a shortage of nurses trained to carry out common physical observations
- Communication difficulties, which may be due partly to the greater number of professionals involved in the care of the patient
- Sometimes it may appear that clarity of thinking, instruction and leadership behaviour is discouraged, and this may even result in a certain amount of confusion and communication difficulties with other colleagues
- Learning to deal with the apparently greater sensitivity of some non-medical (and sometimes medical) colleagues. Little is gained by adopting a superior attitude because of your medical qualifications
- Acquiring a greater knowledge of your patients by talking to non-medical colleagues, such as ward nurses, community psychiatric nurses, social workers, occupational therapists and care workers.

RESPONSIBILITIES AND CLINICAL TASKS OF THE JUNIOR TRAINEE

Although this is a training job and your aim is to learn and gain experience, nevertheless, certain clinical tasks are expected of you. Overall you are expected to help the patient to recover by helping the clinical team in charge of their care. The team is usually consultant led and he or she is likely to be your boss, as well as responsible for your supervision and writing your references.

Your responsibilities include:

- Medical and psychiatric care of the inpatient under the care of your clinical team
- Carrying out admission clerking. If the patient was admitted and initially clerked by a colleague, then to add further relevant history, examinations and assessments

- Collect the necessary patient information from all available sources (e.g. previous psychiatric contacts, nursing staff, GPs and relatives)
- Carry out the necessary medical examination and investigations; refer further if necessary
- Record changes in mental state/symptomatology in the case notes, and keep these up to date
- Institute relevant treatment, e.g. drug treatment, usually under the guidance of senior colleagues
- Write and rewrite drug charts
- Inform nursing colleagues regarding levels of observation/monitoring
- Arrange for referral to members of the multidisciplinary team, such as social workers, occupational therapists, day hospital staff, etc.
- If a detained patient appeals, you may have to prepare reports and attend tribunal meetings (see later)
- Attend care programme approach (CPA) meetings and record proceedings (see page 29)
- Attend ward rounds; present the patient's case and record the proceedings in the notes
- Provide consultation (telephone advice) and attend the patient if needed, e.g. if requested by nursing colleagues
- Deal with medical and psychiatric problems as they occur
- Meet and keep patients' friends and relatives appropriately informed
- Refer for 'super specialist'/second opinion if necessary (for example, treatment-resistant schizophrenia, patient with forensic problems, difficult to treat eating disorders, personality disorders and specialized psychotherapy referrals)
- Begin discharge arrangements as necessary, e.g. Section 117 meetings for detained patients, CPA meetings
- Prepare summaries, both admission and discharge; (Part I/Part II; see examples)
- Communicate effectively with GPs and other professionals.

When the patient is discharged:
- Provide discharge medication prescription
- Discharge letter for the GP
- Ensure that after-care arrangements, such as visits by the CPNs, social workers and outpatient clinic visits, are organized
- Provide or arrange follow-up in outpatient clinics.

Other duties include:
- Attend the day hospital, including the ward rounds
- Attend the outpatient clinics for new and returning patients
- Attend multidisciplinary team meetings if required to do so
- In some jobs community visits may be required
- When on duty, attend casualty and other wards to provide psychiatric consultation/assessments and advice accordingly

- Take part in on-call rota out of hours as well as the normal working hours
- Hand over the care of newly admitted patients to colleagues if appropriate
- In some circumstances it might be worth attending various therapy groups involving your patients, such as those run in the day hospital
- Many trainees are expected to take on at least one psychotherapy patient under supervision for the duration of their post, or longer in some cases.

ORGANIZATIONAL SKILLS

So that you can help your patients effectively and keep your colleagues happy, as well as minimizing the stress on yourself, you will need to have good organizational skills.

Remember it is impossible to please everyone!

Intellectual capabilities, good clinical skills, diagnostic mastery and the knowledge of psychiatry may be not be enough should your organizational and communication skills fail. Being ahead of the game, able to foresee what information will be needed, as well as keeping everyone (including your patient) satisfied can be somewhat difficult, but you should attempt to do your best.

Successful time management remains the cornerstone of good organizational skills

Remember:

- Tasks usually take longer than you think
- It is better to start small and build up, i.e. be realistic
- Pacing yourself usually helps
- Be realistic about what you can do and achieve.

Organizational skills/tasks can be improved: the following may help:

- Identify key persons with whom you need to communicate effectively
- Keep essential names and contact numbers handy: a personal organizer may be useful for this purpose
- Advise and instruct your colleagues, e.g. nursing staff, in a polite and friendly manner
- Write regularly in the patient's case notes. Entries should be clear and concise and should include the current clinical state of the patient (e.g. relevant aspects of the Mental State Examination), the necessary ongoing information regarding their care, and the treatment plans. Alterations in drug treatment should be clearly laid out, and it also helps to explain the reasoning behind the changes
- Instructions regarding observations and monitoring should be clearly communicated to the key nursing staff, as well as recorded in the notes

- Do not forget your hard-working secretarial staff, who are essential to the smooth running of the team: working closely and on the best terms with them will ease your efforts to become organized
- Devise methods of **prioritizing** the non-clinical work and administrative tasks, such as responding to letters, preparing reports and summaries etc.
- Set aside regular time for administrative work
- Your timetable and contactability (e.g. how and when and where) should be available to your secretary as well as relevant colleagues
- Occasionally it may be advantageous to let your secretary answer your bleep/phone to allow you to deal with important tasks undisturbed
- Keep your own diary; it may also be helpful to use a personal organizer for meetings, appointment dates, etc.
- Endeavour to arrange both your annual and study leave well in advance. Also ensure that cover is arranged during your absence and the covering doctor has been well briefed, so that you don't return to find an unfinished pile of work waiting for you
- Seek and use feedback from colleagues to constantly review and update your organizational skills and working methods
- Learning **assertiveness skills** is likely to be helpful. For example, if you said 'yes' to everything that you are asked to do you will soon find yourself overwhelmed. Sometimes it is not easy or appropriate to say a flat no: better instead to use some assertive techniques that will allow you time to think, e.g. 'I will check in my diary and get back to you' (in 5 minutes, 2 hours, next day, or whenever appropriate); 'Can I think about this?'; 'I may need to gather information', or 'I will need to consult with my senior colleagues'
- Attendance on time and other management skills courses may be also be valuable.

Constantly review your working methods to see if further improvements can be made.

WARD WORK

In a general psychiatric hospital post you are likely to spend a fair amount of time on the wards, taking part in ward rounds and assessing, reassessing and examining patients. It is essential that you not only familiarize yourself with the layout of the wards, but also attempt to understand the ward ethos (running and functioning of the ward) as early as possible during your new post.

On your first day make sure that you have the opportunity to spend time with the senior and experienced ward staff, i.e. charge nurse and ward manager. It may also be helpful to talk to a less senior staff member who has been around for a lengthy period.

Ensure that the following are discussed:

- You are taken through the layout of the ward, such as patients' bed areas, patients' meeting rooms, doctors' assessment/interview/examination room, nursing station, and where the ward rounds are held
- Safety and security arrangements are clearly explained
- Emergency procedures are understood
- Observation policies are explained. For example, make sure you understand what the ward staff mean by level I, level II and general observations
- You are introduced to, or initially at least told about, the key staff on the ward
- Each psychiatric unit or ward has its own way of working, and although it may be somewhat difficult to learn it all on your very first day, this issue should clearly be explored
- The times of nursing staff 'handovers'
- Mutually preferred times for daily information exchange between the charge nurse and yourself regarding current inpatients. Many staff prefer to do this first thing in the morning, so that events of the previous night can be discussed
- Policy regarding seclusion: is there a seclusion room on the ward or elsewhere?
- Documentation policy, regarding incidents such as falls, minor injuries, patients going absent without leave (AWOL) etc.
- The number of beds and type of patients on the ward, e.g. whether severely disturbed, with forensic problems or treatment resistant
- It will be helpful for the staff if they are given your availability timetable. This should be clearly displayed in the nursing station, with your contact bleep number. This will hopefully reduce the number of intrusive and non-essential calls (bleeps) to you.

> **Many of you will have patients in your care on more than one ward, as well as having responsibility for some patients attending the day hospital. The advice given here may be appropriate and can still apply in these circumstances.**

CLERKING PATIENTS (FOR DETAILS SEE PATIENT ASSESSMENT, CHAPTER 2)

Essentially this involves the psychiatric and medical evaluation of patients, as well as recording this information in the case notes. It is important that this is done as thoroughly as possible within the constraints of time and circumstances. Occasionally further information will need to be obtained from other sources, such as previous psychiatric notes, GP or relatives.

Clerking in psychiatry is usually completed with a physical examination and few relevant physical investigations, such as urine drug screening, haematological and biochemical measures. This information must be accurately recorded in the case notes and the details should be clear, relevant and legible. You must also ensure that the details of any further investigations are recorded. The preferred as well as the differential diagnosis should also be entered in the case notes where possible.

It is often helpful to record the reasoning behind your preferred and differential diagnostic categories, and this must be followed by a clear and concise management plan. This should include the biological and psychosocial aspects of treatment, and outline any further information that needs to be obtained, such as any treatment already commenced, other drugs in use, and observations needed both at the initial and later stages of admission. Finally, all recordings should be clearly dated, with your signature, name and position, in addition to your contact or bleep numbers.

WARD ROUNDS

Variations exist among psychiatric units and consultants as to how ward rounds are conducted, as well as what is expected from the new trainee. Your aim should be not only to try and establish your role and what is expected from you, but also to turn the ward round into a learning experience.

Psychiatric ward rounds may appear quite different from the conventional medical and surgical ward rounds and can be divided as follows.

MAJOR WARD ROUNDS

These usually occur once a week and apply to all inpatients. Most of the multidisciplinary team (MDT) members attend, as well as medical students, a variety of visiting workers and relatives. Most patients are discussed and many are actually seen/reviewed. However, some consultants prefer to discuss the patient's care first and then see them individually later, in the presence of fewer people, e.g. a nurse and the house officer (i.e. you). Following discussions, decisions regarding investigations, referral to other professionals, drugs and psychobehavioural treatments, leave and discharge arrangements are made. Some wards may also include sessions for CPA and Section 117 meetings. The time taken depends upon a number of factors and may vary from 2 to 4 hours. There may be variations as to how active and involved a new trainee psychiatrist is expected to be. What is certain is that you will have to record, accurately and concisely, the relevant points made during the ward round, such as the patient's clinical state, treatment changes and future plans.

MANAGEMENT WARD ROUNDS

Sometimes referred to as 'mini' ward rounds, these are much more brisk and business-like and may be taken by the senior/specialist registrar. They are in general short, lasting approximately 1 hour, and are usually much more focused. Not all patients are discussed and the emphasis tends to be on acutely ill patients and whatever urgent decisions need to be made regarding investigations, treatment changes, patient leaves, and sometimes discharges.

DAY HOSPITAL WARD ROUNDS

In many units these are conducted by occupational therapists or specific day hospital staff, with the consultant and house officer in attendance. The aim is to keep the medical team aware of the patient's progress as well as assessing the need for medical intervention or changes in medication. Often the day hospital staff keep their own notes and the OT will usually record relevant points or changes made at the end of the ward round.

'NIGHT ROUNDS'

It is highly likely that during your training you will be required to take part in out-of-hours on-call duty. Generally this means being available for consultations on both the medical side (i.e. casualty and other general wards) and the psychiatric wards. However, the likelihood of disturbed sleep will be relatively small compared to your previous posts, and there are always ways of minimizing the chance of being called out unnecessarily (see below). Try to discuss with the day nursing staff any concerns they might have and the need to complete any outstanding tasks before your departure. You should also try to make sure that this information is passed on to the night staff taking over. It might be useful to carry out a short night round of all the psychiatric wards, late in the evening.

Prior to your departure you should ensure the following:

- Drug charts are up to date
- Any emergency medication likely to be required is considered and prescribed if essential or clinically indicated
- Patient leave arrangements are clear
- Patients expected to return from leave have done so, and if not, what should be done about it (in the case of detained patients who break leave arrangements the police are often informed and involved)
- Any instructions (e.g. level of observations) concerning a particular patient are clear and well communicated
- Any urgent reviews have been carried out.

DAY HOSPITAL

The day hospital plays an integral part in modern psychiatric treatment and attendance is determined by:

- The psychiatric needs of the patient
- Diagnostic labels
- Social circumstances (social support availability)
- Range of services offered.

A well staffed and efficiently run day hospital may act as a halfway house, either prior to discharge or following discharge from an acute ward.

Non-medical professionals working in the day hospital

- Occupational therapists (OTs)
- Nursing staff
- Art and drama therapists
- Various other professionals, e.g. music therapists
- Psychologist/psychotherapist
- Counsellors

The range of services offered may include

- Occupational therapy
- Specialized training programmes, such as assertiveness training
- Various psychobehavioural treatments, either individual or group therapies
- Drug treatments
- ECT

PSYCHIATRIC SERVICES

Psychiatric care has developed considerably and continues to evolve. As well as providing the basic hospital wards, rehabilitation wards, outpatient clinics and day hospital facilities, psychiatric units also provide or have available a variety of different services.

Some of these include:

- Community-based multidisciplinary teams
- Crisis intervention teams
- 'On-call' community psychiatric nurses (CPNs)
- Out-of-hours services consisting of a doctor, nurse and social worker
- Emergency psychiatric clinics during normal hours
- Drug dependency centres/clinics.

Other services that may have a connection with the psychiatric service include:

- Telephone helplines
- Self-help groups
- Support hostels/group homes for the mentally ill
- Supervised living quarters
- Outreach teams/intensive home treatment teams
- Social services
- Housing services
- Many other voluntary organizations, such as Alcoholics Anonymous (AA), womens' centres, agencies catering for the needs of ethnic minorities or special groups.

The list continues to expand and evolve.

OUTPATIENT CLINICS

Psychiatric outpatient clinics differ from the usual general medical clinics in a number of ways. In the early days you may find yourself sitting in the clinic, or being supervised closely by senior colleagues. The clinic may be in psychiatric unit premises or run in a community setting. Some clinics are solely for the new referrals, whereas others cater for new referrals as well as returning patients.

You are quite likely to inherit the caseload of your predecessor.

When reviewing returning patients, and in order to do your job effectively, the following procedures may be useful:

- Before seeing the patient read through the most recent letters, relevant previous correspondence and summaries
- Introduce yourself and explain to the patient that you have now taken over from his or her previous doctor, and explain how long you will be staying in your present post
- Establish from the patient what they know of their diagnosis, plus current and previous treatments
- Avoid making sudden or drastic changes to established treatments
- Make a point of exploring other diagnostic and treatment possibilities that may have been missed by previous doctors
- Most returning patients are seen for 15–30 minutes every 4–6 weeks, depending on the clinic and their clinical needs.

NEW REFERRALS

On average you are likely to see one or two new patients in each clinic and, as previously stated, during the initial stages you are likely to be supervised fairly closely. Further into your job, you will be allowed to assess a patient over a period of an hour, and then confer with your senior (who is also likely to be running a clinic at the same time) to discuss diagnostic and management options.

Before you start your assessment, take advantage of all sources of information, such as the referring letter and previous correspondence. Initially you are likely to use the standard (and possibly more rigid) method of history-taking and carrying out a mental state examination (described in Chapter 2), but as you gain in experience you may modify this according to the clinical situation and type of patient.

At the end of the assessment, and having discussed it with your senior colleague, you will need to explain to the patient what their difficulties may be and how you propose to help them. Occasionally an urgent admission may be justified. However, the usual course of action, depending upon the findings, is outpatient management. This may involve:

- Further investigations
- Instigation of appropriate treatment (drugs or psychobehavioural, or even both)
- Referral to other colleagues, day hospital or psychology department
- Further reviews at later dates (4–6 weeks)
- Discharge back to the GP if appropriate.

EMERGENCY PSYCHIATRIC CLINICS

Some units, like the Maudsley Hospital (London) run fairly comprehensive clinics (24 hours), whereas others, such as Charing Cross Hospital (London) have emergency psychiatric clinics available only during normal working hours. Such clinics are open to self-referral but will also accept emergency referrals from GPs and other health-care professionals. They are usually conducted in a multidisciplinary setting and the assessments are usually carried out by a duty psychiatrist, psychiatric nurse and social worker.

Initially many trainee psychiatrists find it difficult to assess/interview the patient in the presence of a nurse and/or social worker. Some may even consider that their authority and competence are being undermined, especially if these colleagues are senior and more experienced. However, you must not allow these feelings to affect your judgement and professionalism, and do remember that you bear a greater responsibility for the clinical needs of the patient, as well as a legal responsibility. No non-medical person should (or is likely to) interfere with your medical or psychiatric treatment, especially if it involves the use of drugs.

Depending on clinical needs and social circumstances it may be worth starting treatment and providing regular review while the patient is waiting to be seen by a particular sector psychiatric team.

One sensible way to deal with your uncertainties is to learn from experienced colleagues such as nurses and social workers. In this way you will soon adapt, and may even enjoy working with the different professionals. You will also find your working experiences richer and more likely to bear fruit. Collaboration with colleagues is also the most effective way of reducing the stresses you are likely to encounter when dealing with psychiatric patients.

Another advantage of working in a multidisciplinary setting is that the non-psychiatric/non-medical issues are more easily and usually immediately dealt with by social workers and nurses.

YOUR ROLE IN THE EMERGENCY CLINIC

- If your unit has one of these clinics, you may be expected to work there for one or two sessions per week
- Aim to be reasonably brief but thorough, and do not waste time with the trivia of a particular problem
- In many instances you may have to provide a psychiatric screening service, and those requiring urgent treatment will need to be referred to colleagues working in the wards or clinics
- With regard to self-referrals, always make sure the GP is informed of the decision and treatment given
- Provide drug treatment, whether initiating it, changing or continuing
- Arrange further reviews, by yourself (or colleagues), in the emergency psychiatric/outpatient clinic
- Discharge back to the GP if appropriate.

MULTIDISCIPLINARY TEAM

In the UK, the following individuals may be members of the MDT (or attend the MDT meetings):

Medical staff

- Senior house officers (SHOs)
- Registrars (being phased out under Calman reforms)
- Specialist registrars (SpRs), previously known as senior registrars (SRs)
- Lecturers, research fellows
- Clinical assistant (part-time and full-time), GPs employed for sessions in psychiatry
- Associate specialists
- Consultant, senior lecturers, readers, professors.

Non-medical staff

- Psychiatric nurses (ward managers, charge nurses, staff nurses)
- Community psychiatric nurses (CPNs)
- Student nurses (general and psychiatric)
- Nursing assistants (previously known as auxiliaries)
- Locum/agency nursing staff
- Occupational therapists
- Psychologists
- Other therapists (art, drama, etc.)
- Social workers (case workers)
- Mental Health Act coordinators (e.g. for Section 117 meetings, managers' hearing, tribunal hearing)
- Organizer and arranger of CPAs
- Voluntary workers
- Secretarial staff.

Some visitors to MDT meetings may include:

- Patients' advocates
- Other specialist workers who may be involved and attend, e.g. ward rounds
- Care workers
- Probation officers
- Drugs and alcohol workers
- Members of voluntary agencies such as MIND, or specialist ethnic groups
- Translators
- Voluntary workers
- Medical/nursing/social work students.

You are likely to encounter the members of the multidisciplinary team (MDT) on your induction day. The role of the team, the specific staff members and their seniority level may vary within each psychiatric unit. As psychiatric patients use and depend upon non-medical services heavily, the smooth and effective functioning of each MDT cannot be overemphasized.

Many psychiatric units run weekly MDT meetings during which the following may be discussed:

- Minutes of a previous meeting
- Outcomes of previous assessments
- New referrals and their allocations to which team member
- OPD arrangements, plus community visit arrangements
- CPA arrangements
- Business matters.

Legally the consultant carries the ultimate clinical responsibility for the patient, which is quite distinct from either leadership or chairmanship of the MDT. The chairmanship may be fixed, or rotate among the more senior members.

Many MDTs have secretarial staff in attendance to take minutes and deal with administrative issues, such as outpatient appointments, community visits and CPA dates.

The team is most likely to function effectively if each member has a clearly defined role which is respected and appreciated. The leader or chairman should ensure that all the tasks are clearly communicated and assigned, and that the cohesiveness of the team is maintained. The development of individual members, as well as the team as a whole, should be fostered and encouraged.

> With regard to your particular role as a new psychiatric trainee in the MDT, it is essential that you take the time to meet and get to know the key members, particularly those with whom you will have regular dealings. It is very also important to observe and learn the working dynamics of the team. You should try to clarify your role and the tasks that are required of you fairly early on in your post.

Your tasks as a member of the MDT may include:

- Reporting back the outcomes of previous assessments that need to be discussed
- Taking on a referral for the outpatient clinic
- Signing of drug charts for CPNs
- Making yourself available for CPA meetings
- Carrying out joint community visits with other MDT members (if required).

PSYCHIATRIC NURSING STAFF

The role of the psychiatric nurse is broad and variable. Unfortunately, the level of contact with the patient seems to follow an inverse relationship with seniority: in other words, the more senior the nurse the less patient contact there appears to be.

You may notice that psychiatric nurses have greater autonomy than their general medical colleagues, playing a more active role in ward rounds and MDT meetings, such as presenting a patient's clinical progress and expressing management views. A typical example of the latter are comments and views regarding leave arrangements for detained patients. You may feel the nursing staff almost take over your role on occasions: do not resent this, but aim to foster a relationship with your nursing colleagues that will promote an active and appropriate role for you in the care of the patient.

Many psychiatric nurses have had a general nursing training and will happily perform basic physical nursing procedures. However, **do not** expect them to monitor i.v. lines or perform ECGs etc. **Do** make sure that the nursing staff are both willing and able to undertake physical procedures such as measuring of temperature, blood pressure and monitoring of fluid charts.

The various roles of the psychiatric nurse include:

- Promotion of mental health
- Monitoring of mental state/health
- Observations of patients, particularly those acutely ill
- Listening, providing support, guidance and reassurance
- At times act to restrict the movement and freedom of patients, such as those being detained. Occasionally act to control a violent patient
- Dispense and monitor drug treatments
- Some will have to act as primary nurse, run support/patient groups and provide supportive psychotherapy and counselling, while others (those trained) provide more specialized forms of psychotherapy
- Provide regularly patient updates for the medical staff
- Contact the duty doctor if necessary
- Take part in ward rounds and MDT meetings.

Specific nursing staff

The following is a guide to the nursing hierarchy and structure, which continues to evolve.

Title	Role/job
Student nurse (general and mental)	To learn; assist others in monitoring and observing patients. The time spent listening to patients is often therapeutic
Nursing assistant	To carry out patient care under the direction of a charge nurse
Staff nurse (RMN)	Act as primary nurse. More senior, likely to take charge of the ward
Charge nurse/sister	Supervise staff and other nurses
Senior charge nurse/sister	Continuous responsibility for ward/caseload
Nurse manager	Responsible for a number of wards and their non-medical staff
Clinical nurse specialist	Senior clinical nurse in specialist area who advises and teaches others

In the UK a registered mental nurse (RMN) is a nurse who has completed either a 3-year training in psychiatric nursing or an 18-month psychiatric nursing training following qualification as registered general nurse (RGN)

- Management of non-medical staff and wards, depending on their seniority; this role is often undertaken by a ward manager or nurse manager
- In an emergency a qualified nurse can exercise a 6-hour nurse holding power under Section 5(4) of the Mental Health Act (1983). He or she may 'prevent an informal inpatient receiving medical treatment for a mental disorder, from leaving the hospital for up to 6 hours, or until a doctor arrives, whichever is the earlier' (MHA 1983)
- Convey to detained patients, their rights and status under the MHA.

SOCIAL WORKERS

Social workers do not just sort out housing and arrange bus passes, but in fact do a very difficult job. Their role is to identify personal, social and environmental difficulties that are affecting patients adversely. Social workers are usually employed by the local authority. By law, a detained patient has the right to a social worker.

Some of the roles of psychiatric social workers include:

- Making the patient (or client, as they tend to refer to them) aware of various community resources, or lack of
- Acquiring and passing on knowledge of voluntary and neighbourhood organizations and community groups
- Providing guidance on how to go about obtaining
  — Social security claims benefits
  — A range of welfare benefits, e.g. disability living allowance (DLA)
  — Housing and rehousing
- Making other members of the MDT, as well as the patient (if appropriate), aware of how social factors can exacerbate the patient's mental illness
- Acting as case worker/key worker, in the case of a patient under a Care Programme Approach (CPA)
- Attending CPA meetings
- Attending ward rounds and MDT meetings.

Many social workers have had the training to provide a wide range of specialized psychotherapies, or to run therapeutic groups.

| Note | Note: Approved social workers (ASW) are involved in mental health assessments. This means organizing and helping to carry out assessments, as well as seeking out Section 12-approved psychiatrists for those being evaluated for detention under the Mental Health Act. |

OCCUPATIONAL THERAPIST

The role of the occupational therapist (OT) in illness (mental or otherwise) has long been recognized. The World Federation of Occupational Therapists defines occupational therapy as a treatment of physical and psychiatric conditions through specific activities in order to help people reach their maximum level of function and independence in all aspects of daily life.

Occupational therapists play an important role in the treatment of a psychiatric patient, whether they are an inpatient, an outpatient (e.g. attending a day hospital) or in a community setting. As such they are an important member of the MDT and may act as key worker (as part of CPA), as well as carrying out joint assessments with other members of the team, including the doctor.

The OT's involvement usually begins as the patient's mental state begins to improve, e.g. following an episode of acute psychosis. Their role is to provide a skilled programme of daily activities for all patients under their care, tailored to each patient's personality, background, habits, likes and dislikes, psychological problems and diagnosis, including medication. This knowledge is acquired by a careful assessment of the patient, by the use of formalized questionnaires, as well as a psychiatric summary from the referrer, usually the psychiatric trainee. Many referrals take place during ward rounds and MDT meetings, but many OTs prefer to gather information regarding their patients from personal contact with the team members.

The OT assesses the patient by looking at all the important aspects of that individual's life. She is likely to explore areas of daily living (activities of daily living, ADL), work and leisure, identify the patient's strengths, areas of difficulty, likes and dislikes, choices and lifestyle. In other words, the aim is to obtain a holistic view of the patient in terms of capabilities during the current illness, and whether these require further investigation and/or treatment.

Patients are specifically helped with their psychological problems by assessing their response to work and by breaking down the components of a particular task.

Patients with severe mental illnesses may be allocated specific tasks designed to alleviate their symptoms. For example, depressives may be helped with self-confidence; the anxious may be taught anxiety management; and hypomanics may be shown ways of channelling aggression and excitement creatively. Imaginative interests and tasks may help reduce apathy, and the psychotic may be shown ways of distracting themselves from delusions and hallucinations.

A wide variety of therapeutic programmes based on domestic life, games and vocational training are also provided. Many OTs work alongside, or use, specialist teachers providing, for example, art and music therapy. Some also take part in providing group psychotherapy and structured social retraining schemes.

Most OTs in a psychiatric setting work in, and run, day hospitals composed of those who are either currently inpatients or who attend on an outpatient basis. A number of patients may have been referred from the community, e.g. by a GP.

Your role is to provide medical/psychiatric support for patients undergoing occupational therapy, usually in the day hospital setting.

You may be required to help the OT in the following ways:

- Provide referrals and medical/psychiatric summaries
- Carry out an initial medical/psychiatric assessment
- Ensure that the necessary drugs are prescribed and drug charts kept up-to-date
- Attend to medical/psychiatric needs, including any emergencies that may arise
- You may have to make medical entries in the OT's day hospital case notes
- Attend day hospital ward rounds
- Keep the GP informed, e.g. with discharge letters
- Educate/inform OTs regarding any relevant medical/psychiatric disabilities patients may have.

In many psychiatric units the trainees follow up their own patients (i.e. those under their firm/MDT) throughout the occupational therapy/day hospital attendance, whereas in others the trainee will have specified sessions for the day hospital and may be medically responsible for *all* the patients attending, both as inpatient and as outpatient.

ART THERAPIST

Art therapists use different media to gain a reflection of patients' thoughts and the issues they brings to the art therapy session. The relationship is one of partnership, trying to understand the art process and the product that comes out of that session.

Art therapists use:	
A Personal statements	art as medium
B Focus of discussion	patient's expression through art
C Analysis of the above	denied, suppressed, erased thoughts
D Self-evaluation	psychotherapeutic approach

In the art therapy session the therapist tries to see thoughts that have been consciously denied, erased or suppressed and which are reflected in the art work. Transference which develops during the art work also plays an important role. Some prefer to call it art psychotherapy.

Art therapists may work with individuals or groups:

- Patients who are admitted to hospital for psychiatric treatment can be referred (usually in the day hospital)
- Adults and children with learning disabilities
- Individuals in prisons, or on probation
- Individuals who feel distressed and could be helped by art therapy
- Emotional and behavioural disturbances in children is a specific area where art therapy is often found to be helpful
- Children with autistic disorder: in trying to understand their perceptions, the acute distress and symbolism may be processed through art therapy.

Most referral's to art therapist are self-referrals or are made by non-medical staff (e.g. nurses and OTs).

CLINICAL PSYCHOLOGIST

Clinical psychologists are most closely connected with mental health care and form an integral part of the multidisciplinary psychiatric team. However, they also work in GP practices, in general medical settings, in the care of the elderly and dying, and in HIV/AIDS services, as well as in social service settings. Some work in specialized services, such as forensic psychiatry. They have an important role in the multidisciplinary team, investigating, assessing and providing treatment for psychological and behavioural disorders.

ROLE OF THE CLINICAL PSYCHOLOGIST IN MENTAL HEALTH SETTINGS

The clinical psychologist contributes to both inpatient and outpatient services, and some even act as key worker for patients under a CPA. Their role can be broadly divided into assessment and treatment.

ASSESSMENT

This means assessing the patient's suitability for whatever psychological treatment is on offer from that particular department. Patients are usually asked to complete a brief questionnaire before the assessment visit.

Other specialist assessment skills include:

- Intelligence testing
- Personality assessments
- Neuropsychological assessment, especially for those suspected of brain damage/dementia.

Psychologists also provide professional reports on patients for civil or forensic purposes.

TREATMENT

Clinical psychologists provide a number of treatment programmes for wide-ranging psychiatric, psychological and behavioural disorders. The treatments offered will usually reflect their interests and training, but most tend to favour a behavioural and cognitive approach. However, some do practise other psychotherapeutic treatments, and many provide supervision for cognitive behaviour treatment groups.

The following disorders may be treated by psychologists, on both an inpatient and an outpatient basis, and either solely or in conjunction with traditional psychiatric treatments.

- Neurotic disorders such as anxiety disorders, various phobias, and obsessive–compulsive disorders
- Depressive disorders, especially when there are suicidal thoughts, self-esteem problems and guilt
- Adjustment disorders, bereavement and loss
- Anger management/control and relationship difficulties
- Assertiveness techniques
- Adjustment to physical illness
- Adjustment/adaptation to organic disorders such as dementia and head injuries (dealing with disabilities as a result of medical conditions)
- Behavioural/habit disorders
- Eating disorders
- Personality disorders
- Post-traumatic stress disorder
- Psychosis – adjusting to/living with treatment-resistant hallucinations and/or delusions
- Stress management
- Tranquillizer withdrawal.

What the MDT requires of you

Nursing staff

Their expectation of you will vary according to the setting in which you work (whether on an acute or a rehabilitation ward, etc.), their own responsibility and seniority, and what they perceive as your responsibility. Overall they will expect to be treated as professional colleagues and not be burdened with unreasonable demands and expectations.

Psychiatric nurses have a very difficult and stressful job. They would like you to:

- Be prompt, courteous and reliable regarding consultation requests
- Give clear but manageable instructions, both verbal and written, in the case notes, regarding observations/monitoring/leave arrangements for the patient
- Not expect them to carry out acute medical nursing procedures, such as the care of i.v. lines or the giving of injections, especially if they have no training or facilities
- Avoid disturbing the nursing handover meetings

What the MDT requires of you *(contd)*

- Take their worries regarding the clinical state and needs of a particular patient seriously
- Offer your timetable giving information regarding your availability
- Write legibly and keep case notes and drug charts up to date
- Fill incidence forms clearly and promptly
- Be aware of what is a nursing responsibility and what is not
- Keep on top of the routine medical 'chores' for the patient, such as writing discharge letters, referral letters, filling and signing investigation forms and, not least, the Parts I and II discharge summaries
- Keep examination rooms clean and tidy
- Be supportive and refrain from undermining the authority of nursing staff unless this is clinically indicated and appropriate
- Avoid taking sides in the event of a confrontation between staff and patient, or between individual staff.

Social workers will expect you to:

- Provide clear, legible and appropriate referrals
- Have some awareness of their role and duties (this includes the specific role of the approved social worker (ASW) who is involved in mental health assessments)
- Not to encourage patients to make unrealistic demands (money, housing) from the social services
- Respond appropriately to their worries concerning the clinical state of the client: for example, the social worker may notice early signs of deterioration in the patient's health
- Advise and educate on the particular medical/psychiatric problems affecting the patient.

Occupational therapists require:

- Clear, legible, concise yet comprehensive referrals which are appropriate: it is both pointless and unsafe to refer an acutely psychotic or suicidal patient
- As much relevant information as possible, and what you hope to achieve for the patient from the occupational therapy
- Your availability for further consultation and advice
- Drug treatments kept clear and up to date, including the charts
- A sympathetic and professional response to concerns about the patient
- Advice and education regarding the relevant medical/psychiatric symptomatology/illness
- Regular review of your patient and attendance at relevant meetings and ward rounds.

What the psychologist requires of you

- Clearly and comprehensively written referrals. It is also useful to enclose a brief psychiatric summary of the patient, including their current treatments (e.g. drugs)
- What your expectations of the psychology service are, as well as what is on offer

What the MDT requires of you *(contd)*

- *Not* to have to treat suicidal or homicidal psychotic patients without medical support or cover
- Your availability for further consultations etc.
- A professional response to their concerns about any medical/psychiatric problems the patient may have
- Appropriate screening, rather than a blanket referral.

PATIENT ADVOCATE

Many psychiatric units are increasingly visited by patient advocates, who are a relatively new addition to the care services. Although they seem to be a good idea the system is still in its infancy, so its usefulness is not yet proven. You may have to see a patient with an advocate, but usually your permission will have been sought prior to the advocate's attendance. Should you feel uncomfortable or uncertain about the presence of a patient advocate, you should discuss the matter with your seniors before agreeing to it.

Theoretically, the *role of patient advocates* is to:

- Help the patient air his or her worries and concerns, which may be difficult for them to do when alone with a doctor
- Make requests that the patient may be likely to forget about
- Discuss treatment and the rationale behind it, especially where the patient finds the doctor difficult to understand.

The advocate should not:

- Make judgements regarding what is in the patient's best interest
- Encourage confrontation between the patient and staff
- Discourage the patient from accepting treatments being offered.

PLANNING FOR DISCHARGE

As the newly admitted patient's psychiatric condition stabilizes and clinical improvement begins to take place, the process of discharge planning commences, which should take account of the support and care available in the community, from both relatives and professionals.

The discharge process is fairly formalized especially for detained patients, in which case Section 117 meetings have to take place (see under Legal issues). You are expected to work closely with your colleagues to ensure that all the necessary arrangements have been made.

All patients with serious mental illness should be part of the Care Programme Approach (see below).

Before the patient leaves the hospital you should ensure that you have written to their GP giving brief details of the admission (e.g. dates, circumstances), the likely diagnosis, the discharge arrangements (e.g. outpatient appointments), and medication on discharge. Many hospitals allow a 2-week supply of medication; it is your responsibility to write the prescription if required.

CARE PROGRAMME APPROACH (CPA)

Every patient who makes significant contact with the psychiatric services should have a CPA.

This means that all their psychiatric, psychological and social needs are identified and highlighted. This administrative requirement was emphasized in the report of the inquiry held into the care of Christopher Clunis (England), and was brought into clinical management planning to ensure that there was a needs-led, clear, written and well communicated discharge plan for each patient.

The range of patients is reflected in the range of tiers, or levels, of CPA. Those who need limited and occasional input are placed in the lower tiers, and those whose needs are more complex and intensive are correspondingly placed higher.

CPA is required for patients who:

- Have suffered and suffer from mental illness or mental disorder (e.g. personality disorders)
- Have a poor prognosis
- Have had more than 3 months' inpatient treatment
- Have had three or more admissions in the past 18 months
- Have dementia and who are at risk and live in their own homes
- Are discharged under Section 117
- Have seriously attempted suicide and suffer from mental illness
- Are difficult or offending patients.

To provide an effective CPA:

- Health and social services must work together to perform psychiatric and social assessments
- A care coordinator is identified who coordinates all the service provisions in the community
- The care plan is clearly documented and circulated among the professionals involved
- Regular reviews are held to ensure continued contact with the patient. The period between each review depends on the level of CPA and changing circumstances in the patient's condition.

Patients' needs must be considered seriously, by referral and the involvement of relevant professionals, e.g. social workers, occupational therapist, art therapist, community nurse, housing and the GP etc. The main purpose is to identify their needs; attempts should be made to meet these and to communicate with relevant community personnel.

SUPERVISION REGISTER

All patients should have a risk assessment to evaluate whether there are significant risks of:

- Harm to self
- Harm to others
- Serious self-neglect.

If any of the above currently applies to a particular patient, then that individual should be placed on a supervision register, usually recommended by the consultant psychiatrist in charge.

For risk assessment the document *Guidance on the discharge of mentally disordered people and continuing care in the community* (HSG (94) 27) may be helpful (see also Chapter 6, psychiatric emergencies). This is another administrative measure to identify patients with any of the significant risks described above as a result of enduring mental illness. The order determines an administrative requirement to have a local register, which is a part of the CPA process. It should have a named key worker, geared to provide coordinated support, for a patient who needs the most serious tier of the CPA in the community.

The supervision register consists of the names of patients needing the above, held by each psychiatric provider unit, and is held locally and usually in conjunction with the local social services. The dates of inclusion in the register, as well as the dates of review, should be stated. Furthermore, there should be locally developed criteria to take patients off the register when appropriate. (**Note:** at the time of writing, abolition of the supervision register is being considered.)

CHAPTER 2

PSYCHIATRIC ASSESSMENT

History taking 32

The Mental State Examination (MSE) 43

Mini Mental State Examination (MMSE) 51

Physical examination 54

Psychiatric assessment usually consists of:

- History taking
- Mental state and physical examinations
- Investigations and formulations.

A complete psychiatric assessment will usually involve a compilation of the relevant information (from the patient and from informants) and an examination of the mental state, which is usually supplemented by further investigations (e.g. laboratory investigations). How much emphasis is placed upon each component will vary according to the patient's circumstances, the presentation, the findings, the setting (whether in the community, outpatient, inpatient, or in an emergency), and of course the availability of time and resources.

A successful psychiatric assessment should normally result in clarification of the patient's problems, the commencement of a therapeutic alliance, consideration of the diagnostic possibilities and a feasible management plan. In fact, in many cases the therapeutic process actually begins with the first psychiatric assessment.

HISTORY TAKING

PREPARATION

Some thought should be given to this issue, as it is likely to facilitate the effectiveness, efficiency and safety of the assessment.

BACKGROUND INFORMATION

Obtain as much background information as possible from all the likely sources, e.g. the referrer, the GP, previous psychiatrist's, nursing staff and other professional carers, as well as friends and family. Be as objective as possible and rely on your own assessment: just because a patient has been given a particular diagnostic label in the past it does not necessarily follow that this will remain true. This is because psychiatric symptomatology may change with the passage of time, and the previous assessment may not have been rigorous enough.

From the referrer (especially health-care professionals) obtain the following information:

- The patient's name, age, address, etc.
- Psychiatric difficulties
- Risk of suicide/homicide
- Forensic history
- Previous psychiatric diagnosis

- Any medical problems
- Medications
- Referrers' involvement/role with the patient
- Name, contact address and telephone number of referrer
- Referrer concerns and expectations
- Future involvement of referrer
- Actions to be taken if patient does not have a psychiatric problem.

The way in which the above information is obtained will vary with the background of the referrer, but you should aim to get as much information as you can before accepting the patient for assessment.

PREPARATION OF THE ASSESSMENT ROOM

Thought also needs to be given to this, and adequate preparations should be made regarding the place where the assessment is to be carried out.
  The issues to consider include:

- Safety (see below)
- Privacy: although the place should be private, colleagues should know of your whereabouts
- Lighting should be adequate for MSE and physical examination (if considered appropriate)
- Seating: ideally the patient should sit beside the writing desk, so that all of his or her body may be observed. The height levels of seating should be similar
- The environment should be calm and quiet so that the patient is put at ease and can be heard properly.

SAFETY

- Safety is essential, especially when seeing a patient who is potentially violent
- Know where the **'panic button'** is and how to use it. If there is none, establish an alternative way of summoning help
- Both patient and doctor should have equal access to the exit, and the door should be easy to open. Avoid blocking the patient's exit
- Remove all objects that could be used as weapons
- Always inform your colleagues of your location, who you are with, and the amount of time you are likely to spend with them
- Avoid seeing a patient alone if there is a history of violence
- Always request a chaperon if you need to carry out an intimate physical examination
- Make yourself aware of local guidelines on dealing with violence
- Attend any training courses for dealing with violence as soon as possible. These usually include breakaway techniques.

DEALING WITH SEXUALLY DISINHIBITED PATIENTS

A sexually disinhibited patient may have a history of cognitive impairment, e.g. frontal lobe dysfunction, mania or personality disorder. Ideally such patients should be seen with a nurse as chaperon, preferably of the same sex as the patient. Sexually disinhibited behaviour should be recorded and dealt with within a defined framework or boundary.

THE INTERVIEW

During the early part of your training you may feel somewhat uncomfortable with certain aspects of the history (e.g. the psychosexual history). You may even be lost for words when the patient exhibits sadness, aggression, and bizarre or psychotic behaviour. You may also find it difficult to pin down certain patients (such as those with mania or psychosis), and from the others (such as those with a thought disorder) it may prove impossible to elicit a reasonable history.

You will obviously need to prioritize the amount of time spent on each section of the assessment. For example, those with a thought disorder, such as schizophrenia, may need more time spent on the mental state examination, whereas those with an anxiety disorder such as obsessive–compulsive disorder (OCD) may need more time spent on the actual history taking.

In general it is a good idea to spend a few minutes during the initial part of the interview concentrating on making the patient feel at ease and establishing trust. You will reap the benefits when compiling the necessary information, as well as carrying out the mental state examination.

You should first introduce yourself, explaining who you are and the purpose of your assessment, as well as the time you are likely to spend. Establish whether or not the patient wishes a friend or relative to be present. There will be times when it is more appropriate to see the patient alone, especially when exploring the psychosexual history and sensitive relationship issues. Explain why you need to take notes, and reassure the patient that these will remain confidential (the only exception being where the interview is for the purpose of a medicolegal assessment).

In the opening few minutes allow the patient to speak freely and avoid taking notes in order to put him or her at ease, and hopefully to gain some insight into the likely course of the interview. Certain techniques, such as the use of **open-ended questions** followed by **closed ones** for further clarification of specific topics, will facilitate the interview and may allow the patient to impart information more readily and accurately.

While taking the history you should attempt to clarify important matters by asking the patient to confirm what you have understood. At the end of the interview it is often useful to ask the patient if there is anything they would like to add, or to allow them to point out any important aspect they may feel you have missed. Non-verbal behaviour, such as nodding or the use of certain phrases (e.g. 'go on') will also help.

If appropriate, end by offering your summary of the assessment and asking the patient if they agree with what you have said and your understanding of their problems.

The mental state examination (MSE) can begin with history taking, but may be conducted more formally at a later stage. Certain aspects of the MSE, such as testing for attention span and memory, usually require a more systematic approach.

Psychiatric history taking is an active and complicated process that involves both verbal and non-verbal communication between doctor and patient. The idea is not just to obtain information, but to understand **why** certain information is needed, e.g. **what** is important; **when**, **where** and **how** such symptomatology arose. You should also show that you are interested by pursuing hints, suggestions and insinuations.

- The use of nods, and phrases such as 'go on' at appropriate times, is usually helpful in facilitating the history taking
- You should try to appear neutral, calm and objective
- You will need to show flexibility, by adjusting the tone of your voice and modifying questions to suit the individual patient
- At appropriate intervals, clarification of what the patient has said by repeating sentences and asking him to confirm your understanding is a useful strategy.

- Certain information will provide added weight to diagnostic possibilities. For example, the patient's date of birth may give more information than just their age: there is evidence that those born during the winter months have an increased incidence of schizophrenia. Also, the incidence of birth and developmental problems is known to be increased among schizophrenics.

THE HISTORY

The following is a standardized form of history taking. It is a good idea to be as systematic as possible, especially during the early part of your training, otherwise essential components may be missed out.

- **Patient's profile/identifying data**
  Name, age, gender, marital status, occupation, religion and racial/ethnic origin should be recorded. These details give one some idea about the patient's place in society.

- **Reason, mode and source of referral**
  — Is the patient suicidal?
  — Informally, or formally (under a Section of the Mental Health Act)?
  — From the GP, A&E Department, or other health-care workers?

- **Complaints by the patient (CO)**
  These should be recorded as closely as possible to the patient's actual description. It may also be helpful to ask the patient to list these issues in order of importance, and how they affect his or her life. Do not be surprised if a manic or schizophrenic patient denies having any complaints or worries; on the other hand, a patient with anxiety disorder may have an endless list of complaints.

- **History of presenting complaint (HPC)**
  This again should be recorded as close to the patient's description as possible. Ask them to be as clear as possible about the relevant psychiatric/psychological complaints. You should also attempt to relate the complaints to the following:
  — Their chronological account
  — Any precipitating and perpetuating factors
  — How they affect the patient psychosocially.

Associated symptoms should be further clarified. For example, if the patient admits to a few depressive symptoms these should be followed up by exploring other depressive symptoms. Where the patient expresses paranoid ideation/complaints, clarification should be made of other symptoms that may constitute a particular syndrome (e.g. schizophrenia). Should the patient admit to obsessive thoughts, then clarify compulsive acts and/or rituals; the symptoms of depression and anxiety should also be explored, as their association is quite common.

- **Past psychiatric history (PPsychH)**
  Ask about and record the following:
  — Any previous contact with psychiatric services
  — Any previous hospital admission
  — The number of previous admissions/illnesses
  — The duration of each admission/illness
  — The treatments? drugs? ECT?
  — Any side effects of treatment
  — Previous outpatient treatment
  — Where previously admitted (hospital name) and treatment received
  — Any previous diagnostic labels.

  If the patient has had, say, 10 previous admissions it may be easier to record details of the first and the most recent, as well as the most significant ones.

- **Past medical history (PMH)**
  This should be asked about and recorded; however, endeavour to make it as relevant to psychiatry as possible. Certain medical illnesses, such as neurological disorders, head injuries, thyroid disorders and AIDS-related infections, may well have a psychiatric symptomatology or significance. An operation to remove a bunion may not be so relevant.

- **Drug history**
  Record all current drug intake, whether prescribed or over-the-counter (OTC). The latter may include St John's Wort (an antidepressant) or a cough mixture containing tyramine (potential for interaction with a MAOI). The list should include both psychiatric and non-psychiatric drugs. It may also be useful to record certain significant drugs used over a lengthy period, as well as the therapeutic and non-therapeutic effects of previous psychiatric medications.

- **Alcohol use** (see also Chapters 4 and 6)
  Record both current and previous significant use of alcohol. Some psychiatrists like to record this under *Social history*.

   It is essential that you record the average number of units of alcohol consumed by the patient in a typical week, and any previous history of alcohol-related problems/consequences, whether medical, psychiatric or psychosocial. These might include injuries resulting from a road traffic accident, driving offences, and work-related difficulties.
   Remember that many patients underestimate the amount of alcohol consumed.
  If you suspect an excessive alcohol intake then use the **CAGE** Questionnaire:

C: Have you ever felt you should **Cut** down the amount you drink?
A: Do you get **Annoyed** by people who criticize your drinking?
G: Have you ever felt **Guilty** about your drinking?
E: Have you ever needed to drink first thing in the morning (an **Eye-opener**) to steady your nerves, or get over a hangover?

   Each point scores 1. A positive answer to more than two questions indicates *problem drinking* and should be further explored.

The *criteria for alcohol dependency syndrome* include:

1. **PR:** **Pri**macy of drink (drinking before all other activities)
2. **CO:** **Co**mpulsion to drink
3. **ST:** **St**ereotypical pattern of drinking, e.g. always the same place, same time
4. **TO:** **To**lerance developing to the effects of drinking
5. **RE:** **Re**lief, that is, drinking to gain relief from withdrawal symptoms
6. **WI:** **Wi**thdrawal symptoms on stopping
7. **RE:** **Re**instatement: a recurrence of serious drinking after a period of abstinence.

Note the mnemonic: PR COST TO REWIRE

   For someone to be given the label of alcohol dependency syndrome, three or more of the above criteria should have been present for at least the previous year.

- **Illicit substances/drugs**
  Significant use of illicit substances may be related primarily to a serious psychiatric disorder (e.g. drug-induced psychosis) or may be secondary to a particular psychiatric syndrome, such as abuse of alcohol and illicit drugs in mania, schizophrenia and borderline personality disorder.

You should record:

(a) The current usage of illicit drugs, e.g. type, quality and source; whether oral or by injection; practice of safe injection
(b) Consequences:
  — medical
  — psychiatric
  — psychosocial
  — legal
(c) Previous significant use, with details as described above.

Record also the use of cigarettes, cigars, pipe tobacco and, for certain cultures, Khat (Somali), Huqa/Hubbly Bubbly (Arabs).

- **Family history (FH)**
  It is useful to draw a family tree and some important events, e.g. father died aged 56 when patient was 23, and mother remarried 2 years ago. (Fig. 2.1).

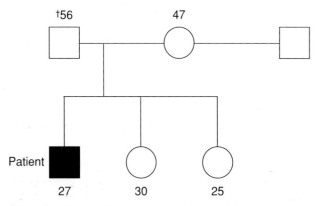

Fig. 2.1 Example of a family tree. (□ = male, ○ = female, † = dead)

Record briefly the kind of relationship with parents and siblings, especially during childhood. It is important to record the details/times of certain important family events, such as death, separation or divorce, and their impact on the patient.

Record details of the patient's own children, wife, partner, etc., and if there are any significant difficulties.

- **Family psychiatric history (FPsychH)**
  If this is positive you should obtain further details. It is especially important to record any history of suicide in the family and of any mental illness with a strong genetic loading, such as bipolar affective disorder and schizophrenia.

- **Personal history (PH)**
  This is a fairly lengthy part of the standard psychiatric history and is usually divided into a number of subcategories, as described below. The extent to which it should be detailed will vary according to the availability of time, the cooperation of the patient, and its relevance to the possible psychiatric problems. However, during the early part of your training you should attempt to obtain as much relevant detail as possible without exhausting the patient or yourself.

– *Birth and development*

  - Date of birth (? Winter birth – higher incidence of schizophrenia)
  - Age
  - Place of birth
  - Birth difficulties: did the patient's mother experience obstetric complications or birth injuries? Apgar scores; some patients may have been told (?schizophrenia ?learning disability)
  - Any prematurity
  - Early developmental milestones.

  Ask: Many children walk and talk at certain ages. Were you told of any difficulties that you might have experienced? (?schizophrenia ?learning disability).

– *Early childhood*

  - Description of their early childhood, family atmosphere
  - Persistent adverse (if any) experiences, such as abuse, either physical, emotional or sexual.

> ⚠ **Caution is required when enquiring about sexual abuse and a gentle, sensitive approach is vital. However, there are times when it may not be appropriate to probe further.**

- Relationship with other children, siblings, parents and relatives
- Any emotional adverse events, such as long hospitalizations, separations or bereavements.

> **Note**   The death of one's mother before the age of 11 is considered a risk factor for depression.

- Any serious health problems, either physical or mental
- The age of starting at nursery and school, and how they coped
- Age at which bladder and bowel control achieved.

– *Adolescence*

Adolescence is an important and potentially stressful period. New experiences such as alcohol use, illicit drugs or sex, if unbalanced or extreme, may lead to adverse consequences. Major events and out-of-the-ordinary experiences should be enquired about and recorded. Many psychiatric illnesses have their onset during adolescence and are often not recognized.

– *Educational record*

The educational record reflects upon the patient's social status, stability and motivation. It is useful to look for an unusual pattern: for example, a schizophrenic patient, at the onset of the illness, may suddenly drop out of the second year at university, even after having had a successful first year.

Record:

- Ages at which education started and finished
- Type of school
- Qualifications achieved
- Relationships with fellow students and teachers
- Any history of truancy
- Further education, such as university, plus qualifications gained.

– *Occupational record*

This also gives certain indications regarding the patient's social background, stability, motivation and success. Once again, look out for an unusual pattern, such as a schizophrenic patient at the age of 35 working as a cleaner, having previously held jobs with a higher socioeconomic status, e.g. teaching. A patient with a dissocial personality disorder may be unable to hold down a job. Enquire about and record the various jobs held, whether he or she faced difficulties with colleagues, or if repeatedly sacked.

– *Psychosexual history*

Many trainees find asking intimate questions regarding the patient's sexual history rather difficult. You will have to gauge how much the patient, is willing to volunteer. Often the use of open-ended and less loaded questions at the beginning will help.

You should enquire about:

- The onset of puberty/menarche
- The age of first sexual experience
- The practice of safe sex
- History of pregnancy and age of menopause
- Sexual orientation, gender difficulties
- Marital relationship and any sexual problems
- Any sexual difficulties and previous treatments
- Any history of sexual abuse, unusual experiences. Ask if he or she has ever been hurt in any way, e.g. sexually.

Note

Obtaining a history of sexual abuse can be fraught with difficulties. You should take an empathetic, non-judgemental and neutral stance regarding memories of sexual abuse. Be careful to avoid prejudging the cause of any sexual difficulties. On occasions the uncovering, or serious probing, of a history of sexual abuse may lead to serious difficulties for the patient: it is therefore important that they are seen by a more senior and experienced colleague, and that contingency support plans are set up.

Avoid directly questioning the reliability of the patient's memory of sexual abuse, but do not accept their account without thinking objectively.

Remember, the reliability of a particular memory may be gauged by its consistency regarding where, how and when it happened.

Forensic history

This important part of the history is sometimes neglected and may not be volunteered by some patient's. Those with certain psychiatric disorders, such as depression, dissocial personality disorder, schizophrenia, and those with alcohol and substance abuse problems, tend to have an increased incidence of forensic problems. For example, a middle aged woman who is financially secure accused of shoplifting may in fact be suffering from depression.

Enquire about:

- Crimes that were discovered and punished, and those not known to the law enforcement agencies
- Any sentences, suspended or otherwise, or time spent in prison
- Attitude towards crime (dissocial personality disorder).

An open-ended and rather less loaded question might be: 'Have you ever done anything that did or might have led to contact with the law?'

- **Premorbid personality**
  This usually refers to the patient's personality before the onset of a particular mental illness. A rather limited and subjective idea about the patient's personality can be obtained by enquiring about enduring characteristics, attitudes, ways of thinking (cognition), feelings (affect/mood) and behaviour (control of impulses and behaviour towards others). Below are some aspects of a patient's premorbid personality (i.e. prior to their mental illness):

  - Attitude towards, or description of self and character, e.g. whether introverted/shy, extroverted/social. Many patients describe themselves as having been 'happy go lucky'
  - Attitude towards others, family, friends, and socio-occupational contacts
  - How others (i.e. those who know patient reasonably well) describe him or her
  - Mood on most occasions
  - Moral and religious beliefs, attitudes
  - Interests and leisure activities (hobbies)
  - Daydreams, fantasy life
  - How he or she tends to react to various stresses, and types of defence mechanisms used.

- **Social history (SH)**
  This should include the following:

  - Marital status, whether separated, divorced or widowed
  - Occupation, and if they have any financial difficulties or debts
  - Unemployed; various benefits, such as Disability Living Allowance
  - Type and suitability of accommodation
  - Social situation/network, where living, the whereabouts of relatives and friends, and whether socially isolated
  - Social and family support available?
  - Social pastimes or hobbies.

  If elderly, ask about:

  - Various social supports
  - Meals on Wheels
  - Home help
  - Attendance at a day centre or other social centre
  - Activities of daily living (ADL), such as personal hygiene, mobility and domestic activity that can be carried out by the patient
  - Carer availability, both professional and non-professional, whether family, friend, or from the voluntary agencies.

- **Informant history (IH)**
  Use all sources to supplement the history taken from the patient. Occasionally it may be necessary or desirable to obtain the patient's permission to do so.

Good sources of information include:

- The GP
- Previous psychiatrist(s) ·
- Nursing staff
- Family and friends
- Other health-care professionals.

Psychiatric history (Summary)

- Patient profile and reason for referral
- Complaints by patient (CO)
- History of presenting complaint (HPC)
- Past psychiatric history (PPsychH)
- Past medical history (PMH)
- Drug history, use of alcohol and illicit drugs
- Family psychiatric history and family history (FPsychH & FH)
- Personal history (PH)
  — Birth and development
  — Early childhood
  — Adolescence
  — Educational record
  — Occupational record
  — Psychosexual history
  — Forensic history
- Premorbid personality
- Social history (SH)
- Informant history (IH)

THE MENTAL STATE EXAMINATION (MSE)

The mental state examination is an essential component of the psychiatric assessment. It consists of a set of standardized questions and observations that allow evaluation of the patient's appearance, behaviour, speech, feelings, thinking, perception and cognition.

It is important that you learn and practise it repeatedly, and know how to modify it according to the clinical situation you are faced with. You may find it helpful to observe a number of different senior colleagues conducting mental state examinations on patients suffering from a variety of psychiatric disorders. You can pick up useful phrases and particular styles, drawing upon the experiences of others initially and eventually developing your own style in conducting the examination.

The examination begins with the first face-to-face contact with the patient (e.g. noting their appearance and behaviour); the other elements are obtained as the assessment proceeds. Certain components can be evaluated purely from observation and the history volunteered by the patient, whereas others will require more formalized and specific questions (e.g. testing of cognitive functioning, exploring for the presence of first-rank schneiderian symptoms).

The time you spend on the mental state examination, in relation to the history, will vary according to the presentation of the particular psychiatric disorder, the particular circumstances and the setting. An acutely psychotic patient with thought disorder may give little history, yet is likely to exhibit many positive findings for the mental state examination, whereas the reverse may be true for someone with chronic obsessive–compulsive disorder. **In an emergency** (e.g. patient threatening violence) you may need to be relatively brief in evaluating the mental state, whereas in an inpatient setting a fair amount of time may be taken.

The MSE can be carried out in a variety of ways and any order, but at least initially you may find it helpful to follow a scheme so as not to miss out anything important. It is advisable to record the examination systematically, perhaps as outlined here.

- The relationship between the MSE and the history is important and a smooth transition between the two is essential.
- The MSE can be woven into the history-taking phase, but may disrupt the structure and flow of the assessment.
- An alternative approach is to note the key points in the history and to introduce them into the MSE, allowing a smooth transition. For example: 'You mentioned that you could not think properly. Did you experience other persons' thoughts being put in to your head?' (thought insertion: a schneiderian first-rank symptom). This approach may have the added advantage of letting the patient know they have been listened to.

Other useful phrases include:

- 'Now, I will be asking you some questions that you may find irrelevant, but which will help me in completing my assessment.'
- 'I would like to ask you some routine questions that will help me to assess your memory' (cognitive part of MSE).
- 'We ask the following questions of all our patients, so please do not be offended if some appear rather strange to you' (asking about auditory hallucinations).

SPECIFIC COMPONENTS OF THE MENTAL STATE EXAMINATION

APPEARANCE AND BEHAVIOUR

The description of the patient's **appearance** should include physical attributes (e.g. tall, short, obese, possible racial origin), facial appearance, description of clothes, and any features which may point to a particular disorder. For example, **self-neglect** with regard to personal appearance (hair and clothes) may occur in disorders such as **depression**, **dementia**, **schizophrenia**, and **drug abuse** (the latter may also have needle marks); **flamboyant clothes** with clashing colours may be worn by a **manic** patient.

Severe **weight loss** may indicate anorexia nervosa, depression or the presence of carcinoma.

The **facial appearance** should be described, as it may also point to a number of disorders as listed below:

- **Anorexia nervosa**: the presence of lanugo (fine) hair, parotid enlargement
- **Bulimia nervosa:** chubby face due to oedema, parotid enlargement
- **Anxiety:** horizontal furrows on the forehead and raised eyebrows
- **Depression:** depressive facies (downcast eyes, and downturning of the corners of the mouth, vertical furrow on the forehead); **T-sign**.
- **Manic:** excited, irritable appearance
- **Parkinsonian** (due to typical antipsychotics); poverty of facial expression
- **Cushinoid**: moon-faced
- **Thyrotoxicosis:** bulging eyes.

Describe the **posture** and **behaviour/movements**, and the presence of any abnormalities, which again may point to different disorders. For example:

- **Anxiety:** restlessness
- **Depression:** hunched shoulders, poor eye contact, downward gaze, psychomotor retardation, depressive stupor
- **Drugs** (e.g. typical antipsychotics): akathisia, acute dystonias, tardive dystonia, parkinsonian tremor and gait (festinant gait)
- **Mania:** increased activity, lack of personal space, sexually inappropriate behaviour
- **Schizophrenia** (especially catatonic type): bizzare posture may be adopted and many abnormal movements can occur (ambitendency, echopraxia, mannerism, negativism, stereotypical movements, waxy flexibility).

You should describe the nature of any **rapport** established with the patient, i.e. the degree of positive interaction between patient and interviewer.

SPEECH/TALK

Speech may reflect a person's thinking. It is essential that you record the presence of physical problems, such as a stroke, causing dysarthria, dysphasia, or any difficulties because English is the patient's second language, or even cultural differences (Italian's may speak more rapidly than the English, for example).

The following should be noted:

- **Rate** The rate of speech may be increased/pressured in manics (who may also exhibit a speech which is emphatic and hard to interrupt), and decreased in those with depression, dementia, schizophrenia

- **Quantity** Anxiety and mania may lead to increased quantity of speech, whereas it may be decreased in those with depression, dementia or schizophrenia
- **Form** The form of speech should also be described, but the **content** is usually recorded under **thoughts**. If an abnormality is detected it is useful to record a verbatim example.

> **Note** Flights of ideas may occur in mania, and echolalia and logoclonia may occur in schizophrenia.

AFFECT, MOOD

Affect refers to the patient's external expression of feelings. It may not always accurately reflect what the patient is really feeling.

Affect may be described as:

- **Restricted:** for example only sad affect is shown (depressed); only euphoria is exhibited (manic); or non-discernible (or flat) affect is seen (schizophrenia)
- **Labile:** affect that shows rapid fluctuation and the ability to regulate it may be lost (delirium, frontal lobe damage, intoxication)
- **Inappropriate:** laughing when the person should be sad (delirium, frontal lobe damage, intoxication), or crying suddenly for no apparent reason (e.g. 'emotional incontinence' in frontal lobe damage and pseudobulbar pathology).

Mood refers to emotion, which is more sustained and pervasive. It should be described:

- Objectively (how it appears to the examiner from the patient's appearance, behaviour and history) and
- Subjectively (the patient's description of his or her own mood).

Other descriptions of mood include:

- Euthymic/normal
- Elated/expansive/grandiose/euphoric
- Anxious/irritable/angry
- Depressed/low.

THOUGHT POSSESSIONS/CONTENT/ABNORMAL BELIEFS AND INTERPRETATION OF EVENTS

These should be explored (a general question might be: 'Have you noticed any interference with your thinking?).

PASSIVITY OF THOUGHTS

Experience of interference with one's thinking by an outside force; it includes:

- **Thought echo:** hearing an echo of one's thoughts
- **Thought withdrawal:** an experience of thoughts being withdrawn from one's mind by an external force
- **Thought insertion:** an experience of thoughts being put into one's mind by an external force
- **Thought broadcasting:** an experience of one's thoughts being broadcast to others, say on the radio, or TV.

Note	Thought echo, withdrawal, insertion and broadcasting are first-rank schneiderian symptoms.

PHOBIAS

Many patients hide these because of embarrassment, even if their lives are significantly affected.

PREOCCUPATIONS/WORRIES

You should record the patient's main preoccupations/worries, especially if they interfere with their life.

OBSESSIONS

These should be clarified, and you should check that the features meet the relevant criteria and are clinically significant. Ask about rituals/compulsions which may also be present.

SUICIDAL THOUGHTS

It is essential to explore these as they occur in many psychiatric disorders and are the main cause of mortality among psychiatric patients. An opening question might be: Do you feel that life is worth living? (see Chapter 6 for details).

HOMICIDAL THOUGHTS

These should also be explored. An opening question might be: 'Do you feel like hurting anyone?' (see Chapter 6 for details).

Note	Suicidal and homicidal thoughts should always be explored.

DELUSIONS

These includes both **primary delusions** (e.g. delusional perception, a first-rank schneiderian symptom and **secondary delusions** (e.g. paranoid, grandiose, nihilistic).

It is important to remember that *delusions are defined as false, fixed, unshakeable beliefs, despite evidence to the contrary, and are out of keeping with the person's educational and sociocultural norms.*

Other types of delusion, which should be explored and recorded if present, include:

● Mood-congruent delusions, as in depression, mania
● Mood-incongruent delusions, as in schizophrenia
● Bizarre delusions, as in schizophrenia.

OVERVALUED IDEAS

These are ideas that are false but which do not reach delusional intensity. They are sustained intense preoccupations and may affect the individual's life. An example is the belief one is fat, held by a thin patient with anorexia nervosa.

ABNORMAL EXPERIENCES/PERCEPTIONS

These include sensory distortions (hyperacusis), sensory deceptions (illusions, hallucinations) and disorders of self-awareness (depersonalization, derealization).

Hallucinations can occur in any modality (auditory, olfactory, somatic, visual). **Second-person auditory hallucinations** ('You should do this; You are a bad man') tend to occur in psychotic depression, whereas **third-person auditory hallucinations** ('He should do this; He is a bad man') are known to occur in schizophrenia. A general opening question might be: 'Do you sometimes hear sound or voices when no one is around?'

COGNITIVE STATE

The cognitive state, i.e. the patient's orientation, attention and concentration, memory, general knowledge, intelligence and abstract thinking, should be checked. If abnormalities are detected they should be further explored with detailed tests of the central nervous system.

It is essential that you adopt a thorough and systematic approach. It may also be useful to explain to the patient that many tests and questions are routine, and that they should not feel anxious.

ORIENTATION

Check the patient's orientation in time, place and person, especially if you suspect problems.

ATTENTION AND CONCENTRATION

This can be tested in a number of ways:

- **Digit span:** ask the patient to repeat digits after you, starting with three, then five, and finally seven. If this is carried out satisfactorily, ask the patient to repeat the digits backwards, starting with three digits.
- **Serial sevens test:** ask the patient to subtract seven from 100 and repeatedly to subtract seven from the remainder as fast as possible. The correct answers are listed below:
  93, 86, 79, 72, 65, 58, 51, 44, 37, 30, 23, 16, 9, 2.

  Many patients find this difficult; if this is the case, then ask the patient to recite the months of the year, or the days of the week, backwards.

MEMORY

This includes short-term and long-term memory.

- **Short-term memory:** this is tested by asking the patient to recite after 5 minutes a given name and address (avoid giving your own address!).

> ⚠ It is conventional to use 5 minutes' recall as a test of short-term memory, but scientifically, and according to neuropsychologists, this is not correct.

- **Long-term memory:** this is tested by asking the patient to describe some autobiographical details, or to recall the date of an important event that might be known to them, such as the year England won the World Cup. (This particular question might not be appropriate for all patients!)

ABSTRACT THINKING

Ask the patient to interpret a proverb, such as: 'People who live in glass houses should not throw stones'.

If the patient suggests that this is because the glass will break, it may indicate concrete thinking as a result of frontal lobe impairment.

> ⚠ It is essential to take account of the person's intelligence and linguistic and educational background, when testing with proverb interpretation.

GENERAL KNOWLEDGE

This may be assessed by asking the patient to name, for example:

- The current Prime Minister
- The Monarch
- Any recent news on the TV.

INTELLIGENCE

This may be assessed clinically (taking account of the patient's educational, linguistic and sociocultural background) from:

- History (the level of education achieved)
- Answers to the general knowledge questions.

INSIGHT

This can be assessed by asking the patient:

- Whether he accepts that he is ill, and, suffering from mental or physical illness?
- If he accepts that he is mentally ill, does he feel that the psychiatric treatment is necessary?

For details of the terminology (psychopathology) used above, see the section on descriptive psychopathology in the Appendix.

The mental state examination (MSE) (Summary)

Appearance and behaviour
General appearance
Facial appearance
Posture and movements
Social behaviour
Rapport with the examiner

Speech
Rate
Rhythm
Quantity
Form

Mood/affect
Objective – anxiety
Subjective

Thoughts/abnormal beliefs
Preoccupations
Obsessions
Phobias
Suicidal and homicidal thoughts
Abnormal beliefs and interpretation of events
Delusions

The mental state examination (MSE) (Summary) *(contd)*

Ideas of reference
Passivity
Thought interference (echo, withdrawal, insertion, broadcasting)

Abnormal experiences
Illusions
Hallucinations (auditory, visual)
Derealization, depersonalization

Cognitive state
Orientation in time, place and person
Attention and concentration
Memory – immediate recall
   short-term,
   long-term
General knowledge and intelligence
Abstract thinking

Insight
Beliefs regarding being ill

MINI MENTAL STATE EXAMINATION (MMSE)

The mini mental state examination is a standardized way of testing and quantifying different aspects of cognition, such as attention, orientation, memory and visuospatial abilities. It is a good screening test with a relatively high inter-rater reliability and is commonly used to assess cognitive impairment in the elderly.

The patient is asked to answer a set of standard questions and perform certain tasks, for which specific scores are given. The maximum score is 30; a score less than 24 may indicate dementing illness.

Mini Mental State Examination (MMSE)

Orientation
Ask the patient:
What is the day, month, date, season, year? (score 5)
Where are you now? (the ward/room, hospital/ building, town, county, country) (score 5)

Registration
Ask the patient to list three objects (e.g. pen, book, watch) and then to recall those objects (score of 1 for each object successfully recalled) (score 3)

Attention and calculation
Ask the patient to perform serial sevens test (subtracting 7 from 100; see MSE) alternatively, ask the patient to spell WORLD backwards (D-L-R-O-W) (score 5)

Mini Mental State Examination (MMSE) *(contd)*

Recall
Ask the patient to recite the three items listed under registration   (score 3)

Language
Show the patient a watch and a pen and ask him to name them   (score 2)
Ask the patient to repeat the following statement:
'No ifs, ands or buts'   (score 1)
Ask the patient to follow these three stage commands:
Take a piece of paper in your right hand (score of 1)
Fold it in half (score of 1)
Place it on the floor (score of 1)   (score 3)

Reading
Write out the following on a piece of paper and ask the patient to read it
CLOSE YOUR EYES   (score 1)

Writing
Ask the patient to write a sentence   (score 1)

Construction
Asked the patient to copy the drawing of intersecting pentagons as
shown below (Fig 2.2)   (score 1)

Total score 30

Regional brain (central nervous system) testing

Frontal lobe
- Rapid sequential movements
- Complex motor behaviours
- Ability to repeat phrases with prosody
- Attention, concentration, judgement, problem solving.

Temporal lobe
- Reading
- Writing
- Naming
- Comprehension of spoken language
- Gnosis: recognition of letters and numbers.

Parietal lobe
- Praxis:
    — Ideomotor: the ability to carry out actions on command
    — Ideational: the ability to carry out acts in a logical sequence
    — Constructional: the ability to arrange shapes and copy diagrams

Regional brain (central nervous system) testing *(contd)*

- Calculations
- Stereognosis
- Right–left and east–west orientation.

Occidental lobe
- Visual memory
- Pattern recognition

Dysfunction of brain regions (lobes)

Frontal lobe
- Impairment of complex motor behaviour
- Inability to repeat phrases with prosody
- Broca's aphasia (non-fluent)
- Impairment of rapid sequential movements
- Impairment of problem solving, judgement, concentration and orientation

Temporal lobe
Unilateral dominant
- Memory difficulties
- Wernicke's aphasia (fluent)

Unilateral non-dominant
- Disorder of speech prosody
- Impaired recognition of sounds

Bilateral
- Korsakoff's syndrome
- Kluver–Bucy syndrome
- Language, memory and emotion are affected

Parietal lobe
Dominant
- Gerstmann's syndrome (agraphia, acalculia, finger agnosia and left–right disorientation)
- Alexia with agraphia
- Astereognosis
- Language recognition and impairment of word memory

Non-dominant
- Disorders of spatial awareness
- Calculation problems
- Impairment of right–left, east–west orientation

Occipital lobe
- Alexia (inability to read)
- Agnosia for faces and colours
- Anton's syndrome – cortical blindness and denial of blindness
- Balint's syndrome – gaze paralysis and abnormal guidance of limbs

PHYSICAL EXAMINATION

A full physical examination is required to be carried out routinely at the time of admission of a psychiatric inpatient. However, only the relevant aspects may need to be carried out in patients being seen in casualty or in the clinics or the day hospital. A physical examination is also required in a psychiatric inpatitis as the need arises, such as development of drug side effects.

When performing an intimate physical examination (especially on a member of the opposite sex) it is essential that you explain its necessity to the patient and asked for the presence of a chaperon.

You should be aware that many physical findings can have possible psychiatric implications (Table 2.1).

TABLE 2.1   The psychiatric physical examination

Feature	Possible implication*
Head and neck	
Altered pupil size	Drug intoxication/withdrawal
Argyll Robertson pupil	Neurosyphilis
Corneal pigmentation	Wilson's disease
Neck mass	Thyroid dysfunction
Dental caries	Eating disorders (repeated vomiting)
Nasal septal defect	Cocaine use
Arcus senilis	Alcohol use
Parotid enlargement	Anorexia/bulimia nervosa
Oesophagitis	Eating disorders (from vomiting)
Skin	
Tattoos	Borderline or antisocial personality
Callus/laceration on knuckles	Eating disorders (due to self-induced vomiting)
Scars from slashing	Borderline personality disorder
Scars from trauma	Antisocial personality, alcohol use
Needle marks/tracks	i.v. drug use/dependence
Piloerection	Opioid withdrawal
Palmar erythema	Alcohol use
Bruising	Alcohol use, seizure disorders
Cigarette burns	Dementia, alcohol use, other neurologic conditions
Dermatitis or excoriated skin	OCD – compulsive handwashing, may occur on knees from cleaning in a kneeling position
Unusual pattern of hair loss	Trichotillomania
Pretibial myxoedema	Graves' disease
Kaposi's sarcoma	AIDS, HIV encephalopathy
Lanugo hair	Anorexia nervosa
Café au lait macules	Neurofibromatosis
Red-purple striae	Cushing's syndrome/disease
Oedema	MAOI drugs, anorexia nervosa
Spider angiomata	Alcohol abuse/dependence
Cardiovascular	
Mitral valve prolapse	Panic disorder, anorexia nervosa
Hypotension	Anorexia nervosa

TABLE 2.1 The psychiatric physical examination (contd)

Feature	Possible implication*
Abdomen and chest	
Enlarged liver	Alcohol abuse
Gynaecomastia	Alcohol abuse/use of antipsychotics (e.g. sulpiride)
Dilated abdominal veins	Alcohol abuse
Decreased motility	Pica (with a bezoar), anorexia nervosa
Genitals	
Chancre	Syphilis (primary)
Mutilation	Psychotic disorder, paraphilia, sexual identity disorder
Testicular atrophy	Alcohol abuse, anabolic steroid use
Musculoskeletal and nervous system	
Gait abnormalities	Normal pressure hydrocephalus
	Dementia paralytica (syphilis)
	High-stepping gait (syphilis)
	Festinating gait (Parkinson's disease)
	Alcohol abuse (cerebellar degeneration)
	Wernicke–Korsakoff syndrome
Tremor	Parkinson's disease, lithium use, caffeine intoxication, alcohol withdrawal, anxiety disorders, antipsychotic (typical) use
Repeated movements	Tourette's syndrome, tic disorders, autism, tardive dyskinesia, OCD, mental retardation
Muscle wasting	Alcohol abuse
General	
Medic-Alert chain or bracelet	

*These implications are speculative: they are not meant to be pejorative or to indicate diagnostic criteria.

Adapted with permission from: David J. Robinson, 1998. Psychiatric Mnemonics and Clinical Guides, 2nd edn. Rapid Psychler Press, Michigan.

Any physical findings of which you are unsure should be discussed with the relevant specialist.

GENERAL PHYSICAL EXAMINATION

- Describe the patient's appearance: whether he looks well or unwell
- Observe for anaemia, clubbing, cynosis, jaundice, facial pallor or flushing, cuts, bruises, needle marks, evidence of movement disorders
- Check the **head** and **neck** for evidence of trauma
- **Eyes** should be examined for pupillary and fundal abnormalities, as well as for evidence of thyrotoxicosis

- **Hands** and **arms** should be examined for nicotine stains, needle marks (drug abusers), cuts (borderline personality disorder), tremor, and some features described above.
- **Cardiovascular system** The pulse rate should be recorded, noting any abnormalities such as tachycardia of thyrotoxicosis. Check the blood pressure (lying and standing if necessary) and note murmurs. In addition, look for evidence of peripheral vascular disease.
- **Respiratory system** *Many psychiatric patients are smokers and are therefore more likely to have respiratory problems.* The chest should be inspected, palpated, percussed and auscultated for evidence of any pathology.
- **Abdomen** Here you need to concentrate on excluding any liver pathology, such as liver enlargement (likely in alcoholics).
- **Neurological system** This has special relevance to the psychiatrist and should be examined as a screening procedure; a head-to-toe lengthy, exhaustive neurological examination is not really necessary in most cases.
- The **handedness** of the patient should be noted.
- Describe the **gait** and the **posture** (effects of medications).
- Check the **reflexes**, which can be tested fairly quickly. Note any abnormalities (e.g. absence of reflexes).
- The test of **power** and **sensation** is only necessary if indicated by the history. Look for evidence of **peripheral neuropathy** in diabetics and alcoholics.

ASSESSING CRANIAL NERVES

Olfactory (I)	May be omitted (ask about changes in smell)
	Importance Impairment possible in Alzheimer's disease or frontal lobe lesions
Optic (II)	Ask about visual acuity. Fields tested by confrontation, both eyes at the same time: 'Which finger is wiggling?'; check pupillary reaction to light and examine discs for swelling or atrophy
	Importance Field defects such as hemianopia imply a contralateral hemispheric lesion. In the presence of visual inattention (tested by simultaneous finger wiggling) check parietal lobe function. *Optic atrophy* has many causes, such as tumours, glaucoma
Oculomotor (III) trochlear (IV) and abducens (VI)	Test eye movements by asking the patient to follow your finger slowly, left to right, up and down. Check pupillary reflexes. Ask about double vision. Look for squint

Importance
Ophthalmoplegias may be present in Wernicke's encephalopathy. Third-nerve (eye down and out) and sixth-nerve (eye cannot abduct) palsies seen post head injury. Acute third-nerve lesion may result from raised intracranial pressure

Trigeminal (V)

Test sensation left and right on mandible, maxilla and forehead. Ask patient to clench the jaw (motor part; difficulty in chewing)

Importance
Herpes zoster infection may lead to *trigeminal neuralgia*, which may cause excruciating pain and can lead to suicide. Lesion of motor part in bulbar palsy

Facial (VII)

Check for facial symmetry (drooping of one angle of mouth). Ask patient to close eyes, purse lips. Check taste

Importance
Lesions of lower motor neurons (polio, Bell's palsy, tumours). Beware of altered facial expression in depression and parkinsonism

Auditory (VIII)

Usually not tested formally (ask about hearing, dizziness, vertigo)

Importance
Congenital rubella can cause deafness, cataract and low IQ. Aspirin and frusemide overdose

Glossopharyngeal (IX) and vagus (X)

Listen to the voice (dysarthria) and inspect the palate as the patient says 'Ah'. Gag reflex

Importance
May occur as a result of trauma, brain-stem lesions and neck tumours

Accessory (XI)

Ask patient to shrug their shoulders

Importance
Polio, tumours near the jugular foramen

Hypoglossal (XII)

Check the tongue for wasting, deviation and fibrillation

Importance
Stroke, bulbar palsy, polio, trauma and TB may cause lesions

Note	Any of the cranial nerve lesions may occur in diabetes, multiple sclerosis, sarcoid, syphilis and HIV. A focused and a relatively brief outline has been described here. You are advised to expand upon the physical examination when necessary and consult appropriate colleagues and suitable medical texts.

SUMMARY AND FORMULATION OF THE ASSESSMENT

It is important to summarize the relevant findings from the history and MSE in order to communicate effectively with colleagues.

The preferred diagnosis and the differential diagnosis (where appropriate) should be recorded and an explanation should be given for the reasoning behind your choice.

Record any biological and psychosocial factors (predisposing, precipitating and perpetuating) that may have had an aetiological role in the development of the particular disorder.

The management plan should consist of a list of all relevant further investigations, as well as both short- and long-term management issues.

DIAGNOSIS AND DIFFERENTIAL DIAGNOSES

Your preferred diagnosis should be based upon the history, MSE and physical examination. You should consider and list the evidence for and against a particular diagnosis. Many patients are considered to have a so-called **dual diagnosis** (e.g. those with alcohol and/or illicit substance abuse, together with mental illness) or **comorbid disorders** (e.g. borderline personality disorder and depression). You should also attempt to list the differential diagnoses, but this may not always be possible. Consideration should always be given to the evidence for and against each diagnosis.

AETIOLOGICAL FACTORS

For each potential psychiatric disorder consider the following:

Biological   Predisposing factors (family history: genetic loading)
                   Precipitating factors (use of illicit drugs, e.g. amphetamines)
                   Perpetuating factors (not taking medication)

Psychosocial   Predisposing factors (?lower social class)
Precipitating factors (adverse life event)
Perpetuating factors (high expressed emotions)

MANAGEMENT PLAN

This should include:

- Supplementing the history from other relevant sources
- Further necessary investigations (psychological, psychometric, neuropsychological, physical, laboratory); these should be listed and arranged as appropriate
- Second opinion, if necessary
- Further observation (e.g. level I, II)
- Precautions that need to be taken: this should include a risk assessment (see Chapter 6) and procedures to prevent self-harm and harm to others
- Implementation of treatment: both long- and short-term treatments should consider biological and psychosocial therapies
- Involvement of other agencies whether voluntary/statutory, medical/social
- For patients admitted involuntarily, Mental Health Act issues such as status, appeals, dates of tribunals, managers' hearings.

INVESTIGATIONS

Investigations play an important part in the completion of a psychiatric assessment and the formulation of an effective management plan. Be guided by the clinical history and err on the side of caution (i.e. do not ignore the need for further investigations). Obviously any *unnecessary* investigations should be avoided.

PRIMARY PHYSICAL INVESTIGATIONS (see Tables 2.2 and 2.3)

These include:

- **Urine** Drug screening, tests for glucose, infection, pregnancy
- **Blood** FBC, U&Es, glucose, liver function tests, thyroid function tests. If clinically indicated, syphilis serology, hepatitis B and C, HIV, folate, B_{12}, serum drug levels (e.g. lithium).

SECONDARY PHYSICAL INVESTIGATIONS

These may be required if indicated by the clinical assessment (specially the physical examination) and include:

- **Blood** Creatinine kinase (investigation for NMS), endocrine investigations, dexamethasone suppression test, genetic tests

- **Others** Chest X-ray, skull X-ray, ECG, EEG, EMG, brain electrical mapping (BEAM), transcranial magnetic stimulation (TMS)
- **Neuroimaging** tests, such as, CT, MRI, functional MRI (fMRI), magnetic resonance spectroscopy (MRS), positron emission tomography (PET) and single photon emission tomography (SPECT)

TABLE 2.2 Haematological values

Venous blood: adult reference values

Analyte	Reference values
Bleeding time (Ivy)	Up to 11 min
Body fluid (total)	50% (obese) – 70% (lean) of body weight
Intracellular	30–40% of body weight
Extracellular	20–30% of body weight
Blood volume	
Red cell mass – men	30±5 ml/kg
– women	25±5 ml/kg
Plasma volume (both sexes)	45±5 ml/kg
Erthrocyte sedimentation rate	0–6 mm in 1 h normal
(Westergren)	7–20mm in 1 h doubtful
	>20mm in 1 h abnormal
Fibrinogen	1.5–4.0 g/l
Folate – serum	2–20 μg/l
– red cell	>100 μg/l
Haemoglobin – men	13–18 g/dl
– women	11.5–16.5 g/dl
Haptoglobin	0.3–2.0 g/l
Leucocytes – adults	4.0–11.0 × 10⁹/l
Differential white cell count	
Neutrophil granulocytes	2.5–7.5 × 10⁹/l
Lymphocytes	1.0–3.5 × 10⁹/l
Monocytes	0.2–0.8 × 10⁹/l
Eosinophil granulocytes	0.04–0.4 × 10⁹/l
Basophil granulocytes	0.01–0.1 × 10⁹/l
Mean corpuscular haemoglobin (MCH)	27–32 pg
Mean corpuscular haemoglobin	
concentration (MCHC)	30–35 g/dl
Mean corpuscular volume (MCV)	78–98 fl
Packed cell volume (PCV) or	
haematocrit – men	0.40–0.54
– women	0.35–0.47
Platelets	150–400 × 10⁹/l
Prothrombin time	11–15s
Red cell count – men	4.5–6.5 × 10¹²/l
– women	3.8–5.8 × 10¹²/l
Red cell life span (mean)	120 days
Red cell life span T (⁵¹CR)	25–35 days
Reticulocytes (adults)	10–100 × 10⁹/l
Vitamin B₁₂ (in serum as cyanocobalamin)	160–925 ng/l

Reproduced with permission from Roger A. Fisken, 1994. Churchill's House Physician's Survival Guide, Churchill Livingstone.

- **Psychological** These may be carried out by psychologists, occupational therapists, social workers and appropriately trained practitioners. They include behavioural analysis, structured instruments to evaluate psychopathology, personality difficulties, psychometric testing (IQ tests) and neuropsychological assessments (e.g. testing for frontal lobe dysfunction)
- **Social** These include assessment of housing, finance and benefits, family/social support, the availability of social resources and activity of daily living (ADL). These are usually carried out by the social worker belonging to the multidisciplinary team.

TABLE 2.3   Biochemical values

Venous blood: adult reference values

Analyte	Reference values	
Acid phosphatase (unstable enzyme)	0.1–0.4 i.u./l	
Alanine aminotransferase (ALT) (glutamin-pyruvic transaminase (GPT))	10–40 i.u./l	
Alkaline phosphatase	40–100 i.u./l	
Amylase	50–300 i.u./l	
α-Antitrypsin	2–4 g/l	
Ascorbic acid – serum	23–57 μmol/l	0.4–1.0 mg/dl
– leucocytes	1420–2270 μmol/l	25–40 mg/dl
Aspartate aminotransferase (AST) (glutamic-oxaloacetic transaminase (GOT))	10–35 i.u./l	
Bilirubin (total)	2–17 μmol/l	
Caeruloplasmin	1–2.7 μmol/l	
Calcium (total)	2.12–2.62 mmol/l	
Carbon dioxide (total)	24–30 mmol/l	
Chloride	95–105 mmol/l	
Cholesterol (fasting)	3.6–6.7 mmol/l	
Copper	11–24 μmol/l	
Creatinine	55–150 μmol/l	
Creatinine clearance	90–130 ml/min	
Creatine kinase (CK) – males	30–200 i.u./l	
– females	30–150 i.u./l	
Ethanol – marked intoxication	65–87 mmol/l	
– coma	>109 mmol/l	
Ferritin – males	6–186 μg/ml	
– females	3–162 μg/ml	
α Fetoprotein	2–6 units/ml	
Glucose (fasting)	3.9–5.8 mmol/l	
γ-Glutamyl transferase (γ-GT) – males	10–55 i.u./l	
– females	5–35 i.u./l	
Immunoglobulins (Ig): IgA	0.5–4.0 g/l (40–300 i.u./l)	
IgG	5.0 –13.0 g/l (60–160 i.u./l)	
IgM – males	0.3–2.2 g/l (40–270 i.u./l)	
– female	0.4–2.5 g/l (50–300 i.u./l)	
Iron – males	14–32 μmol/l	
– female	10–28 μmol/l	

TABLE 2.3 Biochemical values (contd)

Venous blood: adult reference values

Analyte	Reference values
Iron binding capacity (total)	45–72 µmol/l
Iron binding capacity (saturation)	14–47%
Lactate	0.4–1.4 mmol/l
Lactate dehydrogenase (LDH)	100–300 i.u./l
Lead	0.5–1.9 µmol/l
Magnesium	0.75–1.0 mmol/l
5' Nucleotidase	1–11 i.u./l
Osmolality	285–295 mOsm/kg
Phosphatase see acid and alkaline	
Phosphate	0.8–1.4 mmol/l
Potassium	3.3–4.7 mmol/l
Protein – total	62–82 g/l
– albumin	36–47 g/l
– globulins	24–37 g/l
– electrophoresis (% total)	
albumin 52–68	
globulin α_1 4.2–7.2	
α_2 6.8–12	
β 9.3–15	
γ 13–23	
Sodium	133–144 mmol/l
Triglyceride (fasting)	0.6–1.7 mmol/l
Urate – males	0.12–0.42 mmol/l
– females	0.12–0.36 mmol/l
Urea	2.5–6.6 mmol/l

Reproduced with permission from Roger A. Fisken, 1994. Churchill's House Physician's Survival Guide, Churchill Livingstone.

RATING SCALES IN PSYCHIATRY

Many of the rating scales used in psychiatry have been well designed and validated and play an important part in psychiatric research. However, on occasions you may be asked to use a common and relatively simple rating scale in your clinical practice. If such a case arises ask to be trained, so that you can apply the scale correctly. The following are a few examples of rating scales used in psychiatry.

General
- General Health Questionnaire (GHQ)
- Brief Psychiatric Rating Scale (BPRS)
- Present State Examination (PSE)
- Schedule for Affective Disorders and Schizophrenia (SADS).

Alcoholism
- CAGE Questionnaire (C= Cut down, A= Annoyed, G= Guilty, E= Eye opener).

Anxiety
- Hamilton Rating Scale for Anxiety.

Cognitive impairment
- Mini Mental State Examination (MMSE).

Depression
- Hamilton Rating Scale for Depression (HAM-D)
- Beck Depression Inventory (BDI) – 20 items, self
- Montgomery–Asperger Depression Rating Scale (MADRAS)
- Geriatric Depression Scale (GDS).

Mania
- Manic-State Rating Scale (MSRS)
- Rating Scale for Mania (RSM).

Personality disorder
- Personality Assessment Schedule (PAS)
- Structured Interview for DSM-III-R Personality Disorders (SIDP-R).

Schizophrenia
- Scale for the Assessment of Positive Symptoms (SAPS)
- Scale for the Assessment of Negative Symptoms (SANS).

Suicidal behaviour
- Suicide Intent Scale (SIS)
- Reason for Living Inventory (RLI).

PARTS I AND II (DISCHARGE SUMMARY) SUMMARIES

PART I

This should cover all the important aspects of the patient's demographic details, psychiatric history, MSE and physical examination. Most psychiatric hospitals/units require these to be completed within the first week of admission. This task is usually performed by the junior psychiatrist looking after the patient.

PART II

This follows and supplements the Part I summary. It outlines the psychiatric diagnosis, physical diagnosis/findings, physical and psychological investigations, treatment and progress, discharge medications, residual symptoms, prognosis, and date of discharge. It should be completed within 2–3 weeks of patient's discharge and, once again, is usually carried out by the junior psychiatrist caring for the patient.

Both Part I and part II summaries are kept in the patient's case notes and copies are sent to the GP and other relevant professionals.

Examples of Parts I and II summaries are shown below.

REPORT

EXAMPLE PART I CLINICAL SUMMARY: ADMISSION DETAILS

CARING MENTAL HEALTH TRUST

KIND PSYCHIATRIC HOSPITAL LONDON

CONSULTANT: Dr B. Mind   **DATE OF SUMMARY:**

PATIENT DETAILS:

Hospital no:
Title:
Surname:
Forenames:
D.O.B.:
Address:
Telephone:
GP:

DATE OF ADMISSION:

Mode of admission:
Presenting problem:
Past psychiatric history:
Past medical history:
Drug history and allergies:
Family history:
Family psychiatric history:

→

Personal history:
    Psychosexual history:
    Forensic history:
    Pre-morbid personality:
Social circumstances:
    Alcohol and illicit drugs consumption:

MENTAL STATE EXAMINATION:

Appearance and behaviour:
Speech:
Mood/affect:
Thought abnormalities:
Perceptual abnormalities:
Cognitive state:
Insight:
Informant history:

PHYSICAL EXAMINATION:

Dr Brain
SHO to Dr B. Mind, Consultant Psychiatrist

REPORT

EXAMPLE PART II CLINICAL SUMMARY: TREATMENT DETAILS AND POST-DISCHARGE CARE PLAN:

CARING MENTAL HEALTH TRUST

KIND PSYCHIATRIC HOSPITAL LONDON

CONSULTANT: Dr B. Mind

DATE OF SUMMARY:

PATIENT DETAILS:

Hospital no:
Title:
Surname:
Forenames:
D.O.B.:
Address:
Telephone:
GP:

DATE OF ADMISSION:

DATE OF DISCHARGE:

PSYCHIATRIC DIAGNOSIS:

ICD code:
Medical diagnosis:
Treatment and progress:

POST DISCHARGE CARE PLAN:

Physical and psychological investigations:
Full blood count:
Urea and electrolyte:
Glucose:
Liver function:
Thyroid function:
B_{12}, folate:
Syphilis serology:

CT/MRI brain:
Midstream urine:
Residual symptoms on discharge:
Prognosis:
Date of next CPA:

DISCHARGE MEDICATION:

Dr Brain
SHO to Dr B. Mind, Consultant Psychiatrist

TRANSCULTURAL PSYCHIATRY

In any multicultural society the various ethnic groups are as vulnerable to psychiatric disorders as the 'native' population, if not more so. The factors that make them particularly vulnerable include:

- Different skin colour
- Different language
- Different culture
- Apprehension of the host culture
- Fear of assimilation
- Struggle for identity
- Struggle for a place in a different community
- Media stereotyping
- Hostile community
- Racial discrimination.

Despite their training, psychiatrists may suffer from these biases when dealing with patient from an ethnic minority. Racial and cultural generalizations are common in any culture, and psychiatrists are not immune to such influences.

CONSIDERATIONS FOR HISTORY TAKING

Active consideration should be given to an appropriate and respectful assessment of a patient belonging to an ethnic minority. The transcultural aspects should be considered and positively catered for.

'Cultural camouflage' is the notion that the patient may consider his or her symptoms to be culturally appropriate. This can be countered by thorough history taking and objective accounts. A detailed mental state assessment must never be vetoed by the subjective fear of not knowing the patient's culture fully.

An interpreter who is aware of the patient's culture can be of immense assistance.

Pressure from family and relatives should also be considered. No family wishes ill of its members and there may be certain sensitivities of which the psychiatrist must be aware.

Clinical judgement must never be compromised in the face of family pressure.

Community support and other monitoring arrangements may be considered if there is a clear cultural consideration. There should always be multiagency, multidisciplinary discussions attended by the family and advocates of the patient.

Language is a barrier to understanding the symptomatology and the cultural appropriateness of the assessment. An independent interpreter or a close family relative who can interpret can help overcome this. Some beliefs may appear delusional but are normal for the patient: they should be further explored and not used as reasons for detention or treatment, unless supported by other characteristic features of mental illness.

Details of the family and support network in the host country are essential: the patient's view of these and relatives' perceptions should be considered in formulating the diagnosis. Generations may differ in their beliefs and it is important to assess all stakeholder generations involved.

There is some evidence that ethnic minorities do not receive appropriate psychiatric care in the UK and this must be considered when making judgements regarding detention and medication. Some patients are more likely to be detained and feared than others. The patient may be suffering from discrimination, and insensitive treatment attitudes may worsen this perception.

Information to be elicited

- Patient's first language
- Identify group
- Patient's view of the problem
- Family's view of the problem
- Interpreter's impression
- Capacity of the family to deal with the problem
- Patient's religion.

Factors to consider

- Ethnic and cultural sensitivities
- Critical clarification of symptoms
- Developing rapport
- Advocacy
- Domination of the interview by one relative
- Potential for misinterpretation by a relative
- Cultural beliefs about mythology and supernatural experiences.

TRANSCULTURAL PSYCHIATRIC PRESENTATION/ SYNDROMES

In the UK, people from ethnic minorities have tended to cluster in certain defined areas, where life experiences have been recreated that remind them of their own culture. Many areas are reflective of their 'home' life, living in extended families with minimal exposure to the outside culture.

Some culture-bound syndromes include:

DHAT SYNDROME

These men complain of loss of semen in the urine and that this is causing them weakness. It is also considered as an anxiety state and was originally described amongst Indian men.

DJINN SYNDROME

The syndrome implies possession of the patient by a djinn or a genie. The patient will communicate with it, respond and have conversations with it. Sometimes, she may even do bizarre or inappropriate things, attributing them to the djinn. The syndrome is akin to a conversion disorder or dissociative reaction and is usually the result of severe social or familial turmoil, mostly in a female, when she is feeling isolated, unheard and under pressure. The personality transformation is significant, as a previously shy and timid girl may become rude, abusive and disinhibited.

GAS SYNDROME

This also occurs in females from communities where there is little freedom available to women to express their distress. In this syndrome the patient experiences a ball of gas going up from her stomach towards her head, then feeling faint and losing her senses. It is considered a variant of depressive symptomatology, expressed as somatic features. Treatment is as for depressive disorders.

KORO SYNDROME

This describes a fear of the penis shrinking into the abdomen and was originally described in men from south-east Asia. It is regarded as an anxiety state and the affected men fear consequential death.

LATAH SYNDROME

This occurs in the Far East and North Africa. It is an hysterical state consisting of automatic imitative behaviour, namely echolalia, echopraxia and automatic obedience.

SHINKEISHITSU SYNDROME

This has been described amongst Japanese men and consists of obsessionality and anxiety symptoms.

SUSTO OR ESPANTO SYNDROME

This condition has been described as occurring in the Andes mountains of South America. It is considered to be a depressive state in which the individual believes that they have lost their soul.

WINDIGO SYNDROME

This describes a compulsive desire to become a cannibal and was originally described in North American Indians.

CHAPTER 3

SPECIFIC PSYCHIATRIC DISORDERS

Anorexia and bulimia nervosa 72

Anxiety disorders 76

Bipolar affective disorder 83

Depressive disorders 87

Personality disorders 91

Schizophrenia 99

ANOREXIA AND BULIMIA NERVOSA

ANOREXIA NERVOSA

Anorexia nervosa (AN) is diagnosed when there is a morbid **fear of fatness**, self-induced **weight loss** (body weight being maintained below 15% of the norm for that person) and a **body mass index (BMI) of 17.5 or less** (ICD-10). There are also widespread **endocrine disorders**, manifesting as amenorrhoea, raised growth hormone and cortisol, and abnormalities of thyroid hormone and insulin secretion.

CLINICAL FEATURES

The diagnosis is relatively easy: there is the presence of psychiatric symptomatology, as well as physical manifestations, which affect most body systems, e.g. endocrine, metabolic and gastrointestinal.

PSYCHIATRIC SYMPTOMATOLOGY

There are overvalued ideas concerning body weight and physical appearance. This distorted body image leads to the belief that the body (or parts of it, such as the upper arms and thighs) is larger and fatter than it really is. Other symptomatology includes obsessions/compulsions, depression, anxiety and personality disorders. There is also an increased suicide risk.

BEHAVIOURAL FEATURES

These include the avoidance of food, especially carbohydrate-rich foods; overactivity in the form of exercise to produce weight loss; self-consciousness, and social isolation.

PHYSICAL FEATURES

- **General** The patient is thin, pale, emaciated, the skin dry, and lanugo (fine downy) hair covers the face and trunk. Repeated vomiting may lead to pitted teeth, scarring of the knuckles and parotid swelling.
- **Cardiovascular** There may be bradycardia or tachycardia, hypotension, ventricular arrhythmias and other ECG abnormalities.
- **Endocrine** In women there is low LH and FSH, with disturbance of the hypothalamo–pituitary–gonadal axis leading to amenorrhoea. In men the latter leads to poor libido. There may also be elevation of growth hormone and cortisol and disturbance of insulin and thyroid hormone.
- **Gastrointestinal** Constipation, diarrhoea and, less commonly, liver abnormalities and pancreatitis may occur.
- **Haematological** Anaemia and leucopenia can occur.

- **Metabolic** Some of the metabolic abnormalities include hypothermia, hypoglycaemia, hypercholesterolaemia, hypokalaemia and alkalosis.
- **Neurological** Neuropathies and seizures are known to occur.
- **Renal** Renal failure may result from renal calculi, low glomerular filtration rate and low serum magnesium.
- **Skeletal** Osteoporosis.

EPIDEMIOLOGY

The overall prevalence is between 0.5 and 1%, with a higher rate among schoolgirls and female students (1–2%), especially in those from higher social classes. The male:female ratio is 1:10. There is a relatively high mortality, with rates varying between 5 and 15%.

AETIOLOGY

This remains elusive. The **biological** mechanism includes genetic factors (concordance is higher in monozygotic than in dizygotic twins), abnormalities of hypothalamic function, and dysfunction of the 5-HT neurotransmitter system.

Psychosocial explanations include media and peer group pressure, difficulties in interpersonal relationships, and the desire to avoid sexual maturity.

DIFFERENTIAL DIAGNOSIS

Medical disorders
Any disorder that leads to low weight should be considered, these include:

- Addison's disease
- Carcinoma
- Diabetes mellitus
- Inflammatory bowel diseases such as Crohn's or coeliac disease
- Thyrotoxicosis.

Psychiatric disorders

- Bulimia nervosa
- Adjustment disorder
- Depression
- Obsessive–compulsive disorder (OCD)
- Psychotic disorders such as schizophrenia
- Phobic disorders.

MANAGEMENT

See Chapter 4 (p. 130).

PROGNOSIS

The prognosis is variable, with a relatively high mortality rate ranging between 5 and 15%. The early treatment response is good in many, with 20% recovering completely; the remainder follow a chronic and fluctuating course. A third of chronic cases may go on to develop bulimia nervosa (BN).

BULIMIA NERVOSA

As with anorexia nervosa there is a preoccupation with weight and shape **(fear of fatness)**, but **binge eating**, **self-induced vomiting** and the use of **laxatives** or **diuretics** appear to be prominent. The loss of self-control may lead to a trance-like state, especially during episodes of binge eating.

CLINICAL FEATURES

The core features are described above. The weight may be normal or excessive, with marked fluctuations.

PSYCHIATRIC SYMPTOMATOLOGY

Depression, anxiety, obsessions/compulsions, abuse of alcohol and drugs and impulsiveness. Low self-esteem appears to be common.

BEHAVIOURAL FEATURES

Repeated cycles of binge eating (as much as 10 000 kcal may be consumed in one episode) followed by vomiting and purging (laxatives and diuretics). Self-injurious behaviour such as overdosing may also occur.

PHYSICAL FEATURES

These result from purging rather than from starvation as in anorexia nervosa.

- **General** The weight is normal or excessive, with parotid swelling, decalcification of teeth and calluses on the dorsum of the hands (known as Russell's sign).
- **Cardiac** Dysrhythmias due to hypokalaemia can occur.
- **Endocrine** Disturbances of thyroid and cortisol may occur.
- **Gastrointestinal** Oesophageal tears and erosion due to vomiting may be seen.
- **Metabolic** Metabolic disturbance such as alkalosis and hypokalaemia may have serious consequences.
- **Renal** Renal damage may result.

EPIDEMIOLOGY

The onset is usually a little later than that of anorexia nervosa and many will have had a previous history of AN. The prevalence is around 1–3%, with a female:male ratio of 50:1. The mortality rate is somewhat lower than that of AN.

AETIOLOGY

There are a number of similarities between AN and BN; however, in the latter the greater urge to eat and the loss of impulse control appears to be prominent. Genetic factors may also play a part, as there is an excess of relatives with depression, BN and alcohol and drug disorders.

DIFFERENTIAL DIAGNOSIS

Medical disorders

- Klein–Levin syndrome (hyperphagia, hypersomnia)
- Kluver–Bucy syndrome (hyperphagia, hypersexuality, visual agnosias)
- Upper GI disorders (duodenal ulcer, oesophageal strictures).

Psychiatric disorders

- Anorexia nervosa
- Adjustment disorder
- Depression (especially seasonal affective disorder – SAD)
- Bipolar affective disorder
- Obsessive–compulsive disorder
- Personality disorder (borderline PD).

MANAGEMENT

BN itself is usually managed on an outpatient basis. However, admission may be required if there is a worsening of the comorbid disorders, such as severe depression with suicide risk. Occasionally the significant worsening of medical complications (e.g. electrolyte imbalance) will require inpatient treatment.

Medical management involves the identification and correction of medical complications, whereas **psychosocial** treatments include cognitive behavioural therapy aimed at correcting the disorder of eating and impulse control. Comorbid psychiatric disorders should also be actively treated. SSRIs in higher doses have been found to be useful in the treatment of bulimia (see Chapter 4).

PROGNOSIS

The prognosis is better than for AN, but worst in those who progress from AN to BN. It also appears to be better for those whose weight is normal.

ANXIETY DISORDERS

ADJUSTMENT DISORDER

An adjustment disorder results from a maladapted response to a life event or psychosocial stresses. According to ICD-10 it usually occurs within 1 month of the stressful event (note: DSM-IV suggests within 3 months) and the symptoms should not last longer than 6 months. The symptomatology includes depressed mood, anxiety, worries, and inability to cope. Pre-existing medical illnesses may be exacerbated and abuse of drugs and alcohol may result.

EPIDEMIOLOGY

The prevalence ratio varies between 5 and 20%, with increased vulnerability among the medically ill and lower social classes. Males and females are equally affected.

AETIOLOGY

Little is known of the biological factors that may be involved. Psychosocial factors that are suggested include immature coping mechanisms and the nature of the stressful event, especially its symbolism for the patient.

DIFFERENTIAL DIAGNOSIS

These include:

- Anxiety disorders, such as generalized anxiety disorder, acute stress reaction and PTSD
- Affective disorders
- Medical disorders causing anxiety
- Alcohol and drug abuse.

MANAGEMENT

- Exclusion of other medical and psychiatric disorders
- Reassurance
- Psychosocial (supportive psychotherapies/counselling, anxiety management strategies)
- Pharmacological:
  — Short-term use of benzodiazepines, e.g. diazepam 5–10 mg or lorazepam 1–2 mg (avoid in the medically ill)
  — Antidepressants such as paroxetine may be required for a period.

PROGNOSIS

The overall prognosis is good and the majority of patients recover. Poor prognostic factors include abuse of alcohol and drugs, as well as personality difficulties and a previous psychiatric history.

GENERALIZED ANXIETY DISORDER (GAD)

This is a generalized state of excessive and pervasive anxiety, fear and worry, usually accompanied by physical symptoms, which is not specific to a situation.

EPIDEMIOLOGY

Approximately 2–4% of the population suffers from GAD. Over a quarter of GP consultations are for GAD, and 10% of hospital outpatient consultations concern this disorder. Onset is usually before the fourth decade, and two-thirds of patients are women.

AETIOLOGY

The aetiology appears to have both a psychological and a physical basis. The **psychological factors** range from behavioural theories of conditioning and emotional conflicts, childhood separations, to unconscious conflicts between ego and superego.

Biological factors are based on genetic predisposition, as shown by high concordance rates in twins (monozygotic 50%; dizygotic 4%) and in families (up to 15%), as well as autonomic nervous system dysfunction, as reflected by an increased sympathetic tone or parasympathetic abnormalities. It is also noted that habituation to perceived threatening situations is delayed.

CLINICAL FEATURES

These include both physical and psychological symptoms. The **physical** symptoms mostly affect the autonomic nervous system, and include palpitations, tachycardia, breathlessness, dry mouth, perspiration, facial flushing, cold hands and cold sweats, tremulousness, nausea, diarrhoea, fatigue, and urge to urinate. There may also be increased muscle tension and fatigue.

The **psychological** symptoms include apprehension, feelings of fear, hypervigilance, irritability, initial insomnia, lack of patience, mood changes, depersonalization, derealization, illusions and hypnapompic and hypnagogic hallucinations.

Some people have episodes of **hyperventilation** leading to tetany, carpopedal spasm and perioral paraesthesia due to respiratory alkalosis. This can be managed by the use of a paper bag over the nose and mouth for a short period.

DIFFERENTIAL DIAGNOSIS

Anxiety is a common symptom in many psychiatric as well as medical conditions (see Tables 6.1 and 6.2 in Chapter 6). It is present in depression, psychotic, dementing, neurotic, organic and substance abuse disorders, as well as many neurological disorders.

MANAGEMENT

This encompasses both psychological and physical (mostly drugs) treatments (see Chapter 4).

PROGNOSIS

GAD is a mostly chronic and often lifelong disorder. Males recover more often than do females. At 1 year over two-thirds still suffer from the disorder with the same intensity. It is generally resistant to treatment and may give rise to depressive syndromes later in life. However, when the sufferer has a stable personality and the onset is acute with an identifiable cause and relatively short duration, the prognosis is more favourable.

PANIC DISORDER

Panic disorder consists of unexpected, spontaneous and recurrent panic attacks without a medical aetiology, usually not restricted to a defined situation or set of circumstances. The episodic attacks manifest themselves through various autonomic signs and symptoms, together with a dread or fear of losing control, or dying. These patients tend to crowd medical practices and may undergo many investigations before being referred to a psychiatrist.

EPIDEMIOLOGY

The lifetime prevalence of panic disorder is between 1.5 and 3%. Women sufferers outnumber men and the average age of onset is the early 20s. Panic disorder is often associated with agoraphobia; panic attacks seldom occur in the absence of other anxiety disorders.

AETIOLOGY

The **biological** explanations include:

- The contribution of a small but definitive **genetic** basis, as the risk of developing this disorder is increased in first-degree relatives
- Dysregulation of both peripheral and central nervous systems
- Involvement of neurotransmitters, such as noradrenaline, serotonin and GABA
- Functional abnormalities of certain brain regions following the use of panic-inducing agents, as ascertained by neuroimaging studies.

The **psychosocial** explanations include:

- Cognitive behavioural theory, supported by the high success rate of treatment with cognitive behavioural therapy
- Psychoanalytic theories.

DIAGNOSIS

For a definitive diagnosis ICD-10 suggests that, over a month, several unpredictable severe attacks of autonomic anxiety should have occurred, without an objective danger.

CLINICAL FEATURES

Essentially there are recurrent attacks of severe and unpredictable anxiety (panic) which is not restricted to a defined situation or set of circumstances. Symptoms include anxiety, hyperventilation, palpitations, feelings of faintness, fear of imminent death and a desire to escape. Hyperventilation may lead to hypocapnoea, carpopedal spasm, cerebral vasoconstriction and 'pins and needles' in the limbs.

MANAGEMENT

See Chapter 4.

PROGNOSIS

Panic disorder is a chronic disorder with a variable outcome. However, 30–40% of sufferers are symptom free at long-term follow-up; approximately 50% are left with mild symptoms, and 10–20% continue to have significant symptoms.

POST-TRAUMATIC STRESS DISORDER (PTSD)

PTSD is characterized by three subsets of symptoms: **intrusive** symptoms (memories, flashbacks), **avoidance** symptoms and **hyperarousal** symptoms, and in many cases other comorbid (usually depressive) psychiatric symptoms. The disorder can be either acute (duration of symptoms less than 3 months) or chronic (duration of symptoms of 3 months or longer); it can also occur with delayed onset (at least 6 months between the traumatic event and the onset of symptoms). It is one of the few psychiatric disorders where there is little disagreement with regard to the triggering event, as by definition it results from experiencing or witnessing an extremely traumatic event such as a threat to or near loss of life.

CLINICAL FEATURES

These are as described above and may be outlined as below:

- Avoidance; hypervigilance; startle response
- Nightmares; flashbacks; intrusive memories
- Autonomic hyperarousal; symptoms of anxiety, irritability and sleep disturbance
- Comorbid depressive symptoms may also be present.

DIAGNOSIS

Operational criteria based on the above symptomatology and outlined in both ICD-10 and DSM-IV are used for diagnostic purposes.

Other comorbid psychiatric symptoms, especially depression and anxiety, are common and may complicate the clinical picture. Social functioning may become so impaired that the patient may lose his or her job, family, social standing and quality of life.

EPIDEMIOLOGY

Community-based studies have revealed a lifetime prevalence ranging from 1 to 14%, with at-risk individuals (e.g. combat veterans, observers/survivors of civilian disasters, victims of criminal violence and physical attack) showing trauma-specific prevalence rates ranging from 1 to 58%.

In men the highest rates of current or lifetime PTSD are associated with combat experience or seeing someone being injured or killed, whereas in women the highest rates are associated with physical attack and rape.

Over one-third of patients with burn injuries show some from of PTSD and impairment of personal and social functioning.

AETIOLOGY

By definition there should have been a history of a severe stressful/traumatic event; however, this does not imply a simple cause–effect relationship, as many who experience sufficiently traumatic events, do not develop PTSD.

It is suggested that to develop PTSD, there should be presence of certain vulnerability factors, such as:

- A genetic predisposition to psychiatric disorders
- A history of childhood trauma
- The presence of a personality disorder, such as borderline, dependent, dissociate or paranoid
- Recent experience of stressful life changes
- Abuse of alcohol and drugs
- Inability cognitively to rationalize the traumatic event.

MANAGEMENT

See Chapter 4 (p. 136).

PROGNOSIS

The course of PTSD shows variability, with a fluctuation of symptoms over time, worsening during the periods of stress. Approximately 30% show complete recovery, 40% continue to experience mild symptoms, 20% moderate symptoms, and 10% show no improvement or become worse.

In general, those who experience a rapid onset and a shorter duration (<6 months) of symptoms, with a good premorbid personality, effective psychosocial support, early treatment and absence of psychiatric and medical disorders, have a favourable prognosis.

OBSESSIVE–COMPULSIVE DISORDER (OCD)

This is characterized by egodystonic obsessions and compulsions which are not only time-consuming but also interfere with the sufferer's daily functioning.

Obsessions are thoughts, impulses or images, and usually have the following characteristics:

- **R**ecurrent
- **I**ntrusive
- **P**ersistent
- **S**enseless
- **O**wn (i.e. not foreign, as in schizophrenia)
- **U**npleasant
- **R**esistant (but this may wane).

Note	Note the mnemonic RIPSOUR.

Compulsions are repetitive, purposeful and stereotyped behaviours.

Obsessions and compulsions may occur together or alone, and usually follow certain themes. The commonest **obsessions** are as follows (corresponding compulsions in brackets):

- Contamination (repetitive cleaning, handwashing)
- Doubt (repetitive checking, e.g. of locks)
- Intrusive, derogatory, aggressive, sexual thoughts (usually no compulsions, but may involve mental acts)
- Symmetry, neatness, precision (perfection, which may lead to obsessional slowness).

OCD has a high degree of comorbid psychiatric disorders, such as depression, drug and alcohol abuse and other anxiety disorders.

Obsessive–compulsive features may also occur secondarily in many medical (basal ganglia disorders, dementia) and psychiatric disorders, such as schizophrenia, depression, Gilles de la Tourette's syndrome and other tic disorders.

EPIDEMIOLOGY

This disorder has a lifetime prevalence of 1.9–3.2%, but is frequently underdiagnosed owing to patients' reluctance to come forward. There is a bimodal onset, with peaks at 12–14 years and 20–22 years, and males appear to have an earlier onset. Males and females are equally affected.

AETIOLOGY

OCD belongs to a spectrum of disorders which includes Gilles de la Tourette's syndrome and other tic disorders. Genetic factors appear to operate in 50% of cases, and dysregulation of the serotonin system is likely, as SSRIs play a large part in management. Abnormalities of dopamine as well as of other neurotransmitters are increasingly being reported. Studies using neuroimaging techniques point to abnormalities in the basal ganglia and prefrontal, orbitofrontal–subcortical circuits, which is further supported by recent studies using transcranial magnetic stimulation (TMS). **Psychosocial causes** (increasingly being discarded) include psychoanalytic theories (defence against cruel and aggressive fantasies; regression to the anal stage of development) and behavioural theories (compulsive behaviour resulting from learning, and which is maintained by operant conditioning).

DIFFERENTIAL DIAGNOSIS

It is essential to determine that obsessive–compulsive symptoms are not secondary to other serious psychiatric disorders, such as schizophrenia and depression. The symptoms may also occur following damage to the basal ganglia, such as in Sydenham's chorea.

Other disorders to exclude include:

- Gilles de la Tourette and other tic disorders
- Phobic disorders
- Somatoform disorders
- Obsessive–compulsive personality disorder.

MANAGEMENT

This involves **psychobehavioural** management (cognitive behaviour therapy, thought-stopping, response prevention) and **pharmacotherapy**, e.g. use of SSRIs (see Chapter 4). ECT is sometimes used for OCD associated with depression, and in severe cases psychosurgery may be needed (see Chapter 4).

PROGNOSIS

This is a chronic disorder with symptoms that wax and wane, with periods of remission. However, 50% of sufferers appear to recover. Those with anankastic/obsessional personality disorder are predisposed to this disorder and have a poor prognosis. Social stressors and psychiatric illness also worsen the prognosis.

Approximately 75% improve with a combination of SSRIs and response prevention. OCD should be taken seriously, for it may give rise to alcohol and drug abuse, with an associated increased risk of suicide.

BIPOLAR AFFECTIVE DISORDER (MANIC–DEPRESSIVE PSYCHOSIS)

Bipolar affective disorder, also known as manic–depressive psychosis, has a spectrum of presentations and, depending upon the symptomatology and the time course, a number of diagnostic categories have been described.

DIAGNOSIS

Many disorders, both medical and psychiatric, may be confused with mania; these should be excluded and appropriately treated (see Chapter 4).

As there are no laboratory diagnostic tests, the diagnosis rests on the use of a set of operational criteria described in DSM-IV and ICD-10, along with the clinical assessment. It is essential to take a broad view of the patient's symptomatology and take account of the collateral history.

ICD-10 DIAGNOSTIC CATEGORIES

F30.0 HYPOMANIA

Described as a lesser degree of mania in which abnormalities of mood and behaviour are persistent and marked, although not accompanied by hallucinations or delusions. There is mild elevation of mood, increased energy and activity, marked feelings of wellbeing, and physical and mental efficiency.

Increased sociability, talkativeness, overfamiliarity, increased sexual energy, and a decreased need for sleep are often present.

Irritability, conceit and boorish behaviour may take the place of the more usual euphoric sociability, and considerable interference with work or social activity is also common.

To satisfy the diagnosis the presentation should last for several days, and there should be considerable interference with work or social activities.

F30.1 MANIA WITHOUT PSYCHOTIC SYMPTOMS

An elevated mood which is out of keeping with the individual's circumstances and varies from carefree joviality to almost uncontrollable excitement. There is elation, increased energy resulting in overactivity, pressure of speech, and a decreased need for sleep. The usual social inhibitions are lost and attention cannot be sustained. An inflated sense of self-esteem, with expressions of grandiose or overoptimistic ideas, is present.

Perceptual abnormalities may occur, for example appreciation of colours as being especially vivid. There may also be a preoccupation with fine details of surfaces or textures, and subjective hyperacusis. The patient may become extravagant and impractical in schemes, spending money recklessly, becoming aggressive, amorous or facetious in inappropriate circumstances.

The mood is irritable and suspicious rather than elated.

For a *diagnosis* the episode should last for at least 1 week, and be severe enough to disrupt ordinary work and social activities. Mood changes should be accompanied by increased energy and several of the symptoms referred to above, especially the pressure of speech, decreased need for sleep, grandiosity and excessive optimism.

F30.2 MANIA WITH PSYCHOTIC SYMPTOMS

This is described as a more severe form of mania. Inflated self-esteem, grandiose ideas, irritability and suspiciousness may develop into various forms of delusion. In severe cases prominent grandiose or religious delusions of identity or role, and flight of ideas and pressure of speech may result in the individual becoming incomprehensible.

Severe and sustained physical activity and excitement may result in aggression or violence, and neglect of eating and drinking and personal hygiene may result in dangerous states of dehydration and self-neglect.

> **Note**   Approximately 20% of manic patients show schneiderian first-rank symptoms.

For other ICD-10 diagnostic categories see Appendix.

Another way of categorizing bipolar affective disorder is as follows:

- **Type I** describes those with one or more manic or mixed episodes
- **Type II** patients may have had recurrent depressive episodes with subclinical hypomanic episodes
- **Rapid cyclers** are those who frequently present with high and low moods ranging from days to weeks in duration
- Some will present simultaneously with **mixed features** of both mania and depression.

Disorders mimicking a manic episode

Medical causes include:

- **Brain disorder** leading to frontal lobe syndromes, e.g. infections such as HIV, syphilis and encephalitis; degenerative diseases such as Pick's disease, Alzheimer's; tumours, trauma and temporal lobe epilepsy (TLE)
- **Endocrine** (hyperthyroidism)
- **Drugs** (both prescribed and illicit), alcohol (withdrawal phase), amphetamines, cocaine, hallucinogens and steroids.

Psychiatric disorders:

- **Schizophrenia** (Note: 20% of manic patients have schneiderian first-rank symptoms)
- **Brief reactive psychosis** related to an experienced stressful event
- **Adult attention deficit/hyperactivity disorder** (ADHD).

EPIDEMIOLOGY

- Lifetime risk is approximately 1%
- First episode most commonly occurs between the ages of 15 and 30 years, but may occur at any age from late childhood to the seventh to eighth decades
- Average age of onset is the early 20s
- Men and women are equally affected.

AETIOLOGY

Biological theories

Genetic factors play an important part in the development of this disorder, as is shown by family studies and the concordance rate reported for monozygotic twins, which is approximately 70% whereas that for dizygotic twins is around 20%.

    Neuroendocrine abnormalities have also been implicated.

    Medical disorders (neurological, endocrine) and **drugs** (prescribed and illicit) can give rise to the manic syndromes.

Psychosocial theories

Life events, e.g. grief and other emotionally significant experiences, may trigger mania and related syndromes. The **psychodynamic** models of mania suggest that manic defence is a form of protection against depression and loss of superego control.

FEATURES IN MENTAL STATE EXAMINATION (MANIA WITHOUT PSYCHOSIS)

Mood

- Persistent elevation/expansiveness of mood
- Irritability more common than elation
- May be intermingled with depression of mood.

Speech, thinking and cognition

- Speech is pressured, loud, emphatic, and difficult to interrupt
- Increased tempo of thinking, and flight of ideas
- Distractability, attention drawn to irrelevancies
- Inflated self-image, grandiose and expansive ideas
- Up to 20% may have schneiderian first-rank symptoms
- Limitation or loss of insight.

Somatic/biological/behavioural features

- Increased drive and activity
- Increased physical, social and sexual activity
- Excessive risk-taking, inappropriate social behaviour
- Insomnia – often an early sign
- EEG shows a reduction in δ sleep
- Lack of apparent fatigue
- Appetite is good – weight loss due to overactivity in spite of increased appetite.

PROGNOSIS

Overall the prognosis for those who take regular prophylactic mood stabilizers is favourable.

Bipolar I disorder shows an increase in both the frequency and the severity of each episode during the early years, with a subsequent plateau in the later years. The prognosis for **bipolar II** appears to be somewhat better; however, with the former there remains a high suicide risk.

Cyclothymic patients follow a chronic course, with around 30% developing the full-blown bipolar affective disorder.

MANAGEMENT

Psychiatric management consists primarily of mood-stabilizing drugs and psychosocial interventions. For details see Chapters 4, 5, and 6.

DEPRESSIVE DISORDERS

These disorders are characterized by a significant and pervasive lowering of mood, which is inappropriate to the circumstances and usually accompanied by abnormalities of thinking, perception, bodily functions and behaviour. The variations in the symptomatology, temporal factors and presentations have led to a number of varieties of depression being described, and consequently at times resulted in difficulties or even disagreement with regard to the classification.

DIAGNOSIS

This essentially involves the use of criteria as outlined in ICD-10 or DSM-IV, as well as the clinical skills required to make an effective psychiatric assessment. Obviously the medical disorders (including drugs and alcohol) that may cause depressive symptomatology should be excluded and appropriately treated.

ICD-10 uses the following categories to describe some of the varieties of depression (see also Appendix):

- F.32 Depressive episode (mild, moderate and severe)
- F.33 Recurrent depressive disorder
- F.34 Persistent (affective) mood disorders (cyclothymia, dysthymia)
- F.38 Other mood disorders (mixed affective disorder, recurrent brief depressive disorder).

UNIPOLAR DEPRESSION

Clinical depression is defined on the basis of significant and pervasive lowering of the mood, accompanied by physiological, psychomotor and cognitive disturbances. This is considered pathological if its duration and severity exceed normal criteria.

A variety of terminologies have been used to describe depression:

- Unipolar and bipolar mood disorders
- Primary and secondary depression
- Endogenous and reactive depression
- Psychotic and neurotic depression.

CLINICAL FEATURES

Fundamentally, there is a pervasive lowering of mood, accompanied by a range of physiological and psychosocial symptoms. Often there is anxiety, as well as psychiatric symptoms more characteristic of other psychiatric disorders (e.g. psychotic, obsessive–compulsive symptoms).

Significant depression may lead to considerable morbidity (owing to increased vulnerability to other psychiatric and medical disorders) and mortality (mainly because of the increased risk of suicide).

(A) Core symptoms

- **Mood:** lowering of mood – typically *diurnal variation* (depression worse in the mornings)
- **Enjoyment:** lack of interest (anhedonia); lack of pleasure and interest without reason
- **Energy:** lack of energy and tiredness; motor retardation.

(B) Other symptoms

- Suicidal thoughts, plans, self-harm
- Sleep disturbance, e.g. early morning wakening (2 hours or more earlier than usual)
- Self-esteem that is lowered
- Sex – poor libido
- Guilt thoughts
- Attention, concentration, memory difficulties
- Pessimistic – views of self, world and future
- Appetite, weight disturbance (a loss of >5% of body weight over previous month).

> Some symptoms are occasionally described as somatic, vegetative or biological, and include:
>
> - Mood (diurnal variation)
> - Enjoyment: lack of interest/pleasure
> - Energy, lack of
> - Sleep disturbance (early-morning wakening = EMW)
> - Sex – poor libido
> - Appetite: weight disturbance (loss of >5% of body weight over previous month)
> - Amenorrhoea
> - Constipation

F.32 DEPRESSIVE EPISODE

A typical depressive episode is described in terms of core symptoms as well as other symptoms, which should last 2 or more weeks. Depending on the symptoms, the episode can be further subdivided into **mild, moderate** or **severe**:

- A **mild depressive episode** has two features from A and two from B (2A + 2B)
- A **moderate depressive episode** has two features from A and three or four from B (2A + 3 or 4B)
- A **severe depressive episode** has three features from A and four from B (3A + 4B).

A severe episode may have added psychotic symptoms of delusions and hallucinations, which are usually mood congruent.

Note	Severe psychomotor retardation may lead to a depressive stupor.

EPIDEMIOLOGY

Depression is relatively common, with a lifetime risk of 5–12% in men and 9–26% in women in western countries.

Depression appears to be more common among women:

- From the working class
- Who have three or more children under the age of 14
- Who do not work outside the home
- Who lack a confiding relationship
- Who lost their own mother before the age of 11.

The risk of depression is also increased amongst the unmarried, divorced or separated, the unemployed and those from lower social classes and urban areas. The presence of medical or psychiatric disorders and abuse of drugs and alcohol also increases the risk of depression.

The average age of onset is during the late 30s; however, presentations in children and the elderly also occur.

The suicide rate averages around 10% and remains the biggest cause of increased mortality.

AETIOLOGY

The aetiological basis of depression appears to involve a wide range of biological and psychosocial factors, but the exact mechanism remains elusive.

Biological factors
These include:

- **Genetic factors:** the evidence for this (though less strong than for bipolar disorder) comes from adoption and twin studies
- **Neurotransmitters:** studies utilizing biochemistry, molecular science, neuroimaging and treatment with antidepressants point to alterations in neurotransmitters, such as serotonin, noradrenaline and dopamine
- Alterations in **sleep**, **circadian rhythm**, **immunological** and **neuroendocrine systems** also seem to occur among the depressed, though the cause-and-effect relation remains unclear.

Psychosocial factors

The evidence for the role of psychosocial factors comes from epidemiological studies, which identify certain vulnerable groups (see under Epidemiology).

Stressful life events appear to predispose individuals to depression (Freud pointed out the issue of loss as an aetiological basis for depression).

MANAGEMENT

See Chapters 4 and 5 for details.

PROGNOSIS

The prognosis for unipolar depression is variable and depends upon the severity, number of previous episodes, age at onset, psychosocial factors and treatment status.

Most single episodes, left untreated, last around 3–9 months, and. approximately 20% continue to have depressive symptoms for 2 or more years.

Depression recurs in about 50% of cases, rising to 80% in those exhibiting severe symptomatology requiring hospitalization.

The overall suicide risk is around 10%, contributing heavily to increased mortality among the depressed.

F 34.1 DYSTHYMIA

This presents with persistent depressive symptoms (lasting 2 or more years) of insufficient severity to meet the criteria for major depression. It may occur with other psychiatric conditions, such as borderline personality disorder.

Approximately one-third of sufferers go on to develop a more serious mood disorder.

ATYPICAL DEPRESSIVE SYNDROMES

F 38.0 MIXED AFFECTIVE EPISODE

In the mixed affective states there are rapid transitions from mania to depression and vice versa, lasting for at least 2 weeks.

F 38.1 RECURRENT BRIEF DEPRESSIVE DISORDER

By definition this lasts less than 2 weeks (usually 2–3 days), occurring once a month with complete recovery between episodes. The actual symptomatology may fulfil the criteria for mild, moderate or severe depression, except for the duration.

MASKED/ATYPICAL DEPRESSION

The depressed patient may present with somatic or other complaints, instead of a clearly depressed mood.

- **Physical condition:** Chronic pain, hypochondriasis, psychosomatic illnesses, conversion disorders and a poor response to medical treatment.
- **Psychiatric disorders:** Pseudodementia, anxiety states, behavioural changes, (e.g. shoplifting in middle-aged women, sexual disinhibition in middle-aged men etc.).

SEASONAL AFFECTIVE DISORDER (SAD)/SEASONAL MOOD DISORDER

There is a temporal relationship between the onset of depression and the particular season of the year (depression usually commences in autumn/winter and ends in spring/summer). Clinically there are symptoms of depression, carbohydrate craving, fatigue, hyperphagia and hypersomnia (see Chapter 4 for further details and treatment).

PERSONALITY DISORDERS

These are disorders characterized by **maladaptive**, **deeply ingrained** and **enduring behaviour patterns**, manifesting themselves as **inflexible responses** to a broad range of personal and social situations, which are frequently (but not always) associated with subjective **distress** and **impaired social functioning**.

Note	Unlike personality disorders, personality traits or types can be described as flexible, non-pathological and adaptive (e.g. compulsive, histrionic).

Two classification systems are used, namely ICD-10 and DSM-IV.

ICD-10	**DSM-IV**
Paranoid	Paranoid
Schizoid	Schizoid
	Schizotypal
Dissocial (antisocial)	Antisocial
Emotionally unstable	
– Impulsive	
– Borderline	Borderline

Histrionic	Histrionic
	Narcissistic
Anankastic (obsessive–compulsive)	Obsessive–compulsive
Anxious (avoidant)	Avoidant
Dependent	Dependent

Because of the high degree of overlap between many of these disorders, a further subdivision into three broad clusters is described as outlined below:

Cluster A	**Cluster B**	**Cluster C**
Paranoid	Dissocial	
		Avoidant
Schizoid	Borderline	Dependent
Schizotypal	Histrionic	Obsessive–compulsive
	Narcissistic	

EPIDEMIOLOGY

Patients with personality disorders, whether primary or comorbid, are frequently encountered in psychiatric practice. However, in clinical practice you are more likely to deal with certain specific personality disorders (e.g. borderline and dissocial personality disorders), and will no doubt find the management challenging.

An approximate prevalence of personality disorders as a whole is:

- 10% of the general population
- 20% of GP attendees
- 30% of psychiatric outpatients
- 40% of psychiatric inpatients.

COMORBIDITY

There is a relatively high comorbidity (as much as 25–50%) with other psychiatric disorders.

The following psychiatric disorders have some association with specific personality disorders.

- Depression: anxious (anxious), borderline, impulsive, obsessive–compulsive and dependent personality disorders
- Drugs/alcohol abuse: borderline and dissocial personality disorders
- Neurotic disorders:
  — Anxiety: anxious (anxious), borderline, dependent and impulsive personality disorders
  — Eating disorders: borderline personality disorder
  — OCD: obsessive–compulsive personality disorder
  — Somatization: histrionic personality disorder (Briquet's syndrome)

AETIOLOGY

There is strong evidence for the contribution of **genetic factors** in the development of personality disorders. The **early environment** (especially during the first 5 years, when the brain circuitry continues to develop and modify) is also thought to play an important role. For example, the prevalence of dysfunctional families and sexual abuse is quite high among those with borderline personality disorder.

Temperamental factors identified during early childhood may also be associated with personality disorders in adults.

Other **biological abnormalities** associated with various personality disorders include:

- Abnormalities of **sex hormones** (e.g. testosterone) in dissocial personality disorder
- Low **platelet monoamine oxidase** levels have been noted in some individuals with schizotypal personality disorder
- **Smooth pursuit eye movement** abnormalities have been noted in those with traits of introversion, low self-esteem, and schizotypal personality disorder
- **Neurotransmitter** abnormalities, especially of serotonin, have been shown to have some association with aggression, impulsiveness and suicidal behaviour (e.g. borderline personality disorder)
- **EEG** abnormalities (slow-wave activity) have been found in some individuals with borderline and dissocial personality disorders.

PARANOID PERSONALITY DISORDER

This is characterized by excessive **sensitivity to criticism** and, a strong tendency to **bear grudges**. The patient finds **conspiracies** behind innocent events, has a tenacious sense of individual rights and is prone to **suspiciousness** and pathological **jealousy**.

DIFFERENTIAL DIAGNOSIS

Paranoid disorder, paranoid schizophrenia, dissocial personality disorder.

PROGNOSIS

Overall the prognosis for paranoid personality disorders is poor, with many continuing to have marital, social and occupational difficulties.

SCHIZOID PERSONALITY DISORDER

These are **withdrawn, detached** people who rarely experience pleasure, show little emotion towards others (either positive or negative), are uninterested in sexual relationships, prefer **introspection** and **fantasy**, have few or no close relationships, and tend towards eccentric behaviour as they lack social norms.

DIFFERENTIAL DIAGNOSIS

Schizotypal and avoidant personality disorders.

PROGNOSIS

The prognosis is relatively poor and it is unclear how many go on to develop schizophrenia.

SCHIZOTYPAL PERSONALITY DISORDER

These individuals appear odd or strange, show **magical thinking**, **peculiar ideas**, **ideas of reference**, **illusions** and, on occasions, **derealization**.

DIFFERENTIAL DIAGNOSIS

Avoidant personality disorders and schizophrenia.

PROGNOSIS

Many continue to function despite their oddities; however, one study showed that as many as 10% may eventually commit suicide. Schizotypal personality disorder may easily be confused with schizophrenia, and many consider this to be the premorbid personality of schizophrenia patients.

DISSOCIAL PERSONALITY DISORDER

This is also known as antisocial (sociopathic) personality disorder and features **callous unconcern** for others, **irresponsibility** and unconcern for social obligations and rules, **low tolerance**, frustration, and a consequent **tendency to violence**. An **absence of guilt**, a tendency to blame others, and persistent **irritability** appear to be prominent.

DIFFERENTIAL DIAGNOSIS

Borderline personality disorders and schizophrenia.

PROGNOSIS

The prognosis is variable; many improve with age, but comorbid psychosocial problems (e.g. abuse of alcohol, drugs, forensic history) may result in a worse outcome.

EMOTIONALLY UNSTABLE PERSONALITY DISORDERS

These include **impulsive** and **borderline**: both show an inability to control impulses, mood instability and frequent violent outbursts. Borderline personalities show an uncertain self-image and identity, suicidal behaviour, and a tendency to become involved in intense but unstable relationships.

Borderline personality disorder

For the diagnosis at least five of the characteristics outlined below need to be present:

Mood instability
Image/**I**dentity disturbance/**I**mpulsiveness
Suicidal behaviour
Emptiness (chronic feeling)
Relationship instabilities
Abandonment (fear of)
Boredom (chronic feeling of)
'**L**oony' (brief psychosis)
Emotionally 'charged'

Note	Note the mnemonic **MISERABLE**.

DIFFERENTIAL DIAGNOSIS

Many other personality disorders and major psychiatric disorders (e.g. depression and substance abuse).

PROGNOSIS

The short-term prognosis is relatively poor. Many improve with age; however, the abuse of alcohol and drugs usually leads to a less than favourable outcome.

HISTRIONIC PERSONALITY DISORDER

The prominent features include **self-dramatization**, **suggestibility**, **shallow emotions**, **egocentricity**, **longing for appreciation**, **craving to be the centre of attention**, and **persistent manipulative** behaviour. In the USA the diagnosis of **narcissistic personality disorder** is described: this overlaps with the histrionic personality disorder, but also includes the notion of special entitlement and excessive self-involvement with the disorder.

DIFFERENTIAL DIAGNOSIS

Borderline personality disorder and somatization disorder, which may coexist.

PROGNOSIS

There is an apparent improvement with age; however, abuse of alcohol and drugs may lead to a poorer prognosis.

ANANKASTIC PERSONALITY DISORDER

In the USA this is called obsessive–compulsive personality disorder and is characterized by excessive **caution, conscientiousness, perfectionism** and **preoccupation with detail, pedantry** and **limited emotional expression**, a desire for conformity associated with **rigidity**, a tendency towards **obsessional modes of thinking**, and a need to **plan ahead in meticulous detail**.

DIFFERENTIAL DIAGNOSIS

Obsessive–compulsive disorder.

PROGNOSIS

These individuals may do well in certain jobs requiring obsessional behaviour.

Unfortunately, many may go on to develop OCD and therefore have a poor prognosis.

ANXIOUS (AVOIDANT) PERSONALITY DISORDER

Features include **persistent tension**, **self-consciousness**, feelings of **insecurity**, yearning to be accepted and liked, **hypersensitivity to criticism**, a wish for uncritical acceptance in relationships, a tendency to avoid everyday situations and a restricted lifestyle.

DIFFERENTIAL DIAGNOSIS

Schizoid personality disorder.

PROGNOSIS

A protected environment may lead to a favourable outcome, but some may develop social phobia and are therefore likely to have a poorer prognosis.

DEPENDENT PERSONALITY DISORDER

These individuals need encouragement to take over the major responsibilities of life, show **subordination** of their own needs to those of others, unwillingness to make demands on others, a self-perception of **inadequacy**, a fear of being abandoned, and devastation when close relationships end.

DIFFERENTIAL DIAGNOSIS

Agoraphobia, borderline and histrionic personality disorders.

PROGNOSIS

Treatment leads to a favourable outcome; however, loss of the person upon whom the sufferer is dependent is likely to lead to depression and a poor prognosis.

NARCISSISTIC PERSONALITY DISORDER

Described in DSM-IV and characterized by an **elevated sense of self-importance** and **grandiose feelings**.

DIFFERENTIAL DIAGNOSIS

Borderline, dissocial and histrionic personality disorders, which may coexist.

PROGNOSIS

These individuals are difficult to treat and have a poor prognosis.

ASSESSMENT OF PERSONALITY DISORDERS

The assessment of personality disorder should be based on a comprehensive evaluation of the individual by a psychiatric history and MSE, as well as acquiring relevant information from all other sources. There is a need to take a **longitudinal history** and demonstrate the **pervasiveness** of symptoms and behaviours, covering most aspects of an individual's life. Special attention should also be paid to:

- Cognition (how they perceive)
- Affectivity
- Gratification of needs, control over impulses
- Manner of relating to stress.

When clarifying specific personality disorders, some helpful questions include:

Paranoid

- How do you **get on** with other people?
- Do you find you can **trust** people?
- Do you sometimes feel that you are **picked upon**?
- Do you think people like you generally?
- Are you **self-conscious**?
- Are you mostly **treated fairly**?

Schizoid

- Do you have many **friends**?
- Can you **mix** easily?
- Do you prefer to be **alone** or in company?
- Would you describe yourself as **shy**?

Dissocial

- Have you been in much **trouble with the police**?
- How do you get on with **authority**?
- Do you **dislike being told** what to do?
- Do you have **impulses to hurt** others?

Borderline

Questions based on the mnemonic **MISERABLE** (see p. 95).

At least five of these characteristics should be present for the diagnosis to be made.

Individuals with borderline personality disorder commonly display the defence mechanism called **splitting**, which may cause disagreements between staff and lead to management difficulties.

Histrionic

- Do you tend to be **overemotional**?
- Do you like to be the centre of **attention**?
- Do you tend to **rely** on other people a great deal?

Anankastic (obsessive–compulsive)

- Do you always try to follow a **set routine**?
- Do you prefer things to be **very neat and tidy**?
- Are you always **punctual**?
- Do you tend to **check things** more than once or twice?

Anxious (avoidant)

- Do you tend to feel **very tense** and **self-conscious**?
- Do you **live cautiously** and avoid taking unnecessary **risks**?
- Are you concerned that you might not be **popular**?

Dependent

- Do you tend to **rely on others excessively**?
- Do you prefer others to **make decisions for you**?
- Do you often **feel helpless** on your own?

> ⚠ **To avoid diagnostic pitfalls you will need to be flexible in the way you ask these questions, and the answers should be supplemented by information from history.**

MANAGEMENT

See Chapter 4 for details (p. 170).

SCHIZOPHRENIA

Schizophrenia is a relatively common mental disorder with a lifetime prevalence of nearly 1%. It occurs throughout the world, with an onset that is earlier in men (average age 21) than in women (average age 27).

It is a syndrome characterized by disturbances in thinking and communications, with delusions and hallucinations, set against a background of gradual cognitive decline as well as social deterioration.

Not all the above features need be present and, depending upon the symptomatology, the presentation and the time course of the illness, various clinical categories are described. However, it is not always easy to place a patient in one of the subcategories of schizophrenia, and the diagnosis rests heavily upon the clinical skills of the physician as there are no laboratory diagnostic tests. Some of the diagnostic categories in ICD-10 (see also Appendix) are given below.

F20.0 PARANOID SCHIZOPHRENIA

The commonest subcategory, characterized by the presence of paranoid delusions, delusions of reference, delusional jealousy and hallucinations.

F20.1 HEBEPHRENIC SCHIZOPHRENIA

Characterized by incoherence, incongruous mood, silly/irresponsible behaviour, often with giggling, and by the absence of systematized delusions. This particular subcategory presents earlier than others and in general has a poorer prognosis.

F20.2 CATATONIC SCHIZOPHRENIA

Characterized by a pronounced psychomotor disturbance that may involve rigidity, stupor, negativism, posturing or excitement.

F20.6 SIMPLE SCHIZOPHRENIA

This form is insidious in onset and the negative symptoms appear to develop without preceding clear positive symptoms.

F20.5 RESIDUAL SCHIZOPHRENIA

This particular form is dominated by the presence of negative symptoms and is preceded by one of the subcategories described above.

Another way of subdividing schizophrenic symptomatology is by the use of:

- *Positive symptoms*. These include symptoms relating to **hallucinations**, **delusions**, **incongruity of affect** and **disturbance of thinking**, as outlined elsewhere.
- *Negative symptoms*. These consist of **poverty of speech**, **blunting** or **flattening of affect**, **lack of drive**, **psychomotor** and **emotional inertia**.

Many patients present with a mixture of both positive and negative symptoms.
Liddle has described yet another subdivision, into three different syndromes based upon the correlation of clinical symptoms with the findings from functional imaging.

- **Psychomotor poverty syndrome** This is characterised by poverty of speech, affective flattening, and a decrease in spontaneous movement, with blood flow abnormalities in the prefrontal cortex.
- **Disorganization syndrome** Here, there is disorder of the form of thinking and the affect, which is inappropriate, and the blood flow abnormalities are found in the anterior cingulate cortex.
- **Reality distortion syndrome** Characteristically there are delusions and hallucinations, with blood flow abnormalities in the medial temporal lobe.

DIAGNOSIS

As stated earlier, making of the diagnosis rests heavily upon the clinical skills of the physician, using criteria from either DSM-IV or ICD-10. Both of these classification systems employ operational criteria, specifying the presence of specific symptoms for certain lengths of time, and exclude the presence of other disorders such as depression.

Diagnostic criteria – ICD-10

Symptoms should have been clearly present for most of the time during a period of 1 month or more; one of the following should be clearly present, or two if not so clear cut:

(a) **Thought echo**, thought **insertion or withdrawal**, and thought **broadcasting**

(b) **Delusions** of **control**, **influence** or **passivity**, clearly referred to body or limb movements or specific thoughts, actions, or sensations; delusional perceptions

(c) **Hallucinatory voices** giving a running commentary on the patient's behaviour or discussing the patient among themselves, or other types of hallucinatory voices coming from some part of the body

(d) **Persistent delusions** of other kinds that are culturally inappropriate and completely impossible, such as religious or political identity, or superhuman powers and abilities, e.g. being able to control the weather, or being in communication with aliens from another world

(e) **Persistent hallucinations** in any modality, when accompanied either by fleeting or half-formed delusions, without clear affective content, or by persistent overvalued ideas, or when occurring every day for weeks or months on end

(f) **Breaks or interpolations in the train of thought**, resulting in incoherence or irrelevant speech, or neologisms

(g) **Catatonic behaviour**, such as excitement, posturing, or waxy flexibility, negativism, mutism and stupor

(h) **'Negative' symptoms** such as marked apathy, paucity of speech, and blunting or incongruity of emotional responses, usually resulting in social withdrawal and lowering of social performance; it must be clear that these are not due to depression or to neuroleptic medication

(i) A significant and consistent change in the overall quality of some aspects of **personal behaviour**, manifest as loss of interest, aimlessness, idleness, a self-absorbed attitude and social withdrawal.

Many of the above features encompass the schneiderian first-rank symptoms outlined below:

● **Delusional perception:** a delusional meaning (usually bizarre) is attached to an apparently normal perception

- **Auditory hallucinations:** thought echo, running commentary, third-person auditory hallucinations
- **Disturbance of thinking:** thought withdrawal, insertion, broadcasting
- **Passivity phenomenon:** the individual believes that his or her actions, emotions, feelings, impulses and body are controlled by an external agency.

Bleuler's Four As

Classically Bleuler described features that also cover most schizophrenic symptomatology

Autistic thoughts (withdrawal from reality into an inner world of fantasy)
Affective incongruity (e.g. smiling when describing a sad event)
Loosening of **A**ssociations (thoughts are disordered, lacking logical connections)
Ambivalence (presence of conflicting ideas, feelings)

AETIOLOGY

The aetiology remains uncertain. There is evidence from twin and adoption studies and family history of a **genetic** basis which is often positive for schizophrenia.

The evidence for a possible **neurodevelopmental** basis comes from studies showing increased reports of obstetric complications, fetal brain injuries and abnormalities reported on brain imaging, and a plethora of research evidence exists for abnormalities of a number of **neurotransmitters**, such as dopamine and serotonin and glutamate.

The **psychosocial factors** (the evidence for these is rather shaky) implicated in this disorder include abnormal family processes, such as **double-bind** (parents conveying simultaneous conflicting messages to the child), **skew** (mother is dominant while the father is submissive), **schism** (hostility between the parents) and **adverse life events**. However, the research evidence does point to the presence of **high expressed emotions** in the family, which are detrimental and increase the likelihood of the illness relapsing.

PROGNOSIS

About one-quarter of schizophrenics recover from the first episode without ever experiencing a relapse. Around 50% recover but experience several relapses, and, 25% fail to recover at all and develop a chronic form of the illness.

This disorder has a severe psychosocial impact which is not limited to the sufferer and has significant mortality, with around 10% dying as a result of suicide.

Prognostic factors in schizophrenia	
Good	**Bad**
1. Old	1. Young
2. Female	2. Male
3. Married	3. Unmarried
4. No history	4. History ++
5. No family history	5. Family history
6. Good personality	6. Personality problems
7. Good intelligence	7. Poor intelligence
8. Precipitant	8. No precipitant
9. Active onset	9. Insidious onset
10. Positive symptoms	10. Negative symptoms
11. Affective symptoms	11. No affectivity
12. Good response	12. Poor response
13. Compliance	13. Poor compliance
14. Soft neurological symptoms	14. No neurological findings

MANAGEMENT

The management of schizophrenic disorders needs to be tailored to the individual and is usually composed of drug treatment and psychosocial interventions (see Chapter 4 for details).

PHARMACOTHERAPY AND OTHER TREATMENTS

Pharmacotherapy 106

Pharmacology 118

Specific psychiatric disorders: drug treatments and some management issues 121

Other physical treatments 191

Future treatment methods in psychiatry 199

PHARMACOTHERAPY

Drug treatment remains the cornerstone of the therapeutic options available in psychiatric practice. With advances in neuroscience and drug development psychiatrists face a choice of drugs that continues to increase in both numbers and sophistication. At the start of your training you may find this choice bewildering and their use in various psychiatric conditions confusing. Do not be surprised therefore, if it takes some time before you begin to feel comfortable with prescribing.

PRESCRIBING

The guidelines below should ease your passage through the minefield of pharmacotherapy.

- The old maxim remains true as ever: **First do no harm**.
- Try to familiarize yourself with a few of the more commonly used drugs, especially those used by your seniors. You should know about their mode of action, indications, contraindications and side effects, both acceptable and toxic. It is far better to know a few drugs well, rather than a great many only slightly.
- You may find booklets produced by the local pharmacy, with guidelines and recommendations, useful.
- Revise the basic pharmacodynamic and pharmacokinetic concepts that you learned during your medical training, i.e. receptor profile, half-life, metabolism, modes of clearance, and effects of hepatic and renal problems etc.
- Prescribe an adequate dose of a particular drug for a sufficient time before deciding to change.
- Be aware of the interaction between drugs (use as few as possible and generally avoid combinations, if at all possible).
- The choice of drugs will also depend on the diagnosis and the symptoms that need treatment.
- Tailor medications to the individual patient:
  — Take account of the patient's physical (weight, height, body mass index) and medical status (hepatic and renal failure), and even the ethnic origin in some cases.
  — Enquire about the patient's previous response to a specific drug, both therapeutic and adverse. It may also be useful to know what any other genetically related family member's response was to specific drugs (if appropriate).
- Use the appropriate time interval between doses.
- Learn about the use of drugs in special circumstances/patient groups, e.g.:
  — pregnancy, lactation
  — elderly
  — children
  — those with serious medical conditions, e.g. renal or hepatic failure.

Although it is useful to know the receptor profile of a particular drug (especially for its mode of action and side effects), you must remember that the clinical effects do not result just from its effects on certain neurotransmitters/receptors.

A specific neurotransmitter/receptor system does not work in isolation. In reality it is likely to be influenced by other neurotransmitter/receptor system(s), and is more than likely to influence others in return, through the number of neural circuits that connect the various brain regions.

The end clinical effects result from the brain's adaptive processes (e.g. gene expression), the pharmacological interactions and modification within the neural circuitry. Hence a sudden stoppage of a particular drug, or its substitution by another drug, may lead to sudden alterations in the adaptive process (sometimes in reverse), with possibly deleterious effects.

COMPLIANCE

- Consider the patient's viewpoint.
- Does the patient **forget** to take medication? In such cases it may be better to use drugs with a longer half-life, or depot medication.
- Does the patient **refuse** medication? In such cases depot drugs may be more appropriate.
- Is the patient **dangerous** with drugs? What about suicide potential? (Is there a previous history?); avoid drugs that are toxic in overdose (most tricyclics are!).
- Does the patient have a tendency to, or history of, **drug abuse** or **addiction**? Avoid drugs with abuse and/or addictive potential.
- Is the patient **cognitively impaired**? Someone else should take responsibility for dispensing, or dispensing devices could be used that cater for those with memory difficulties, for example.
- Is the patient **aware** of his or her **condition** and the **purpose** for which the drugs are being prescribed? Try to explain and educate in lay terms.
- Is the patient aware of common **side effects** and possible **toxic effects**, as well as what to do if these occur? Inform both verbally and in writing.
- Does the patient feel an active partner in the treatment plans? Encourage active participation in the therapy.
- **Offer a whole treatment package, not just a prescription**.

REVIEW OF DRUG TREATMENT

Drug treatment should be regularly reviewed for:

- Appropriateness of prescribing and dosage
- Efficacy (e.g. reduction of symptomatology) and improvement in mental state
- Side effects/iatrogenic effects
- Possibility of toxic effects, therapeutic monitoring
- Interaction with other drugs
- Compliance
- The need for continuous use.

> **Drug features suggesting therapeutic monitoring may be useful**
>
> - Multitude of interactions
> - Small therapeutic index (e.g. lithium, where toxic side effects are dangerous)
> - Large interindividual variability of metabolism
> - Difficult early detection of toxicity (e.g. early thyroid/renal damage by lithium)
> - Long delay in onset of therapeutic action (e.g. lithium)
> - Well defined plasma concentration and response relationship between the beneficial effects, the nuisance effects and the toxic effects.

Some examples of drugs which have a small therapeutic index with potentially dangerous side effects and need monitoring are:

- Lithium
- Phenytoin
- Digoxin
- Gentamicin.

THERAPEUTIC WINDOW

Certain drugs (e.g. nortriptyline) have a fairly defined therapeutic window (range). Dosages above or below this are usually clinically ineffective.

In the management of drug treatment failure consider the following:

- Review the **diagnosis/symptomatology**; the accuracy? Are there comorbid disorder(s)? Is there use of illicit or prescribed drugs?
- Review the therapeutic response: is it objective enough? i.e. do not rely solely on the subjective opinion of the patient regarding treatment failure.
- Was the dosage, as well as the time span used for the drug, sufficient?
- Compliance: is the patient really taking the drugs as prescribed?
- The presence of intolerable side effects, or toxic effects
- Poor education about treatment issues
- Take into account specific patient issues, i.e. age, gender, race, disease state.
- Specific pharmacokinetic and pharmacodynamic issues.

WITHDRAWING PATIENTS FROM PSYCHOTROPIC DRUGS

Benzodiazepines
See section on benzodiazepine withdrawal below (pp. 137–138).

Selective serotonin reuptake inhibitors (SSRIs)
The occasional occurrence of withdrawal symptoms (most likely after 24–48 hours) after a sudden stoppage is largely dependent upon the half-life of the drug, the length of treatment and the dosage used. Symptoms are more likely with **paroxetine** (relatively short half-life) and least likely with **fluoxetine** (longer half-life). They include:

- **Somatic symptoms:** dizziness, incoordination, lethargy, nausea, headache, fever, sweating, insomnia and vivid dreams

- **Neuropsychiatric symptoms:** dyskinesias, paraesthesia, 'electric-shock-like' sensations, anxiety, agitation, irritability, confusion and, on rare occasions, aggression, impulsivity and hypomania.

Tricyclics (TCAs)

The possible occurrence of withdrawal symptoms varies with individual drugs and patients.

They are most likely to occur within 24–48 hours after withdrawal and are dependent upon the half-life of the drug and the period of treatment. Symptoms include:

- A 'flu-like' syndrome consisting of anxiety, fever, sweating, malaise, myalgia, headache, dizziness and nausea
- Rebound depression and paradoxical mood changes have also been reported following abrupt withdrawal.

MAOIs

Irreversible

Withdrawal symptoms occur occasionally and usually after 1–4 days following abrupt withdrawal. They include: agitation, irritability, nausea, headache, vivid nightmares, REM rebound and, on occasions, acute organic psychosis with hallucinations.

Dietary and drug restrictions should be maintained for at least 10 days after stopping MAOIs.

Reversible

Little information is available at the time of writing.

Antipsychotics

Generally symptoms are more likely to occur 24–48 hours after withdrawal and may even follow a large dose decrease. They include nausea, vomiting, gastritis, dizziness, headache, insomnia and autonomic disturbance. Rebound neurological symptoms (akathisia, dystonia and parkinsonism) and psychosis may also occur.

The likelihood of the occurrence of withdrawal symptoms depends upon the half-life of the specific drug, the dosage, and the period of treatment.

SWITCHING PSYCHIATRIC DRUGS

Antidepressants

It is possible to switch to another class of drug within 24 hours following the use of a drug with a shorter half-life. However, this should not be done following the use of MAOIs, where a 2-week interval is required before commencing on alternatives such as TCAs or SSRIs (see section on MAOIs). For those who fail to respond to two classes of antidepressant a revision of the diagnosis should be considered, and a second opinion may be required.

In general, the first antidepressant should be reduced over a period of 3–7 days before the second antidepressant is started. It is often helpful to start the second drug at a reduced dose. See Table 4.1 for further details.

Anxiolytics

When a switch from one anxiolytic to another is necessary the following factors should be taken into consideration:

- The equivalent dosage
- The class of the drug
- The half-life
- The period of usage.

TABLE 4.1   Switching antidepressants

From		To	Washout period
Tricyclics	→	Tricyclics	No washout: use dose equivalents for switching
	→	SSRI	5 half-lives of cyclic antidepressant (caution required)
	→	SNRI	No washout – taper for 3–7 days before commencing 2nd antidepressant
	→	Irrev. MAOI	5 half-lives of cyclic antidepressant
	→	RIMA	5 half-lives of cyclic antidepressant
SSRI	→	Tricyclics	5 half-lives of SSRI (caution with fluoxetine owing to long half-life of active metabolite
	→	SNRI	5 half-lives of SSRI (caution with fluoxetine)
	→	Irrev. MAOI	5 half-lives of SSRI (caution with fluoxetine) – DO NOT COMBINE
	→	RIMA	5 half-lives of SSRI (caution with fluoxetine)
	→	SSRI	No washout: taper first drug over 2–5 days then start second (use lower doses of second drug if switching from fluoxetine; longer taper may be necessary if higher doses of fluoxetine used)
Irreversible MAOIs	→	Tricyclics	10 days – CAUTION
	→	SSRI	10 days – DO NOT COMBINE
	→	SNRI	10 days – DO NOT COMBINE
	→	NaSSA	10 days – DO NOT COMBINE
	→	RIMA	Start the next day if changing from low to moderate dose; taper from a high dose Maintain dietary restrictions for 10 days
	→	Irrev. MAOI	10 days – DO NOT COMBINE
RIMA	→	Tricyclics	2 days
	→	SSRI	2 days – CAUTION required
	→	SNRI	2 days – CAUTION required
	→	Irrev. MAOI	Can start the following day at a low dose
SNRI	→	Tricyclics	No washout – taper for 3–7 days before commencing 2nd antidepressant
	→	SSRI	3 days – CAUTION required
	→	Irrev. MAOI	3 days – DO NOT COMBINE
	→	RIMA	3 days – CAUTION

Adapted with permission from K. Bezchlibnyk-Butler and J.J. Jeffries (eds), 1998. *Clinical Handbook of Psychotropic Drugs*, 8th edn. Hogrefe & Huber Publishers, Göttingen.

Consult local/national drug formularies and senior colleagues.

Drug dosage equivalents – benzodiazepines

Approximate equivalent dose of 5 mg diazepam:

Alprazolam	0.5 mg
Chlordiazepoxide	15 mg
Lorazepam	500 μg
Lormethazepam	0.5–1 mg
Nitrazepam	5 mg
Oxazepam	15 mg
Temazepam	10 mg

(Adapted from the *British National Formulary*)

Mood stabilizers

Changing from lithium to another mood stabilizer (e.g. anticonvulsants such as carbamazepine and valproate) is possible. Lithium has a half-life of 8–35 hours, but you should be aware that this may increase up to 58 hours after 1 year's therapy. Hence, a longer washout period may be required following chronic use.

Switching between carbamazepine and valproate is also possible. Once again be guided by the pharmacological factors, such as half-life and length of treatment, and of course by your senior colleagues.

Antipsychotics

Switching from one antipsychotic to another may be necessary for several reasons:

- The persistence of extrapyramidal side effects, despite the dosage decrease, may require a change to a less potent typical (conventional) or atypical (novel) antipsychotic.
- Other side effects (such as galactorrhoea, in the case of sulpiride) may also require a switch to an antipsychotic less likely to cause those particular effects.
- In the case of non-compliant patients, depot preparations may be required.
- The patient with persistent negative symptoms may require change to an atypical antipsychotic, whereas, patients suffering from persistent positive symptoms may require a switch back to a typical antipsychotic.
- In the case of treatment-resistant psychosis the patient may require clozapine therapy.

The first drug should be withdrawn gradually and the second commenced following the washout period. However, this may not be practical when the patient is experiencing symptoms. In such cases, one approach is to reduce the dose of the first drug and start the second at a lower dose, and continue decreasing the dose of the first while increasing the dose of the second gradually over 2–4 weeks. Remember to take into account the withdrawal effects of discontinued medications, the risk of relapse, and the need for antiparkinsonian drugs during the conversion period.

When switching from one typical antipsychotic to another, consider:

- The equivalent dosage (Tables 4.2 and 4.3)
- The mode of delivery (?oral/i.m./i.v.)
- The side effects of each drug and the need for others, such as antiparkinsonian drugs.

TABLE 4.2   Equivalent doses of antipsychotics

Drug	Equivalent dose (consensus) (mg/day)	Range of values in literature (mg/day)
Chlorpromazine	100	—
Clozapine	50	50–90
Droperidol	4	1–4
Flupenthixol	3	2–3
Fluphenazine	2	2–5
Haloperidol	3	1.5–5
Loxapine	10	10–25
Pimozide	2	2
Risperidone	2	not yet known
Sulpiride	200	200–270
Thioridazine	100	75 – 100
Trifluoperazine	5	2.5–5
Zuclopenthixol	25	25–60
Depot preparations		
Flupenthixol	10/week	10–20/week
Fluphenazine	5/week	1–12.5/week
Haloperidol	15/week	5–25/week
Pipothiazine	10/week	10–12.5/week
Zuclopenthixol	100/week	40–100/week

These values are only approximate as variations will occur because of a number of pharmacodynamic and pharmacokinetic factors.

TABLE 4.3   Oral/parenteral dose equivalents for psychotropic drugs

Drug	Oral dose (mg)	Equivalent i.m. or i.v. dose (mg)
Benzodiazepines		
Diazepam	10	10
Lorazepam	4	4
Anticholinergics		
Procyclidine	10	7.5
Antipsychotics		
Chlorpromazine	100	25–50
Droperidol	10	7.5
Haloperidol	10	5
Promazine	200	200

It is essential to specify one route of administration when prescribing.

When switching from low- to high-potency antipsychotics, consider:

- Reducing the first drug gradually as the second is added
- The occurrence of cholinergic and sedative effects.

When switching from high- to low-potency antipsychotics, consider:

- Continuation of antiparkinsonian drugs well after the transition period, to avoid the occurrence of extrapyramidal side effects.

When switching from a typical to an atypical antipsychotic:

- Reduce the dose of the typical drug gradually while increasing the atypical dose
- The equivalent doses do not usually apply
- The onset of action of an atypical antipsychotic appears to be more gradual.

When switching from an atypical to a typical antipsychotic:

- Gradually reduce the dose of the first drug as the second is added
- Special precautions are needed when withdrawing (especially abruptly) from **clozapine**, as there is high incidence of rebound psychosis.

DRUG INTERACTIONS

Drug interactions may cause potentiation or antagonism of one drug by another, or occasionally some other effect. It can lead to serious problems, which may be pharmacodynamic or pharmacokinetic in nature. The **adverse drug interactions** should be reported to the Committee on Safety of Medicines (CSM), as well as recorded in the individual patient case notes.

The seriousness of an adverse drug reaction, as well as its frequency, tends to vary from patient to patient. Adverse reactions are more likely with drugs that have a small therapeutic index and those that require careful monitoring. Patients at increased risk from drug interactions include the elderly, children, and those with impaired renal or liver function.

> ⚠ **For specific drug interactions the reader is advised to consult the *British National Formulary* or appropriate local or national drug formularies.**

IDIOSYNCRATIC DRUG INTERACTION

Drug reactions are unpredictable and may depend upon genetic variance, i.e. inborn error of metabolism (handling a drug in a different way), for example:

- Suxamethonium sensitivity
- Neuroleptic malignant syndrome
  - which cannot be predicted
  - which is dose independent.

DRUG TREATMENT IN SPECIAL PATIENT GROUPS

ELDERLY

The elderly differ in their capacity for drug absorption, metabolism and distribution. Cardiac output and renal perfusion are also substantially reduced, and tissue sensitivity is usually increased. Adverse drug effects, such as postural hypotension with neuroleptics, greater sedation with hypnotics, and increased sensitivity to anticholinergic side effects, are also known to occur twice as commonly in those over the age of 70. For all these reasons it is essential that extra care is taken when prescribing psychotropic drugs to the elderly.

General guidelines

- Do not withhold drugs because of age
- Use the lowest effective dose (with many drugs start with 50% of the adult dose)
- Use fewer drugs (avoid polypharmacy)
- Keep the prescribing regimen simple and explain clearly
- Make sure of the diagnosis, then prescribe
- Take account of special medical, pharmacological and psychosocial factors.

Specific classes of drugs and special precautions

Antipsychotics/neuroleptics

- Use one-half to one-third of the adult dose
- The elderly are more prone to parkinsonian and other side effects and these are often harder to treat
- Tardive dyskinesia is more likely to occur.

Anticholinergics

- The elderly are especially sensitive: monitor for constipation, urinary retention, glaucoma and memory difficulties
- Avoid two or more drugs with anticholinergic actions
- Procyclidine is best given b.d. instead of t.d.s.

Anticonvulsants and mood stabilizers

- Avoid drugs excreted by the kidneys, such as *vigabatrin* and *gabapentin*
- The dose of *phenobarbitone* should be reduced
- With *carbamazepine* no change in dosage is required (use lower dose for a mood-stabilizing effect), but associated cardiac arrhythmias are more likely
- For *valproate* the dosage increase should be more gradual
- *Lithium:* lower plasma levels (hence lower dosages) are sufficient for a mood-stabilizing effect; monitor for renal function and other side effects, which are more likely to occur
- Care is required with all the *benzodiazepines* because of the enhanced side effects (especially CNS effects such as sedation).

Antidepressants (Table 4.4)

- Reduce the initial dose of TCAs and take special care with sedating types
- Lofepramine appears to be a safe choice
- With fluoxetine, fluvoxamine and sertraline no change in dosage is required, whereas with proxetine and citalopram a 50% reduction in the initial dose is recommended
- MAOIs appear to cause more problems and are best avoided
- SNRI: no change in dosage is required in healthy elderly patients
- NaSSA (Mirtazapine): reduce the initial dose by 50% (i.e. 7.5 mg).

TABLE 4.4   Drugs and the elderly

	Lower risk	Moderate risk	Higher risk
Anticonvulsants	Carbamazepine	Barbiturates Benzodiazepines Lamotrigine	Acetazolamide Phenytoin Vigabatrin
Antidepressants	Desipramine Lofepramine Nortriptyline? SSRIs Trazodone Tryptophan	Most tricyclics MAOIs Mianserin Flupenthixol	
Anxiolytics and hypnotics	Alprazolam Buspirone Clobazam Lorazepam Oxazepam Oxprenolol Zopiclone	Chlormethiazole Benzodiazepines long-acting Flunitrazepam Flurazepam Propranolol Temazepam Zolpidem	Nitrazepam
Neuroleptics	Risperidone?	Butyrophenones Loxapine Phenothiazines Thioxanthenes	Clozapine
Others	Orphenadrine	Benzhexol Lithium Procyclidine	Paraldehyde

PREGNANT AND LACTATING WOMEN (Table 4.5)

- Drugs should only be prescribed in pregnancy if the expected benefit to the mother is thought to be greater than the risk to the fetus.
- If at all possible drugs should be avoided during the first trimester; no drug is safe beyond doubt in early pregnancy.
- Before prescribing, always exclude the possibility of pregnancy in women of childbearing age.

- Always seek further information concerning specific drugs with regard to their use in pregnancy.
- Some drugs given to a nursing mother can cause toxicity in the infant.
- Lithium is present in milk in significant amounts and may cause toxicity in the infant.
- Consult the *British National Formulary* or appropriate local/national drug formularies for information on individual drugs.

CHILDREN

Children, and especially neonates, differ from adults in their response to drugs. They are especially sensitive to psychotropics and more prone to side effects (e.g. dystonia).

The dosage should be adjusted for weight until a weight of 50 kg or puberty is reached.

Consult the *British National Formulary* or appropriate local/national drug formularies for information on individual drugs.

TABLE 4.5   Drugs and pregnancy (see also *BNF*)

	Lower risk	Moderate risk	Higher risk
Anticonvulsants		Carbamazepine Clonazepam Ethosuximide Gabapentin?	Acetazolamide Benzodiazepines Phenobarbitone Phenytoin Valproate Vigabatrin
Antidepressants	Flupenthixol Tryptophan	MAOIs Mianserin Moclobemide SSRIs Trazodone Tricyclics	Amitriptyline Nortriptyline
Anxiolytics and hypnotics	Zopiclone	β-blockers Buspirone Chloral Chlormethiazole Promethazine	Benzodiazepines Zolpidem
Neuroleptics	Flupenthixol Sulpiride	Butyrophenones Clozapine Loxapine Phenothiazines Risperidone	Prochlorperazine
Others		Antimuscarinics Disulfiram Methadone Paraldehyde	Diethylpropion

PATIENTS WITH SERIOUS MEDICAL CONDITIONS

Renal impairment (Table 4.6)

- Special care is needed, depending upon the degree of impairment, whether the drug is eliminated entirely by renal excretion or is partly metabolized, and its toxicity.
- Nephrotoxic drugs (e.g. lithium) should, if at all possible, be avoided in patients with significant renal impairment; if their use is essential use the dose regimen based on glomerular filtration rate.
- The total daily dosage of a drug can be reduced either by reducing the size of the individual dose or by increasing the interval between doses.
- Consult the *British National Formulary* or appropriate local/national drug formularies for information on individual drugs.

TABLE 4.6   Drugs and renal impairment (see also *BNF*)

	Lower risk	Moderate risk	Higher risk
Anticonvulsants	Phenytoin Valproate	Barbiturates Benzodiazepines Carbamazepine Ethosuximide Gabapentin Vigabatrin	
Antidepressants	Mianserin Moclobemide Tricyclics Tryptophan	MAOIs Fluvoxamine SSRIs Trazodone	Amoxapine
Anxiolytics and hypnotics	Zopiclone	Benzodiazepines β-blockers Buspirone Chlormethiazole Zolpidem	Chloral
Neuroleptics	Loxapine	Clozapine Phenothiazines Risperidone Sulpiride	
Others		Antimuscarinics Disulfiram	Lithium

Liver disease (severe) (Table 4.7)

- Keep drug prescribing to a minimum.
- Avoid drugs which are **hepatotoxic**, highly protein bound, likely to enhance hepatic encephalopathy (e.g. CNS depressants), and which are mainly metabolized by the liver.
- **Antidepressants:** reduce the dosage of TCAs, with fluoxetine being given on alternate days; avoid MAOIs.

- **Antipsychotics:** avoid clozapine; reduce the dosage of phenothiazines and risperidone.
- **Anticonvulsants and anxiolytics:** reduce dosage and use with caution.

TABLE 4.7   Drugs and liver disease (see also *BNF*)

	Lower risk	Moderate risk	Higher risk
Anticonvulsants	Gabapentin Vigabatrin	Benzodiazepines Carbamazepine Phenytoin LD	Barbiturates Ethosuximide Paraldehyde Valproate
Antidepressants	Mianserin Tryptophan	SSRIs Moclobemide Trazodone Tricyclics	Lofepramine MAOIs
Anxiolytics and hypnotics	Benzodiazepines (short acting) Propranolol (low dose)	Benzodiazepines (long acting) Buspirone Chlormethiazole Zolpidem Zopiclone	Chloral Benzodiazepines (high dose) Propranolol (high dose)
Neuroleptics	Loxapine Pimozide Sulpiride Zuclopenthixol	Clozapine Phenothiazines Risperidone	
Others	Lithium	Antimuscarinics Disulfiram Paraldehyde	

PHARMACOLOGY

This is a vast and complicated subject: however, some understanding of the basic concepts is essential for safe and rational prescribing. It is beyond the scope of this book to deal with this subject comprehensively, but a few concepts will be outlined and an attempt should be made to understand these and their relevance.

Pharmacology encompasses pharmacodynamics and pharmacokinetics. The clinical effects of a particular drug result from interaction between these pharmacological parameters.

PHARMACODYNAMICS

This is the study of what drugs do to the body, and involves some of the concepts outlined below.

You are advised to have some understanding of these concepts:

- Receptors
- Neurotransmitters/neuromodulators
- Binding of drugs and endogenous neurotransmitters to receptors
- Agonists
- Partial agonists
- Antagonists
- Non-competitive antagonists.

Some important neurotransmitters implicated in psychiatric disorders
(see Tables 4.8, 4.9)

Acetylcholine (Ach)
Dopamine (DA)
δ-Amino butyric acid (GABA)
Glutamate
Noradrenaline (NA)
Nitric acid
5-Hydroxytryptamine (serotonin)

Note: each of above has many subclasses (e.g. D1, D2 for dopamine)

PHARMACOKINETICS

This is the study of what body does to the drug (i.e. drug handling or drug disposition) and it involves some of the concepts outlined below. Once again, you are advised to have some understanding of these for effective and safe prescribing.

Absorption

- Routes of drug administration (oral, intramuscular, etc.)

Distribution

- Blood–brain barrier
- Body compartments
- Protein binding.

Metabolism and excretion

- Sites of metabolism
- Biotransformation (oxidation, hydroxylation, etc.)
- First-pass metabolism
- Elimination half-life of the drug
- Bioavailability

- Steady state
- Zero-order kinetics
- First-order kinetics
- Loading dose
- P450 (CYP) enzyme system
- Lipid/water solubility
- Routes of excretion.

TABLE 4.8   Pharmacological effects on neurotransmitters/receptors

Block	Effect
NA reuptake block	Antidepressant Side effects: tremors, tachycardia, sweating, insomnia, erectile and ejaculation problems Potentiation of pressor effects of NA (e.g. sympathomimetic amines) Interaction with guanethidine (blockade of antihypertensive effect)
5-HT reuptake block	Antidepressant, antiobsessional Can increase or decrease anxiety, depending on dose Side effects: GI distress, nausea, headache, nervousness, akathisia, sexual side effects, anorexia Potentiation of drugs with serotonergic properties (e.g. L-tryptophan); caution re 'serotonin syndrome'
DA reuptake block	Antidepressant, antiparkinsonian Side effects: psychomotor activation, aggravation of psychosis
H_1 blockade	Most potent action of cyclic antidepressants Side effects: sedation, postural hypotension, weight gain Potentiation of effects of other CNS drugs
ACh blockade	Second most potent action of cyclic antidepressants Side effects: dry mouth, blurred vision, constipation, urinary retention, sinus tachycardia, QRS changes, memory disturbances Potentiation of effects of drugs with anticholinergic properties
α_1 blockade	Side effects: postural hypotension, dizziness, reflex tachycardia, sedation Potentiation of antihypertensives acting via α_1 blockade (e.g. prazosin)
α_2 blockade	May lead to increased release of acetylcholine and increased cholinergic activity CNS arousal; possible decrease in depressive symptoms Side effect: sexual dysfunction, priapism Antagonism of antihypertensives acting as α_2 stimulants (e.g. clonidine, methyldopa)
5-HT_1 blockade	Antidepressant, anxiolytic and antiaggressive action
5-HT_2 blockade	Anxiolytic, antidepressant, antipsychotic, antimigraine effect, improved sleep Side effects: hypotensive, ejaculatory problems, sedation, weight gain

Adapted with permission from K. Bezchlibnyk-Butler and J.J. Jeffries (eds), 1998. Clinical Handbook of Psychotropic Drugs, 8th edn. Hogrefe & Huber Publishers, Göttingen.

TABLE 4.9   Pharmacological effects on neurotransmitters/receptors

Block	Effect
Dopamine blockade	Additive or synergistic interactions occur between various dopamine receptor subtypes
D_1	May mediate antipsychotic effect
D_2	In mesolimbic area – antipsychotic effect: correlates with clinical efficacy in controlling positive symptoms of schizophrenia; an inverse relationship exists between D_2 blockade and therapeutic antipsychotic dosage (i.e. potent blockade = low mg dose)
	In nigrostriated tract – side effect: extrapyramidal (e.g. tremor, rigidity, etc.)
	In tuberinfundibular area – side effect: endocrine prolactin elevation (e.g. galactorrhoea etc.)
D_3	May mediate antipsychotic effect on positive and negative symptoms of schizophrenia
D_4	May mediate antipsychotic effect on positive symptoms of schizophrenia

Adapted with permission from K. Bezchlibnyk-Butler and J.J. Jeffries (eds), 1998. Clinical Handbook of Psychotropic Drugs, 8th edn. Hogrefe & Huber Publishers, Göttingen.

SPECIFIC PSYCHIATRIC DISORDERS: DRUG TREATMENTS AND SOME MANAGEMENT ISSUES

ALCOHOL-RELATED PSYCHIATRIC DISORDERS AND WITHDRAWAL

The harmful use of alcohol can lead to medical, psychiatric and psychosocial complications that affect not only the patient but their family and associates. Some of the psychiatric complications include:

- Alcohol dependence syndrome
- Alcohol hallucinosis
- Alcohol dementia and cognitive impairment
- Anxiety
- Depression
- Paranoia and pathological jealousy
- Wernicke–Korsakoff syndrome.

Harmful alcohol use may also be a secondary feature of a primary psychiatric illness, such as in bipolar affective disorder, depression, schizophrenia, borderline personality disorder, etc. The use of alcohol in a particular psychiatric disorder has management and prognostic implications and should therefore always be enquired about.

When alcohol-related disorders occur in association with other psychiatric disorders, the term dual diagnosis is increasingly being used.

ALCOHOL DEPENDENCE SYNDROME

A cluster of physiological, behavioural and cognitive phenomena has been described for an entity called **alcohol dependency syndrome** (these may also applied to any other addictive substance).

According to ICD-10, three or more of the criteria outlined below should have been present during the previous year before a person can be described as having alcohol dependency syndrome: *[3 or MORE in prev year]*

These criteria include: *[ICD-10 as Diagnos Criteria]*

PR	**Primacy:**	the drinking of alcohol takes precedence over all other activities
CO	**Compulsion:**	there is a compulsion to drink alcohol
ST	**Stereotype:**	there is a tendency to drink alcohol in a stereotyped way, such as at the same place and at the same time
TO	**Tolerance:**	an increase in the amount of alcohol is required to achieve the effects originally produced by a lower amount
RE	**Relief:**	alcohol is drunk to provide relief from withdrawal symptoms
WI	**Withdrawal:**	abstinence leads to withdrawal symptoms
RE	**Reinstatement:**	a return to the original dependence type of drinking after a period of abstinence.

> **Note** | Note the mnemonic PR COST TO REWIRE.

MANAGEMENT

In general, a patient with a history of alcohol dependence should receive both medical and psychiatric work-up. You should also ensure:

- Adequate hydration *[Hydration]*
- Correction of any nutritional deficiencies *[N. Deficiencies]*
- Medical and psychiatric conditions are treated actively
- Support is provided for psychosocial difficulties by enlisting the help of other members of the multidisciplinary team
- Not only are the acute problems dealt with, but the long-term management issues are also addressed. *[Medical Psychiatric Psychosocial]*

Psychosocial
See Chapters 3 and 5.

Pharmacological

This will depend upon the clinical presentation, the problems (medical and psychiatric) faced by the patient, and his or her motivation with regard to the treatments being provided.

The various pharmacological treatments involve:

- Treatment of medical complications
- Treatment of psychiatric complications
- Detoxification programmes
- The use of drugs such as disulfiram to help maintain abstinence.

ALCOHOLIC HALLUCINOSIS

- The patient is orientated and may realize that the voices are hallucinations
- Vivid auditory hallucinations, usually threatening and accusatory, but without other cognitive impairment
- Hallucinations may occur in other modalities and while drinking, between episodes, or during withdrawal
- Persecutory delusions may also occur.

MANAGEMENT

- Admit, and detain if necessary.
- Ensure the patient is protected from harm to either himself or others as a result of the voices.
- Drug treatment: for serious hallucinations treat with antipsychotics but make sure there are no serious contraindications, such as liver failure.
- Hallucinations generally clear within a month.

> ⚠ **Antipsychotics can lower the seizure threshold and should therefore be used with caution.**

ALCOHOLIC DEMENTIA AND COGNITIVE IMPAIRMENT

Cognitive impairment and the presence of alcohol dementia are serious complications. They usually follow chronic abuse, resulting from the direct effect of alcohol on the neural tissue, or as a result of secondary problems such as repeated head injury.

MANAGEMENT

This is best carried out in specialist units.

ANXIETY

Approximately one-quarter of alcoholics suffer from anxiety disorders, especially generalized anxiety disorder (GAD). Anxiety disorders may be either primary or secondary to alcohol abuse.

MANAGEMENT

This usually involves:

- A detoxification programme
- Psychosocial measures to deal with anxiety and help keep off alcohol
- Drugs such as buspirone 10 mg t.d.s. and antidepressants such as paroxetine 20 mg o.d. may also be useful, especially when there are few depressive symptoms.

DEPRESSION

Depression may affect one-third of alcoholics and may be primary or secondary to alcohol abuse. The history may help to decide, although it is often difficult to be sure.

MANAGEMENT

This usually involves:

- A detoxification programme
- Other psychosocial measures to help keep off alcohol
- The use of antidepressants.

SSRIs, such as citalopram are safer to use in those with a history of alcohol abuse, but do make sure there are no major medical contraindications to the use of antidepressants. Antidepressants may also help prevent a relapse to drinking.

> **Note** Many alcoholics present with features of both anxiety and depression. This condition is common in the community and is usually managed by GPs.

WERNICKE–KORSAKOFF SYNDROME

Although not all are necessarily present simultaneously, the essential features of this syndrome include:

Confusion, confabulation (as a consequence of memory impairment)
Ataxia
Nystagmus
Ophthalmoplegia
Neuropathy (peripheral)

Note the mnemonic **CANON**.

MANAGEMENT

- Urgent treatment in a medical setting
- Initially thiamine 100 mg i.v. (slowly, i.e. over 10 minutes) and folate 1 mg i.v., followed by oral thiamine 100 mg daily for several weeks.

NB: Potentially serious allergic adverse reactions may occur during or shortly after the parenteral administration of thiamine.

Committee for Safety of Medicines (CSM) advice regarding the parenteral use of thiamine includes:

(i)   Restricting its use to patients in whom parenteral treatment is essential
(ii) i.v. injections should be given slowly (over 10 minutes)
(iii) There should be facilities for treating anaphylaxis

- Clonidine 0.3 mg b.d. has been reported to improve memory.

PARANOIA AND PATHOLOGICAL JEALOUSY

Features (especially while on alcohol) include paranoia, suspiciousness, hostility and full-blown pathological jealousy. The latter may have serious consequences, usually for the partner.

Pathological jealousy may have other psychiatric causes, such as:

- Paranoid schizophrenia
- Depressive disorder
- Neurosis
- Personality disorder
- Organic disorder.

MANAGEMENT

This varies with the severity of the symptomatology and whether there is the likelihood of serious psychosocial consequences.

Management measures include:

- A detoxification programme
- Other psychosocial measures to deal with the alcohol dependency, aggression, paranoia and jealousy

- Drugs: neuroleptics such as haloperidol 2–5 mg b.d., but make sure there are no medical contraindications
- In the case of pathological jealousy consider the safety of the person the jealousy is directed against (consider warning the potential victim)
- Admission may be necessary (this allows separation from the target of their jealousy).

> **Note** Neuroleptics can lower the seizure threshold, therefore the risk of withdrawal fits should be borne in mind.

ALCOHOL WITHDRAWAL, UNPLANNED

- Minor withdrawal
- Major withdrawal (delirium tremens)
- Alcohol withdrawal seizures.

MINOR WITHDRAWAL (ABSTINENCE)

Sudden discontinuation of alcohol (and other sedatives) in those with chronic use can lead to withdrawal syndrome. The features include:

- Anxiety, irritability
- Autonomic disturbance, i.e. sweating, tachycardia and hypertension
- Coarse tremor of the hands and tongue
- Craving for alcohol
- Insomnia, vivid dreams
- Morning shakiness and hangover.

These features usually appear within 8 hours following the cessation of alcohol and usually peak between 24 and 36 hours.

MANAGEMENT

- Reassure the patient.
- Provide supportive measures.
- Use cross-tolerants such as benzodiazepines, but antihistamines and β-blockers should be avoided. Alcohol may be used in an emergency and when benzodiazepines are not available.
- Chlordiazepoxide 25–100 mg orally every 4–6 hours on the first day, decreasing by 20% per day over 5 days.
- Lorazepam is preferred in the elderly, where there may be liver impairment and metabolic problems.
- Diazepam may also be used: 2–20 mg orally every 3–6 hours on the first day, reducing by 20% daily over 5 days.
- Give thiamine 100 mg i.v. immediately (but slowly, i.e. over 10 minutes) and continue orally for at least 3 days.

NB: Potentially serious allergic adverse reactions may occur during or shortly after the parenteral administration of thiamine.

> ⚠️ **Committee for Safety of Medicines (CSM) advice regarding the parenteral use of thiamine includes:**
> - **Restrict its use to patients in whom parenteral treatment is essential.**
> - **i.v. Injections should be given slowly (over 10 minutes).**
> - **There should be facilities for treating anaphylaxis.**

- Magnesium sulphate (because of frequent hypomagnesaemia) 1 g i.m. or i.v. every 6–12 hours for 48 hours.

MAJOR WITHDRAWAL (DELIRIUM TREMENS – DTs)

There are certain risk factors for the development of DTs:

- Previous history
- Presence of head trauma, infection and poor nutritional state
- Chronic and severe use of alcohol
- Recent binge followed by abrupt cessation.

Features include:

- Autonomic disturbance, such as tachycardia and hypertension
- Confusion and agitation
- Hallucinations – visual, tactile and auditory
- Pyrexia and sweating
- Tremulousness
- Seizures, usually preceding delirium
- Weakness.

These features usually appear 24–72 hours following cessation or reduction of alcohol, but the onset can be delayed for as long as 7 days.

MANAGEMENT

DTs is a medical emergency and should be treated in a medical setting. It carries a mortality rate as high as 20%, and therefore the treatment should be regarded as urgent and given top priority.

Involve and hand over to medical colleagues.

Medical management usually involves:

- Supportive measures for autonomic disturbances – this may need intensive care management
- Benzodiazepines: chlordiazepoxide 50 mg, or lorazepam 2 mg, or diazepam 10 mg i.v. or i.m. initially, and repeated until symptoms subside

- Monitoring for the development of focal neurological signs
- High-calorie, high-carbohydrate diet
- The psychiatrist may have to play a role in advising on the management of severe hallucinations. Cautious use of neuroleptics should be considered, along with long-term management issues
- Those at risk while still on the psychiatric ward should be closely monitored for changes in pulse, blood pressure, respiration and temperature.

ALCOHOL WITHDRAWAL SEIZURES

Withdrawal seizures usually occur within 8–48 hours after cessation of drinking and usually precede delirium.

MANAGEMENT

- Administer diazepam 5–10 mg i.v. and repeat if necessary at 10–15-minute intervals. Maximum dose is 30 mg.
- Contact medical colleagues who should be involved in the management.
- Look for a possible aetiology, such as brain disorders and use of seizure threshold-lowering drugs.

PLANNED ALCOHOL WITHDRAWAL (DETOXIFICATION)

Planned alcohol detoxification may be carried out in an inpatient or a community setting.

Inpatient detoxification is suitable for those:

- With coexisting medical problems or a history of seizures and DTs
- With serious coexisting psychiatric illness
- With severe dependence
- With previously failed community detoxification
- Who lack home support.

All patients admitted for alcohol detoxification should be:

- Screened for medical complications
- Given a physical examination followed by the appropriate investigations, including haematology (FBC), urea and electrolytes, liver function tests, calcium and phosphate
- Given a psychiatric evaluation for the presence of a coexisting psychiatric disorder.

Many psychiatric units use a written contract, to be signed by the patient, agreeing to adhere to the rules and regulations of detoxification programme.

Patients should also be given:

- Psychological support, e.g. through the key nurse
- Nutritional support in the form of hydration and prophylactic vitamins such as thiamine (vitamin B), to prevent Wernicke's encephalopathy. If the latter is suspected the patient should be immediately started on high-potency thiamine (100 mg i.v. slowly: see CSM advice, p. 126) and then continued orally for 3–5 days

USE OF BENZODIAZEPINE (BZD) FOR WITHDRAWAL SYMPTOMS

The severity of withdrawal symptoms can be wide-ranging, therefore a broad range of drug dosages may be required. The following are guidelines, which should be tailored to the individual patient, taking into account factors such as their previous exposure to benzodiazepines.

- **Mild to moderate withdrawal symptoms:** Chlordiazepoxide 5–10 mg orally t.d.s. or q.d.s., reducing by 20% daily, usually over a 5-day period
- **Moderate withdrawal symptoms:** Chlordiazepoxide 15–20 mg orally t.d.s. or q.d.s., reducing by 20% daily, usually over a period of 5 days
- **Severe withdrawal symptoms:** Chlordiazepoxide 40–60 mg orally t.d.s. or q.d.s., reducing by 20% daily, usually over a period of 5–10 days.

In addition it is useful to prescribe PRN chlordiazepoxide 5–10 mg orally b.d. The use of prophylactic antiepileptics is controversial, so be guided by the patient profile, e.g. previous history of seizures, and by your seniors.

Chlormethiazole is also occasionally of use in the management of withdrawal symptoms.

The success of the detoxification programme may be measured by the extent to which, or the length of time, the patient remains abstinent, as well as by the successful avoidance of medical and psychosocial complications.

Some of the psychosocial measures that may help to maintain abstinence include:

- Helping the patient to avoid the environmental cues that lead to drinking, e.g. a drinking partner or a particular place of drinking
- Attendance at a voluntary organization such as Alcoholics Anonymous (AA)
- Attendance at the day hospital, e.g. for group therapy or occupational therapy
- Education of friends and relatives
- Rehousing and employment training if appropriate.

Pharmacological measures that may help include the use of:

- Acamprosate
- Disulfiram (Antabuse)
- Drug treatment for coexisting psychiatric disorders.

DISULFIRAM (ANTABUSE)

This should be instituted by those with experience and requires specialist supervision.

- Ensure the suitability of the patient, i.e. that he or she is motivated and able to understand the medical rationale and the risks involved
- Ensure that no alcohol has been consumed during the 24 hours prior to starting treatment
- On the first day start with 800 mg in a single dose and reduce over 5 days to 100–200 mg daily
- Review regularly and reconsider its continuation at 6 months.

Contraindications include:

- Ischaemic heart disease, cardiac failure, history of cerebrovascular accidents and hypertension
- Suicide risk
- Psychosis
- Severe Parkinson's disease
- Pregnancy and breastfeeding.

Side effects include:

- Drowsiness and, initially, fatigue
- Halitosis
- Hepatic cell damage
- Nausea and vomiting
- Peripheral neuritis
- Psychiatric symptoms
- Reduced libido.

ANOREXIA AND BULIMIA NERVOSA

ANOREXIA NERVOSA (AN)

Treatment may be either on an inpatient (in severe cases) or an outpatient basis, and generally includes a mixture of psychiatric, psychological and medical treatments. Hospital admission is necessary if the weight loss is rapid or severe (>30%) and in extreme life-threatening circumstances the use of the Mental Health Act may be required. Other disorders should be excluded and comorbid psychiatric symptomatology/disorders such as depression should be actively treated.

Overall, the aim should be the correction of low body weight causing medical complications (the latter should always be sought and corrected).

Psychosocial treatments include a behavioural reward programme (to increase weight), cognitive behavioural therapy and family therapy.

See section on anorexia nervosa for diagnosis, medical complications, laboratory screening and treatment strategies (Chapter 3, pp. 72–75).

USE OF DRUGS

- Appetite stimulants have questionable value
- Nutritional feeding: in severe cases, but be guided by the local pharmacy
- Antidepressants are often used, especially if there are depressive symptoms and some obsessive features:
  — Tricyclics: clomipramine 150 mg/day or more over 4–6 weeks may produce a clinical response
  — SSRIs: fluoxetine and paroxetine, even though they may cause initial anorexia in some, have also been used with some success
  — Neuroleptics in low doses have been found useful in some cases.

BULIMIA NERVOSA (BN)

A condition considered less serious but more prevalent than anorexia nervosa, this is usually managed using psychological treatments or with added pharmacotherapeutic measures. Medical complications and comorbid psychiatric disorders should be identified and appropriately treated (see also Chapter 3).

DRUG TREATMENT

- Antidepressants: SSRIs in doses relatively large (e.g. fluoxetine 40–60 mg), have been found to have a significant effect on binge eating and purging
- Monoamine oxidase inhibitors (MAOIs), both reversible (moclobemide 150–600 mg/day) and irreversible (phenelzine 15–30 mg t.d.s)
- Tricyclics: especially clomipramine (150 mg/day or more), which has significant effect on serotoninergic reuptake.

ANXIETY DISORDERS

As a trainee psychiatrist you are less likely to deal with patients with anxiety disorders, as these are generally more common in the community and managed largely by GPs. The patients you are likely to encounter are those who present in A & E, the ones with severe disorders, or those with other psychiatric illnesses where the anxiety symptoms are a secondary feature.

In general, anxiety disorders are managed by a combination of psychological (usually behavioural and/or cognitive psychotherapy) and drug treatments. A brief account of various anxiety disorders and their management follows.

PANIC DISORDER

Panic disorder is described as episodic attacks of extreme anxiety that manifest in various autonomic signs and symptoms, together with a dread or fear of losing control, or dying (see Chapter 3).

MANAGEMENT

- Exclude medical causes (see Chapter 6)
- Look for and treat comorbid psychiatric disorders, e.g. depression, generalized anxiety disorder (GAD), post-traumatic stress disorder (PTSD)
- Consider non-pharmacological options, such as cognitive behavioural therapy.

DRUG TREATMENT

- Benzodiazepines (for details see Chapter 6) are useful for emergency short-term treatment, especially in acute presentations
- Alprazolam (favoured in the USA) 0.25–0.5 mg t.d.s. Maximum 3 mg/day (Note: This will need to be withdrawn slowly)
- Antidepressants: imipramine in low doses (25 mg/day); SSRIs such as fluoxetine in low doses, e.g. 10 mg/day, and paroxetine.

GENERALIZED ANXIETY DISORDER (GAD)

Those with GAD suffer from excessive anxiety and worry most of the time. Other problems include fatigue, muscle tension and difficulties with concentration and sleep (see Chapter 3).

MANAGEMENT

- Exclude medical disorders and drug use (for those causing anxiety see Chapter 6)
- Treat comorbid psychiatric disorders such as depression and somatoform disorders
- Non-pharmacological treatments such as relaxation therapy, anxiety management, e.g. in the day hospital, and cognitive behaviour therapy (CBT).

DRUG TREATMENT

- For short-term treatment use a low-dose benzodiazepine such as diazepam 2–5 mg t.d.s.
- Buspirone 20–40 mg/day (less in the elderly)
- Antidepressants (tricyclics and SSRIs) are especially useful when there are some depressive symptoms.

PHOBIA(S)

A phobia is an irrational fear that interferes with a person's normal behaviour, such as work or other activities. Phobias are more common in the community and are largely managed by GPs. They are often underdetected, as many sufferers are too embarrassed to seek treatment.

SIMPLE PHOBIA

A **simple phobia** is usually a specific fear, for example heights, flying, animals or needles. The fear of animals appears to be more common in women, whereas the fear of height affects men more often.

Management

- Exclude primary medical or psychiatric disorders such as depression, PTSD, OCD, schizophrenia
- Behavioural therapy: this usually entails a combination of relaxation and desensitization, e.g. the treatment of needle phobia would involve a specific number sessions of behavioural therapy
- Drug treatment includes low-dose benzodiazepine, e.g. 5–10 mg diazepam, for a short period in conjunction with behavioural therapy.

SOCIAL PHOBIA

A person suffering from a **social phobia** is inappropriately and usually extremely anxious in circumstances in which he is observed and could be criticized, e.g. public speaking.

Management

- Exclude primary psychiatric disorders such as depression and schizophrenia
- Behavioural therapy by desensitization through exposure.

Drug treatment

- β-Blockers, e.g. propranolol 20–40 mg, especially for performance anxiety, 45 minutes beforehand
- Low-dose benzodiazepine
- Antidepressants (MAOIs), e.g. phenelzine 45–90 mg/day.

AGORAPHOBIA

Agoraphobics suffer from extreme anxiety when away from home, in crowds, or in situations they cannot leave easily. This may occur with or without panic attacks.

Management

- Exclude medical disorders

- Look for and treat primary psychiatric disorders such as major depression, schizophrenia, other phobic and panic disorders
- Behaviour therapy: exposure to phobic situations and training to cope with panic attacks.

Drug treatment

May be used in addition and may include benzodiazepines for short periods, antidepressants (MAOIs) such as phenelzine 40–90 mg/day, and SSRIs such as paroxetine 20 mg/day.

MIXED ANXIETY AND DEPRESSIVE DISORDER (ANXIETY–DEPRESSION)

Here symptoms of both anxiety and depression occur, with neither predominating. It is common in the community and largely managed by GPs.

MANAGEMENT

- Exclude medical disorders
- Identify and treat primary psychiatric disorders such as depression, schizophrenia and other anxiety disorders
- Mild forms may be treated with counselling, cognitive behavioural therapy or other forms of psychotherapy
- Avoid misdiagnosing generalized anxiety disorder (GAD).

DRUG TREATMENT

Benzodiazepines should only be used for a short time. Antidepressants are more effective than anxiolytics, and include SSRIs such as paroxetine 20 mg/day.

Anxiety disorders and some suitable drug treatments	
Anxiety disorders responsive to pharmacotherapy	**Drugs of choice**
Panic disorder with and without agoraphobia	High-potency benzodiazepines Tricyclic antidepressants SSRIs (e.g. paroxetine) MAOIs
Generalized anxiety disorder (GAD)	Sedative tricyclics (e.g. dothiepin) Benzodiazepines Buspirone SSRIs (e.g. paroxetine)
Obsessive–compulsive disorder (OCD)	SSRIs in relatively high doses (sertraline, paroxetine, fluoxetine) Tricyclics (clomipramine)

Anxiety disorders and some suitable drug treatments (contd)	
Post-traumatic stress disorder (PTSD)	Tricyclics SSRIs, SNRIs MAOIs Nefazadone
Social phobias	β-blockers High-potency benzodiazepines MAOIs SSRIs (e.g. fluoxetine)
Anxiety secondary to psychosis	Benzodiazepines

Note: Benzodiazepines should be avoided in patients with a clear history of substance abuse.

OBSESSIVE–COMPULSIVE DISORDER (OCD)

This disorder comprises obsessive thoughts and compulsive rituals which may occur either together or alone (see Chapter 3).

MANAGEMENT

- Exclude medical disorders (e.g. Sydenham's chorea)
- Explore and treat primary psychiatric disorders, as OCD symptomatology may be a secondary feature in major depression (30%); Gilles de la Tourette syndrome (30–50%), which is now considered to be part of the OCD spectrum of disorders; dementia; schizophrenia; and phobic disorders.

Psychobehavioural treatments include:

- Exposure and response prevention
- Thought stopping
- Desensitization procedures
- Various psychotherapies
- Family therapy.

DRUG TREATMENT

- Tricyclics such as clomipramine (which has a potent serotonin reuptake blocking profile), in relatively high doses of 250 mg/day
- SSRIs in relatively high doses: fluoxetine 40–80 mg daily and paroxetine 40–60 mg daily
- Augmentation of SSRIs with buspirone 5–15 mg t.d.s. or lithium may also help in partial responders
- Anxiety symptoms can be helped by short-term use of benzodiazepines.

Common anxiolytic drugs

Drug	Usual dosage
Benzodiazepine anxiolytics	
Alprazolam	4–6 mg/day (panic disorder)
	1–2 mg/day (GAD)
	1–2 mg/day (social phobia)
	1–6 mg/day (anxiety in psychosis)
Chlordiazepoxide	20–40 mg/day (GAD)
	20–100 mg/day (anxiety in psychosis)
Clonazepam	2–4 mg/day (panic disorder)
	0.5–1 mg/day (GAD)
	0.5–1 mg/day (social phobia)
	2–6 mg/day (anxiety in psychosis)
Diazepam	6–40 mg/day (GAD)
Lorazepam	1–6 mg/day (GAD)
	2–10 mg/day (anxiety in psychosis)
Oxazepam	30–90 mg/day (GAD)
Non-benzodiazepine anxiolytics	
Buspirone	20–40 mg/day (GAD)
Antidepressants	
Clomipramine	50–250 mg/day (OCD)
Other tricyclics	Same antidepressant dose as in panic disorder, GAD and PTSD
SSRIs	
Fluoxetine	20–60 mg/day (panic disorder)
	20–60 mg/day (OCD); once in morning
Paroxetine	20–60 mg/day (panic disorder); once in morning
	20–60 mg/day (OCD); once in morning
Sertraline	50–200 mg/day (panic disorder); once in morning
	50–250 mg/day (OCD); once in morning
MAOIs	
Phenelzine	Same antidepressant dose as in panic disorder, social phobia and PTSD

POST-TRAUMATIC STRESS DISORDER (PTSD)

This results from experiencing extremely traumatic event(s), such as a threat to or near loss of life (see Chapter 3).

MANAGEMENT

- Screen for comorbid primary psychiatric disorders such as depression, psychotic disorders (where disturbing thoughts may relate to many events rather than just one) and other anxiety disorders
- Early psychological intervention (e.g. crisis counselling, debriefing) following the traumatic event may play a preventative role
- Referral to support groups (e.g. Medical Foundation for Victims of Torture in the UK) (**Note:** Those working in catchment areas with a high proportion of refugees are more likely to encounter such patients)
- Specialized psychotherapies: a number of psychotherapies have been used and are effective to varying degrees.

Controlled reliving through **'rehearsal'** and **'trauma story'** has been used: these are based on **cognitive behavioural therapy**. **EMDR** (eye movement desensitization and reprocessing) has also been found to be effective in many cases.

DRUG TREATMENT

The literature is rather limited but a number of drugs have been found to be useful, especially in conjunction with psychobehavioural treatment and where there is comorbid depression.

- Antidepressants:
  — SSRIs: fluoxetine and paroxetine
  — Tricyclics: amitriptyline
  — MAOIs: phenelzine is especially helpful for avoidance and intrusive symptoms
- Buspirone
- Benzodiazepines: low dose for short periods
- Carbamazepine: helps with hyperarousal, hostility and intrusive symptoms.

BENZODIAZEPINE DEPENDENCE AND WITHDRAWAL

Benzodiazepine (BDZ) dependence/abuse is a serious problem and therefore the prescribing of BZD, although acceptable for the short-term management of anxiety disorders, should always take this into account.

Features suggestive of abuse/dependence include:

- 'Addictive personality'
- Use of multiple prescribers, e.g. GPs and hospital doctors (who may be unaware of each other)
- Claims of regularly running out and losing medications
- Demanding and difficult behaviour
- Purchasing drugs from non-prescribers ('street sellers').

Withdrawal symptoms can occur within hours (short-acting BDZ) or as late as 3 weeks (long-acting BDZ) and include:

- Anxiety
- Anorexia
- Autonomic symptoms
- Blurred vision
- Dizziness
- Headache
- Hyperthermia
- Insomnia
- Seizures
- Tremor
- Tinnitus
- Psychosis

MANAGEMENT OF WITHDRAWAL

- Assess the urgency and validity (i.e. is it real?) of withdrawal
- Clarify usage features, i.e. whether high dosage, lengthy/chronic use or use of short-acting BDZ
- Discuss and develop partnership for planned withdrawal. Assess the patient's motivation, which is essential. Form a contract like that used for alcohol detoxification. Make plans for long-term abstinence.

WITHDRAWAL FROM RELATIVELY LONGER-ACTING BDZ, E.G. ALPRAZOLAM, LORAZEPAM AND TEMAZEPAM

Use cross-tolerants with a longer half-life, e.g. diazepam in doses sufficient to eliminate withdrawal symptoms. Dosage should be tapered off gradually, taking account of individual variations, e.g. the length of time taken, either weeks or months.

SUGGESTED WITHDRAWAL PROGRAMME FOR SHORT-ACTING BDZ

- Substitute with the equivalent dose of diazepam.
- Reduce diazepam by 2–2.5 mg in fortnightly steps.
- The above reduction dosage can be varied to suit individuals.
- Total withdrawal period may vary from 4 weeks to a year, or even more.

Approximate equivalent doses of 5 mg diazepam	
Chlordiazepoxide	15 mg
Lorazepam	500 µg
Lormethazepam	0.5–1 mg
Nitrazepam	5 mg
Oxazepam	15 mg
Temazepam	10 mg

(Adapted from the *British National Formulary*)

BIPOLAR AFFECTIVE DISORDER (MANIC DEPRESSIVE PSYCHOSIS)

Bipolar affective disorder (BAD), also known as manic depressive psychosis, has a spectrum of presentations and a number of diagnostic categories have been described (see Chapter 3).

MANAGEMENT

These patients present fairly regularly in general psychiatric settings and quite often those with manic episodes are a difficult management problem. For those who comply, the drug treatment is quite effective (60–80%).

MANAGEMENT GUIDELINES FOR MANIC PATIENTS

- Aim to exclude and, if appropriate, treat other causes that may mimic a manic episode (see Chapter 3).
- Use all your negotiation skills and involve others to ensure patient compliance.
- Educate the patient and ensure that he or she understands why regular psychiatric supervision is necessary. Monitor their state of mental health and the treatment programme so as to minimize the chance of a relapse.

Suggested guidelines for initial stabilization of the manic patient

When presented with an acutely psychotically agitated manic patient

↓

Start a high-potency neuroleptic (e.g. haloperidol 5 mg orally or i.m. (first 24 h. 4-hourly)
Add or substitute neuroleptics with BDZ (e.g. lorazepam 1–2 mg orally or i.m., max. 4-hourly)
As soon as clinically possible carry out pre-lithium (or other mood stabilizer) screen

↓

Alternate the neuroleptic with benzodiazepine (e.g. lorazepam 2–4 mg orally or i.m. 4-hourly, or clonazepam 1–2 mg 6–8-hourly PRN for agitation or psychosis)

Start lithium at 300 mg mg b.d. and titrate to serum level

↓

If lithium is contraindicated or has been ineffective, initiate alternative mood stabilizers (CBZ, valproate or clonazepam)

↓

Once the patient is on a stable regimen, gradually reduce the neuroleptic and 24–48 hours later begin to taper the benzodiazepine slowly

> ⚠ **Lithium should be commenced as soon as possible with manic patients; however, it takes between 7 and 15 days for it to alleviate the typical manic symptoms. Therefore, you should start with faster-acting drugs such as neuroleptics and benzodiazepines, and then add lithium (or alternative) therapy.**

Acute manic episode

This is usually managed initially by the use of benzodiazepines and antipsychotics, followed by mood stabilizers, e.g. lithium. (For details see 'Manic patients' in Chapter 6).

LONG-TERM MANAGEMENT

This essentially involves the use of mood-stabilizing drugs, their monitoring, and regular clinical follow-up to ensure that the patient remains well. The psychiatrist plays a central role and, depending on the clinical state of the patient, it is likely that the other members of the MDT, such as a social worker, CPN or occupational therapist, will also be involved. Efforts should also be made to advise on and protect patients from other potential psychiatric problems, such as abuse of alcohol and illicit drugs, and psychosocial problems such as forensic and sexual-related problems.

TABLE 4.10 Mood stabilizers and their effectiveness in subtypes of bipolar affective disorder

Disorder	Lithium	Carbamazepine	Valproate	Clonazepam
Typical manic episode	+++	++	++	?
Rapid cycling mania	+	++	+++	+
Hypomania with rapid episodes of depression	+++	++	?	?
Schizoaffective disorder (manic or mixed)	+++	++	?	?
Acute mania with psychosis and agitation	?	?	?	?

NON-DRUG MANAGEMENT

Appropriate psychosocial therapies, if suitable, should also be offered; these include:

● Sessions with the occupational therapist, e.g. at the day hospital
● Group therapy and/or counselling
● Cognitive behaviour therapy (CBT).

TABLE 4.11 Mood stabilizers and dosages

Mood stabilizer	Initial dose	Maintenance dose	Maximum dose
Lithium carbonate (or citrate; also available as syrup)	300 mg b.d	300–600 mg b.d.[1]	3000 mg/day[2]
Carbamazepine	200 mg b.d	400 mg b.d.[3]	1200 mg/day
Sodium valproate	250 mg b.d	1000–1500 mg/day[4]	3000 mg/day

Initial stabilization involves the use of neuroleptics (usually typical) and benzodiazepines (e.g. lorazepam), usually in combination, to sedate and calm the patient.

Maintenance refers to the treatment period following initial stabilization of the acute episode.
[1] The maintenance dosage needs to be titrated to serum levels of lithium, 12 hours after the last dose (trough levels). Most agree on a **serum level of 0.8–1.2 mmol/l** during initial treatment, whereas during long-term maintenance treatment **levels of 0.4–1.0 mmol/l** are usually adequate to prevent the recurrence of a manic episode.
[2] The maximum dosage for lithium should not exceed 3000 mg/day. However, this is hardly ever reached because of the limiting side effects, such as tremor, GI irritation and weakness.
[3] Anticonvulsant therapeutic serum levels for carbamazepine usually do not correlate to its use as a mood-stabilizing agent; however, often it is titrated to a **serum level of 17–54 μmol/l**. Some suggest a higher level is needed for antimanic effects. More importantly, it is essential that FBC is monitored once 2–3-weekly initially, then once every 3–6 months.
[4] Some recommend titrating valproate to a **serum level of 350–700 μmol/l** (trough level).

Note: Approximately one-third of bipolar patients (manic or mixed) fail to respond to lithium alone. A significant proportion of these non-responders will improve with either the substitution or the addition of other mood stabilizers, as listed above.

SPECIFIC MOOD STABILIZERS

LITHIUM

This is the drug of choice in bipolar affective disorder, but its mode of action is not fully understood. In 60–80% of classic bipolar patients it reduces the frequency and severity of both the manic and the depressive components of the disorder. Its other uses include:

- As an augmenter for antidepressants in treatment-resistant depression
- Treatment of aggressive, agitated patients
- Treatment of borderline personality disorder (BPD).

PHARMACOLOGY

- Because of its narrow therapeutic index and the possibility of toxic build-up, it is usually recommended that lithium should be initiated by the psychiatrist following medical screening.
- Regular serum level monitoring is essential.

- Litium is excreted by the kidneys, with an elimination half-life of approximately 24 hours.
- Renal function should be established prior to its commencement.
- Its reabsorption in the proximal tubules is influenced by sodium levels. Anything that affects sodium levels, e.g. diarrhoea or vomiting, can lead to toxicity.
- It is available in many formulations, including syrup (lithium citrate), but only oral preparations are available.

Dosage
The usual dose varies between 600 and 1200 mg/day.

Therapeutic serum levels

- Usually checked 12 hours after the last dose
- For treatment of **acute episode** 0.8–1.2 mmol/l
- For maintenance **prophylaxis** 0.4–1.0 mmol/l (lower end for the elderly).

Drug interactions
Drugs likely to increase lithium levels:

- Thiazide diuretics
- Erythromycin
- Metronidazole
- NSAIDs such as indomethacin.

Drugs likely to decrease lithium levels:

- Theophylline.

Drugs likely to increase toxicity when prescribed with lithium:

- Digoxin
- α-Methyldopa
- Haloperidol.

Side effects

- **General:** weight gain and fine tremor (5%) (**Note:** With higher serum levels coarse tremor may develop, followed by myoclonus and seizures or toxic levels)
- **GI tract:** initial discomfort; at toxic doses nausea, vomiting and diarrhoea
- **Renal:** nephrogenic diabetes insipidus
- **Endocrine:** hypothyroidism; calcium abnormalities owing to the effect on parathyroid function
- **Cardiac:** T-wave inversion occasionally
- **Haematological:** leucocytosis
- **Teratogenicity:** Ebstein anomaly has been reported from its use in the first trimester of pregnancy.

Initiating lithium treatment

You are likely to do this in consultation with your seniors, especially during the early part of your training. It is essential that you acquire a knowledge of:

- Pretreatment laboratory investigations (Table 4.12)
- Contraindications and side effects (Table 4.13)
- The appropriate dosage
- Serum level monitoring procedures.

Side effects

Nausea: take lithium with meals, or milk; use sustained-release formulations; spread out the dose (e.g. from b.d. to t.d.s)

Diarrhoea: reduce dose; use antidiarrheals (e.g. lomotil) briefly; change to lithium citrate

Hypothyroidism: add thyroxine 0.05–0.20 mg/day (be guided by T_4 and TSH)

Nephrogenic diabetes insipidus: increase fluid intake (dilutes lithium); decrease lithium dose

Tremors: use smaller, more frequent doses; reduce total dosage; titrate very slowly if necessary; propranolol 10–20 mg t.d.s; use sustained-release preparations

Incoordination/ataxia: reduce lithium dose

TABLE 4.12 Laboratory investigations during lithium therapy: pretreatment and maintenance

Pretreatment investigations
1. FBC: lithium sometimes causes a benign increase in WBC values
2. Urea and electrolytes and renal function to ensure normal renal function and clearance. (Note: the presence of dehydration, renal failure and serum creatinine over 1.5 mg/dl represents a relative contraindication to lithium therapy)
3. Thyroid function tests (including TSH) for baseline, and to rule out thyroid dysfunction as a cause of symptoms
4. Pregnancy test (lithium use during the first trimester has been associated with serious fetal cardiac abnormalities, e.g. Ebstein's anomaly)
5. ECG to rule out sinoatrial node dysfunction, bradycardia and ST/T changes, all of which may be aggravated by lithium
6. Medication screen: NSAIDs (with the exceptions of aspirin) decrease renal clearance of lithium and increase toxicity risk. In addition, angiotension-converting enzyme (ACE) inhibitors are contraindicated with lithium therapy.
   Low-salt diets can lead to increased lithium retention and hence an increased risk of toxicity.

Investigations during maintenance treatment
1. Check plasma lithium levels twice during the first 10 days of treatment, and then at least every 3 months during maintenance treatment. It is advisable to check serum level approximately 5 days after each dosage change, or change in other drugs that potentially interact with lithium
2. Thyroid (T_4 and TSH) and renal function tests (creatinine*) every 4 months for patients under 18 years of age

*If serum creatinine is significantly above normal, 24-hour urine for creatinine should be checked. Adjust the dosage, or consider changing to another mood stabilizer.

TABLE 4.13   Relationship between lithium serum levels (toxic and non-toxic) and signs and symptoms

Lithium serum level	Signs and symptoms
Initial therapy (0.6–1.4 mmol/l)	Fine tremor of hands, dry mouth, mild increase in thirst, mild polyuria, mild nausea (usually transient)
1.5 mmol/l	GI effects: nausea, vomiting, diarrhoea
2.0 mmol/l	Polyuria, dizziness/light-headedness, blurred vision, slurred speech, confusion, blackouts, muscle weakness and fasciculations, exaggerated deep tendon reflexes
2.5 mmol/l	Agitation, choreoathetoid movements, incontinence (urine and faeces), myoclonic twitches and movements, followed by stupor and coma
3.0 mmol/l	Cardiac dysrrhythmias, epileptiform seizures
4.0 mmol/l	Hypotension, vascular collapse

Note: It is essential that regular laboratory investigations be carried out during lithium therapy. These include U&Es, creatinine (to monitor potential renal toxicity), calcium, and thyroid function (including TSH). Long-term use of lithium often results in hypothyroidism, which is reversible or treatable with thyroid supplementation. You should also note that the above are **trough levels**. **Side effects** result from much higher levels, i.e. if the trough level is 1.4 mmol/l peak levels are much higher, and are responsible for side effects.

Duration of therapy

There are no absolute rules regarding the duration of lithium treatment in bipolar affective disorder: a patient may stay on the drug for years without serious side effects. The decision to discontinue lithium in normal circumstances should be made by a senior psychiatrist and should not be taken lightly. Unfortunately, all too often it is the patient who decides to discontinue, possibly leading to a relapse of the manic episode.

Partial or non-responders to lithium:[a] augmentation strategies and alternative mood stabilizers

Consider augmentation if lithium is ineffective[b] or leads to only a partial response by adding:

Carbamazepine
200–600 mg b.d.[c]

or Valproic acid[c]
500–750 mg b.d.

or Clonazepam
2–3 mg b.d.

or Thyroid supplementation

Partial or non-responders to lithium:[a] augmentation strategies and alternative mood stabilizers *(contd)*

or Haloperidol
    2–5mg q.d.s.

[a] Lithium monotherapy is the preferred choice for all bipolar–manic patients in the acute and maintenance phases. However, 20–40% of patients relapse within 2 years and less than 50% achieve complete remission.
[b] Before concluding that lithium is ineffective ensure that serum levels between 0.6 and 1.2 mmol/l have been reached for 2–3 weeks. Try to treat any benign side effects before switching to another mood stabilizer.
[c] In some cases carbamazepine or valproate have been used as first-line drugs if the patient exhibit features of rapid cycling, dysphoric mania, or mixed states involving both depression and mania.

> **Note**
> ECT has been shown to be highly effective in manic patients and should be considered as an alternative to failed pharmacotherapy, or even in situations when an urgent antimanic response is required.

CARBAMAZEPINE (CBZ)

Carbamazepine is used in bipolar affective disorder, usually when lithium is not considered appropriate, and occasionally as a first-line drug in rapid cycling mania. As with lithium, it is not clearly understood how it reduces the frequency and severity of both the manic and the depressive features.

Its other indications include the treatment of:

● Aggressive, agitated patients
● Borderline and psychopathic personality disorder
● Chronic pain such as trigeminal neuralgia
● Seizures, as an anticonvulsant.

PHARMACOLOGY

● Its absorption is rather unpredictable.
● The peak plasma levels are reached 2–6 hours after the dose.
● Its half-life is 13–17 hours and a steady state is reached in 2–4 days, therefore a therapeutic level is reached in approximately 4 days.
● It is 80% protein bound, therefore only 20% crosses the blood–brain barrier (BBB). A low albumin level may lead to toxic doses being reached earlier.
● Serum plasma levels required for anticonvulsant effects do not correlate with those needed for its therapeutic clinical effect in bipolar disorder.
● Serum plasma levels are usually measured to check for toxic levels being reached, and sometimes to exclude compliance problems.

- Starting dose is 100–200 mg t.d.s., increasing by 100–200 mg increments every 5 days.
- Dosage varies between 800 and 1200 mg/day.
- CBZ is an autoinducer of metabolic enzymes (P450 system), therefore 1 month later its own levels may need to be increased.

DRUG INTERACTIONS

Drugs likely to increase CBZ levels:

- Calcium channel blockers
- Cimetidine
- Erythromycin
- Fluoxetine
- Isoniazid.

Drugs likely to decrease CBZ levels:

- Phenobarbitone
- Phenytoin.

Drug levels likely to be decreased by CBZ:

- Haloperidol
- Oral contraceptives
- Theophylline
- Tricyclic antidepressants
- Valproic acid.

SIDE EFFECTS

- Initial **relatively common** side effects include ataxia, double vision, lethargy, nausea, vomiting and tremor.
- **Haematological:**
  - Aplastic anaemia (1 in 500 000). Advise patient to report fever, easy bruising, sore throats and rashes
    Note: Avoid combining CBZ with other drugs that affect white cell production, e.g. clozapine
  - Leukopenia: usually not below 3000. May occur transiently in approximately 10%
- **Hepatic reaction** (usually during the first month):
  - ALT and AST show a mild increase
  - Life-threatening hepatic reaction in only 1 in 10 000
  - The presence of liver disease is therefore a relative contraindication
- **Gastrointestinal tract:** abdominal pain, anorexia, nausea and vomiting
- **Cardiac:** may slow cardiac conduction
  - Pretreatment ECG should be carried out to check for pre-existing A-V delay, which is a relative contraindication for the use of carbamazepine
  - It may suppress ventricular automaticity

- **Renal:** Antiduretic action can lead to hyponatraemia (water intoxication, seizures)
- **Skin:** Generalized rashes (10–15%); stop the drug and investigate (e.g. FBC) for serious consequences
- **Teratogenicity:** 1% risk of spina bifida has been reported.

For laboratory investigations for carbamazepine, pretreatment and maintenance treatments see Table 4.14. For comparisons with other moods stabilizers see Table 4.15.

SODIUM VALPROATE (VALPROIC ACID)

Sodium valproate is usually considered third in line, following lithium and carbamazepine. However, it may be used as a first-line drug in so-called **rapidly cycling bipolar affective disorder**. It is also effective in dysphoric or mixed mania and mania due to medical disorders. Occasionally it is combined with lithium or carbamazepine in treatment-resistant mania. Like lithium and carbamazepine its effectiveness in mood instability is not clearly understood.

Its other indications include:

- Treatment of agitated, aggressive patients
- Treatment of borderline personality disorder
- As an anticonvulsant in a variety of seizure disorders (e.g. primary generalized epilepsy)
- Schizoaffective disorder.

PHARMACOLOGY

- It is highly protein bound, and so caution is needed when plasma albumin is low and toxic levels may be reached quickly.
- The elimination half-life is 12–16 hours and metabolism is through the P450 system.
- Plasma levels for its effective anticonvulsant actions do not appear to correlate with its positive clinical response in mania.
- The plasma levels may be checked to monitor compliance and toxicity, and are usually maintained between 350 and 700 μmol/l.
- Available as syrup, capsules and tablets.

Dosage
Initially 300 mg b.d., increasing by 200 mg/day at 3-day intervals. Usual maintenance dose is 1–2 g daily; maximum dose is 2.5 g/day in divided doses.

DRUG INTERACTIONS

It inhibits liver enzymes involved in the metabolism of:

- Diazepam
- Phenobarbital.

Monitor closely (or avoid concomitant use) when used with highly protein-bound drugs, as toxicity can occur at therapeutic levels, e.g.:

● Carbamazepine
● Phenobarbital
● Phenytoin.

> ⚠️ **When anticonvulsants are used in combination, plasma monitoring is especially important.**

SIDE EFFECTS

● **General:** lethargy
● **GI tract:** nausea, vomiting, gastric irritation, pancreatitis (rare) and weight gain
● **Neurological:** tremor (up to 10%)
● **Haematological:** thrombocytopenia
● **Hepatic:** usually during the first few months a transient rise in LFTs (40%); if this persists, stop the drug and seek advice
● **Dermatological:** alopecia (usually transient)
● **Teratogenicity:** 1–2% cases of spina bifida have been reported following its use in the first trimester of pregnancy.

TABLE 4.14   Anticonvulsant/mood stabilizers: suggested guidelines for laboratory investigations pretreatment and maintenance

Mood stabilizer	Pretreatment	During maintenance treatment
Carbamazepine	FBC Liver function tests LFTs Serum iron ECG Pregnancy test	Check FBC and LFTs every 2 weeks for the first month, than every 3 months Stop the drug if the WBC drops below 3000 mm³, or if LFTs increase threefold Check serum levels every 2 weeks for the first month, then 3-monthly (aim for 17–54 µmol/l)
Valproate	FBC Liver function tests ECG Pregnancy test	Check FBC and LFTs every 2–4 weeks for the first 6 months of treatment, then 3–6-monthly if no abnormalities appear. Check serum level approximately 5 days after each dosage change (aim for 350–700 µmol/l)
Clonazepam	Liver function tests	LFTs 6–12 monthly, especially if high dosages are used

TABLE 4.15   Mood stabilizers and comparison of their side effects

Side effects	Lithium	Carbamazepine	Valproate	Clonazepam
Cardiovascular				
Hypotension		+		+
Hypertension		+		
Dizziness	+	+	+	+
Central nervous system				
Parkinsonism	+			
Muscle cramps	+	+		
Muscle rigidity	+			
Seizures	+			
Headache	+	+	+	+
Ataxia/incoordination	+	+	+	+
Sedation		+	+	+
Memory impairment	+			+
Insomnia	+		+	
Nightmares	+			
Dermatological				
Psoriasis	+			
Allergic rash	+	+	+	+
Alopecia	+	+	+	
Photosensitivity		+	+	
Endocrine				
Hypothyroidism/goitre	+			
Hyponatraemia		+		
Gastrointestinal				
Increased appetite	+		+	+
Dry mouth/thirst	+	+		+
Nausea/vomiting	+	+	+	+
Diarrhoea	+	+	+	+
Constipation		+	+	+
Hepatitis/jaundice		+	+	+
Abdominal cramps	+	+	+	
Oedema	+		+	
Pancreatitis		+	+	
Haematological				
Leucopenia		+	+	
Leucocytosis	+			
Eosinophilia	+	+	+	
Agranulocytosis		+	+	
Anaemia		+	+	
Thrombocytopenia		+	+	
Ophthalmic				
Blurred vision	+	+		+
Diplopia		+	+	+
Otological				
Tinnitus		+		
Vertigo	+			
Renal				
Polyuria	+			

TABLE 4.15 Mood stabilizers and comparison of their side effects *(contd)*

Side effects	Lithium	Carbamazepine	Valproate	Clonazepam
Urinary frequency	+	+		
Diabetes insipidus	+			
Interstitial nephritis	+			
Sexual				
Impotence	+	+		+
Amenorrhoea	+			

CLONAZEPAM

Used occasionally for its mood-stabilizing effects (see Table 4.15).

DEPRESSION

Depression presents in many different guises and a number of diagnostic categories are described (see Chapter 3). A patient suffering from a depressive disorder is more likely to be admitted if he or she is suicidal, psychotic, suffering from agitation, or motor retardation, and/or lacking in social support. You are also likely to have to deal with patients referred to the outpatient clinic for assessment by GPs or other health workers, liaison referrals, or those referred on as suicide risks (see Chapter 3).

MANAGEMENT

Appropriate management involves the following:

- Clarification of depressive symptoms (especially the suicide risk) and depressive categories
- Looking for underlying medical causes, including drugs
- Exploration of psychosocial issues
- Providing a treatment package, which should include:
  — psychosocial treatments
  — drug treatments
  — other treatments, including ECT in severe cases.

CLARIFICATION OF DEPRESSIVE SYMPTOMS AND DEPRESSIVE CATEGORIES

ICD-10 uses the following categories to describe some of the varieties of depression:

- F.32 Depressive episode (mild, moderate and severe)
- F.33 Recurrent depressive disorder
- F.34 Persistent (affective) mood disorders (cyclothymia, dysthymia)
- F.38 Other mood disorders (mixed affective disorder, recurrent brief depressive disorder).

When clarifying depressive symptomatology use an approach where open-ended questions are asked first, followed by closed question. Look for the pervasiveness of the symptoms, deviations from the normal for that particular person (for example a milkman usually gets up very early in the morning, and so caution is required in the interpretation of his reported time of waking). Enquire how these symptoms affect all the important facets of the patient's life.

Some psychiatrists regularly use specially designed rating scales, such as the Hamilton Depression Scale, the Beck Depression Inventory or the Montgomery–Asperger Depression Rating Scale (MADRAS), formally to evaluate depressive symptomatology.

UNDERLYING MEDICAL CAUSES (INCLUDING DRUGS)

When evaluating a patient with depressive symptomatology you must also consider medical causes, as correcting these may resolve the symptomatology without the need for further antidepressant treatment.

How extensive the medical evaluation need be may be determined by the medical history. For example, a patient with a history of thyroid problems and depressive symptoms should have his or her thyroid status carefully evaluated and corrected before antidepressant therapy is considered.

Nevertheless, a patient with a medical disorder under treatment, and who also has depressive symptoms, should not be denied antidepressant treatment. The choice of drug should be carefully evaluated for the possibility of interaction with the disease status and other drugs being used. Furthermore, it is not good practice to assume that someone with diagnosed cancer should feel depressed owing to psychosocial stresses and decline to offer any further

Medical disorders causing depressive symptoms	
Cardiac:	Ischaemic heart disease
Cancers:	Many cancers and brain metastases
Endocrine:	Diabetes mellitus, hypothyroidism, hypercortisolism
Hepatic:	Liver failure
Infections:	HIV, syphilis
Metabolic:	Hypercalcaemia, hypokalaemia
Neurological:	Brain metastases, tumours, dementia, multiple sclerosis, Parkinson's disease, stroke (especially affecting the dominant hemisphere)
Renal:	Renal failure
Respiratory:	Hypoxia

evaluation and appropriate treatment: That particular patient may well have depressive symptoms as a result of severe anaemia, hypercalcaemia and the presence of brain metastases.

When drugs are causing depressive symptoms, you should first consider a change to an alternative which is less likely to cause depression. You must also remember that depression in medical disorders may also benefit from psychological treatments, in addition or as an alternative to antidepressant therapy.

Drugs causing depressive symptoms	
Alcohol	Propranolol
Anticholinergics	Ranitidine
Anticonvulsants	Reserpine
Barbiturates	Sedatives
Benzodiazepines	Steroids
Cimetidine	Stimulant (withdrawal)
Clonidine	Thiazides
Oral contraceptives	

PSYCHOSOCIAL ISSUES

Some depressive symptoms may result from or be exacerbated by psychosocial problems, such as stressful life events (e.g. loss of partner, job etc.). When appropriate criteria are satisfied these may be described as an adjustment disorder. Furthermore, where psychosocial issues play a major part, and there are no severe biological symptoms of depression, an appropriate form of psychotherapy, such as supportive counselling, or cognitive behavioural therapy, may be more beneficial. If it is at all possible, helping a patient with psychosocial stresses, such as poor housing, may help to alleviate milder forms of depressive symptomatology.

PROVISION OF A TREATMENT PACKAGE

Psychosocial treatments include:

- Cognitive behavioural therapy (CBT)
- Psychodynamic psychotherapy
- Supportive psychotherapy
- Other forms of psychotherapies (see Chapter 5 for details).

DRUG TREATMENTS: ANTIDEPRESSANTS

A large variety of antidepressants are available. The choice is usually dictated by the clinical profile of the patient, familiarity with a particular drug and its availability (unfortunately this is sometimes dictated by the cost).

The following may help in choosing an appropriate antidepressant:

- Use the general prescribing guidelines described earlier
- Clarify the previous successful or unsuccessful use of a particular antidepressant, even among first-degree relatives
- Give the antidepressant a good trial – at least 3–4 weeks – before considering changing to another
- Changing drugs because of intolerable side effects should be documented in the case notes
- Abruptly stopping drugs with a shorter half-life (e.g. paroxetine) may lead to withdrawal symptoms and should be avoided
- Switching to another class of drug within 24 hours is possible following the use of a drug with a shorter half-life; however, this should not be done following the use of MAOIs, where a 2-week interval is required before commencing on alternatives such as TCAs or SSRIs (see section on MAOIs).

When prescribing a particular antidepressant consider the following:

Drug factors

- The side-effect profile (e.g. sedating or non-sedating, troublesome anticholinergic effects, effects on libido)
- Pharmacological parameters, such as half-life, drug interactions etc.
- Cost: generic drugs are cheaper, but this should be balanced by factors such as side-effect profile (SSRIs are in general better tolerated than TCAs), toxicity in overdose (most TCAs), and indirect savings made by of keeping patients out of hospital.

Patient and illness factors

- Age, sex, special situations (e.g. pregnancy) and disease status
- Compliance, previous use
- Suicide risk by overdose (avoid TCAs and irreversible MAOIs)
- The depressive symptoms to be targeted.

For those who fail to respond to two classes of antidepressant a revision of diagnosis should be considered and a second opinion may be needed; you should also consider:

- Augmentation with drugs such as lithium, L-thyroxine and buspirone
- Other therapies, such as ECT, psychosurgery, specific cocktails of drugs used in special units.

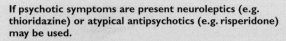

> **If psychotic symptoms are present neuroleptics (e.g. thioridazine) or atypical antipsychotics (e.g. risperidone) may be used.**
>
> **Always consider psychological treatment as an alternative or in addition to drug treatments.**
>
> **Patients should be educated and encouraged to take an active part in their treatment programme.**
>
> **Always be alert to a suicide risk as the depressive symptoms begin to lift in a severely depressed patient.**

TIME PERIOD FOR ANTIDEPRESSANT THERAPY

The duration of antidepressant treatment should be that which is sufficient. In general it is recommended that those with a **first clinical** presentation should be treated with antidepressants for at least 6–9 months, and then tapered off under careful clinical supervision. Those with **previous depressive episodes** should be kept on antidepressants for longer than a year, perhaps several years.

The classes/groups of antidepressants available include (see Table 4.16):

- Tricyclics (TCAs)
- Selective serotonin reuptake inhibitors (SSRIs)
- Serotonin and noradrenergic reuptake inhibitors (SNRIs)
- Noradrenergic and specific serotonergic antidepressants (NaSSA)
- Monoamine oxidase inhibitors (MAOIs), both irreversible and reversible (RIMAs)
- Others.

TRICYCLIC (AND TETRACYCLIC) ANTIDEPRESSANTS

These are relatively cheap and effective and are in no way inferior to other classes of antidepressants. They do, however, cause troublesome side effects and are toxic in overdose, with a few exceptions such as lofepramine.

Indications

- Depressive disorders, especially in moderate to severe forms, and with somatic features
- Anxiety disorders such as GAD, mixed anxiety–depression, phobic disorders, post-traumatic stress disorders, obsessive–compulsive disorder
- Chronic pain, such as trigeminal neuralgia
- Nocturnal enuresis (imipramine)
- Chronic fatigue syndrome/ME (in lower doses).

TABLE 4.16   Antidepressant summary

Medication	Anticholinergic effects	Sedative effects	Hypotension	Possibility of seizures	Half-life (hours)	Dose range (mg)
● Tricyclics						
Amitriptyline	4+	3+	3+	+	20–46	100–300
Clomipramine	4+	2+	3+	+	20–40	50–250
Desipramine	2+	1–2+	2+	+	10–32	100–300
Imipramine	3+	2+	3+	+	4–34	100–300
Nortriptyline	2+	2+	1+	+	18–88	50–150
Protriptyline	4+	1+	2+	+	53–124	10–60
Trimipramine	3+	3+	3+	+	9	100–300
Lofepramine						70–210
Dothiepin						75–225
● MAOIs						
Irreversible						
Isocarboxazid						10–60
Phenelzine						45–90
Tranylcypramine						10–30
Reversible (RIMAs)						
Moclobemide						300–600
Brofaromine						
Cimoxatane						
● SSRIs						
Fluroxramine	1+				15	100–300
Fluoxetine	0	0	0	+	5–7 days	20–60
Paroxetine	1+	0–1+	0	0	24	20–60
Sertraline	1+	0	0	+	26	50–200
Citalopram						20–60
● SNRIs						
Venlafaxine	0	0	0	+	9–11	75–375
● NaSSA (Noradrenergic and specific serotonergic antidepressant)						
Mirtazapine					20–40	15–45
● Others						
Amoxapine	2+	2+	1+	+++	8–33	100–300
Trazodone	0	3+	2+	+	6–14	100–600
Nefazodone	0	1+	1+	?	6–14	200–600

Contraindications

● Cardiac: arrhythmia, e.g. conduction defects, recent myocardial infarction
● Liver disease
● Glaucoma
● Psychiatric: mania

Pharmacology

● Half-life (see Table 4.16). Most given once a day, but some b.d. or t.d.s.
   (e.g. lofepramine)

- Commencing dose should be 50–100% of lower end of dose range to avoid side effects
- Serum monitoring of drug levels is usually not required, with the exception of cases of overdose.

Drug interactions

Side effects (see Table 4.16) see also *British National Formulary* or local formularies

- **Antiadrenergic:** postural hypotension
- **Anticholinergic:** drowsiness, weight gain
- **Antimuscarinic:** blurred vision, precipitation of narrow-angle glaucoma, constipation, dry mouth, urinary retention (especially the elderly with enlarged prostate)
- **Cardiac:** arrythymias, tachycardia, cardiotoxicity, conduction delay, other ECG changes, postural hypotension, syncope
- **Endocrine:** galactorrhoea, gynaecomastia, testicular enlargement, blood glucose changes
- **GI tract:** black tongue, paralytic ileus, reflux
- **Haematological:** agranulocytosis, eosinophilia, leukopenia, thrombocytopenia
- **Hepatic:** liver function test abnormalities
- **Metabolic:** hyponatraemia (especially the elderly)
- **Neurological:** cognitive impairment, lowering of seizure threshold, movement disorders, e.g. akathisia, dyskinesia, tremor
- **Psychiatric:** hypomania
- **Sexual:** anorgasmia (especially women), erectile or ejaculatory dysfunction (30–40%)
- **Others:** Facial oedema, photosensitization, skin rashes, neuroleptic malignant syndrome (rare), pyrexia

SELECTIVE SEROTONIN REUPTAKE INHIBITORS (SSRIs)

These are increasingly replacing TCAs in terms of the amount being prescribed. Although still relatively expensive, they have the advantage of fewer side effects and relative safety in overdose (see Table 4.16).

Examples include:

- Citalopram
- Fluvoxamine
- Fluoxetine
- Paroxetine
- Sertraline.

Indications

- Depressive disorders
- Anxiety disorders (mixed anxiety depression, GAD, phobic disorders, PTSD, panic disorders), obsessive–compulsive disorder (in relatively higher doses), chronic fatigue syndrome (in lower doses)
- Other psychiatric disorders with comorbid depressive symptoms.

Contraindications

- Severe renal and hepatic failure
- Dehydration
- Mania.

Pharmacology

SSRIs vary with regard to their half-life (fluoxetine has the longest at around 7–14 days, owing to its active metabolite), serotonin specificity, drug interactions and the few the side effects specific to a particular SSRI. Citalopram is considered to have the greatest specificity for serotonin among current SSRIs.

Dosage (see Table 4.16)

All are given once a day (in the case of fluoxetine missing a dose is less crucial because of its long half-life). With the exception of fluoxetine, withdrawal symptoms may be experienced on sudden cessation of the drug (worst in the case of paroxetine).

Drug interactions

The following drugs, which are metabolized by the P450 system, will have their *plasma levels raised* if given concurrently with fluoxetine and paroxetine:

- Alprazolam
- Carbamazepine
- Diazepam
- Digoxin
- Haloperidol
- Tricyclics
- Valproic acid.

Side effects

- **GI tract:** abdominal discomfort, nausea, vomiting and diarrhoea (these are usually transient and occur during the early part of the treatment)
- **Metabolic:** hyponatraemia
- **Neuropsychiatric:** anxiety, headache and restlessness
- **Sexual:** lowered libido, orgasmic difficulties.

SEROTONIN–NORADRENERGIC REUPTAKE INHIBITORS (SNRIs)

Sometimes described as 'cleaner' TCAs because they have fewer side effects than TCAs, these drugs inhibit the reuptake of both noradrenaline and serotonin.

Venlafaxine

Indications

- Depressive disorders
- Depressed phase of bipolar disorder
- Anxiety disorders (GAD, panic disorder, social phobia)
- Other psychiatric disorders with comorbid depressive symptoms.

Contraindications

- Hypertension (in a small proportion of patients there is a dose-dependent rise in blood pressure, and BP monitoring is therefore required
- Severe renal and hepatic failure
- Mania.

Pharmacology

Its active metabolite has a half-life of approximately 5–12 hours. The **dose** ranges from 75 to 375 mg/day, given in divided doses. However, a once daily formulation is now also in use. Avoid abrupt withdrawal following > 1 week's treatment because of withdrawal symptoms.

Side effects

The side-effect profile resembles that of the SSRIs.

- **Cardiac:** hypertension (in doses > 200 mg), palpitations
- **GI tract:** nausea (dose dependent), abdominal pain, vomiting, weight changes, constipation and anorexia
- **Hepatic:** reversible increase in liver enzymes
- **Neuropsychiatric:** agitation, anxiety, abnormal dreams, headache, insomnia, somnolence and convulsions
- **Metabolic:** hyponatraemia
- **Skin:** rashes.

NORADRENERGIC AND SPECIFIC SEROTONINERGIC ANTIDEPRESSANTS (NaSSA)

NaSSA are selective antagonists of α-adrenergic receptors, regulating the release of noradrenaline (NA) and serotonin (5-HT). They increase the release of NA and 5-HT and block $5\text{-}HT_2$ and $5\text{-}HT_3$ receptors.

Mirtazapine

Indications
Depressive disorders.

Contraindications

- Severe hepatic, renal or cardiac failure
- History of closed-angle glaucoma
- Mania.

Pharmacology

- The **dose** range varies from 15 to 45 mg daily and it may be given once (at bedtime) or twice daily. Commence at 15 mg daily for 4 days, increase to 30 mg daily, and then to 45 mg daily after 10 days if required.
- The half-life is between 20 and 40 hours.
- The drug is 85% protein bound.

Side effects

- **Cardiac:** postural hypotension and, on rare occasions, oedema
- **GI tract:** dry mouth, constipation, increased appetite and weight gain
- **Haematological:** rarely reversible agranulocytosis and leucopenia
- **Hepatic:** elevated liver enzymes (uncommon), jaundice
- **Neuropsychiatric:** agitation, insomnia, sedation (30%) and seizures (very rare).

Overdose
Low toxicity in overdose

MONOAMINE OXIDASE INHIBITORS (MAOIs)

MAOIs are divided into two major groups, irreversible and reversible.

Irreversible MAOIs
These are further subdivided into:

- Hydrazine group: phenelzine and isocarboxazide
- Non-hydrazine group: tranylcypromine.

> ⚠ **With irreversible MAOIs the avoidance of tyramine-containing compounds is essential, otherwise hypertensive crises may ensue.**

Indications

- Depressive disorders, especially of the atypical variety. These are characterized by hyperphagia, weight gain, and mood changes which worsen as the day progresses
- Anxiety disorders, panic disorders, phobic disorders (e.g. social phobia) and PTSD
- Depression unresponsive to other antidepressants.

Contraindications

- Cerebrovascular disease
- Abnormal liver function tests or hepatic impairment
- Phaeochromocytoma
- Mania.

Pharmacology

Dosage

- Phenelzine 45–90 mg/day in divided doses t.d.s.
- Isocarboxazide 10–60 mg/day in divided doses o.d. or b.d.
- Tranylcypromine 10–30 mg/day in divided doses b.d.
- These drugs should be avoided at bedtime
- 3–5 weeks are needed to judge the therapeutic response.

> ⚠️ **After stopping MAOIs, allow a 2-week drug-free period before starting another antidepressant. MAOIs should not be started for at least 1 week (2 weeks in the case of phenelzine) after stopping a tricyclic, SSRI or related antidepressant (2 weeks for paroxetine and sertraline, but 5 weeks for fluoxetine).**

Side effects

- **Cardiovascular:** postural hypotension in 10–15% (treat with support stockings and adequate hydration), arrhythmias
- **GI tract:** increased appetite, weight gain and constipation
- **Hepatic:** hepatotoxicity, increased liver enzymes
- **Neuropsychiatric:** dizziness, insomnia, euphoria, blurred vision, nystagmus and convulsions. Pyridoxine deficiency may develop with phenelzine leading to paraesthesia and peripheral neuropathy. Hypomania
- **Metabolic:** Hyponatraemia
- **Sexual:** Anorgasmia.

Other, potentially fatal, side effects:

- **Hypertensive crises** caused by mixing MAOIs with tyramine-containing compounds (see Chapter 6).
- **Serotonin syndrome:** this results from combining MAOIs with serotonin-augmenting drugs such as TCAs, SSRIs, SNRIs and nefazadone (see Chapter 6).

Drugs and food interactions with MAOIs (see Table 4.17)
Many food and drugs interact with MAOIs: patients should therefore be educated and supplied with written information to that effect. They should also carry a card indicating that they take MAOIs.

Note: Many over-the-counter preparations contain tyramine.
Directly acting sympathomimetics (bronchodilators) are safe to use with MAOIs.

TABLE 4.17   Dietary advice for patients taking MAOIs

Foods not allowed
Broad beans, fava beans
Beer
Cheese, aged/matured
Fish, smoked/pickled
Liver, beef or chicken
Sausages
Red wine, especially chianti
Yeast extracts

Foods allowed in small quantities
Alcohol (except as noted above)
Avocado, ripe
Banana, ripe
Soy sauce
Yoghurt

Foods allowed in moderate quantities
Caffeine (coffee, tea, soft drinks)
Cheese, cottage or cream
Chocolate
Figs
Meat tenderizers
Raisins

General advice for patients taking MAOIs
- Eat fresh food
- Avoid food that has fermented or 'gone off'
- Avoid sauces, gravies and soups at restaurants

Drugs which should be avoided with MAOIs
All OTC drugs (seek advice from doctor or pharmacist)
Anaesthetics (check with anaesthetist)
Anticonvulsants (e.g. carbamazepine)

TABLE 4.17   Dietary advice for patients taking MAOIs *(contd)*

Appetite suppressants
Buspirone
Dopaminergic drugs (e.g. L-dopa)
Inhalers and decongestants
Narcotic painkillers (e.g. pethidine)
Oral hypoglycaemics
Sympathomimetics

Antidepressants: TCAs (e.g. clomipramine), SSRIs, SNRIs
Wait for 2 weeks after stopping MAOIs before starting the above antidepressants

Before commencing MAOIs
Wait 5 weeks following stoppage of fluoxetine
Wait 2 weeks following stoppage of paroxetine and sertraline
Wait 1 week following stoppage of citalopram, fluvoxamine, TCAs and venlafaxine

Drug interaction with MAOIs
Drugs causing hypertension with MAOIs
Adrenaline
Aminophylline
Amphetamines
Caffeine
Carbamazepine
Cocaine
Direct-acting sympathomimetics
Ephedrine
Guanethidine
L-dopa
Methyldopa
Methylphenidate
Phenylethylamine
Phenylpropranolamine
Pseudoephedrine
Theophylline
Tyramine

Drugs causing hypotension with MAOIs
Calcium channel blockers
Diuretics
Hypoglycaemic agents
Prazosin
Propranolol

Drugs whose activity is enhanced with MAOIs
Anticholinergics
Anticoagulants
Succinylcholine

Drugs that may lead to serotonin syndrome when taken with MAOIs
Buspirone
Nefazedone
SSRIs
TCAs
Tryptophan

TABLE 4.17   Dietary advice for patients taking MAOIs (contd)

Other drugs that should be avoided with MAOIs
Aldomet
Clonidine
Guanethidine
Reserpine

MAOIs and anaesthesia (consult with the anaesthetist)
● A 2-week washout is recommended before elective general anaesthesia but is not absolutely essential
● Avoid curare, as it has indirect sympathomimetic effects
● For hypotension, volume expansion or direct-acting sympathomimetics (e.g. noradrenaline) should be used instead of indirect-acting agents (e.g. metaraminol)
● Avoid droperidol because of reports of cardiac and respiratory depression with MAOIs.

Reversible inhibitors of monoamine oxidase A (RIMAs)
These drugs are safe with tyramine-containing foods/drugs, but excessive consumption should be avoided to minimize the risk of hypertension.

Moclobemide is the only drugs currently in use. Others being assessed are brofarmine, cimoxatone and toloxalone.

Moclobemide

Indications

● Depressive disorder
● Chronic dysthymia
● Seasonal affective disorder
● Social phobia.

Contraindications

● Acute confusional state
● Mania (thyroxicosis may precipitate mania)
● Phaeochromocytoma
● Severe hepatic impairment
● Thyrotoxicosis.

Pharmacology

● Dose is 300 mg daily in divided doses; usual range is 150–600 mg daily.
● Dosing is not affected by ageing or renal function, but should be lowered in hepatic disease.
● It has low protein binding and an elimination half-life of 1–3 hours.

Side effects

- **GI tract:** nausea
- **Hepatic:** rarely, raised liver enzymes
- **Metabolic:** hyponatraemia
- **Neuropsychiatric:** agitation, confusion, dizziness, headache, restlessness and sleep disturbance
  Hypomania/mania may be precipitated in bipolar disorder.

OTHER ANTIDEPRESSANTS

Amoxipine
Second-line drug which has some dopamine-blocking actions: consequently it may cause extrapyramidal side effects.
Dosage: 100–300 mg daily in divided doses.

Trazodone
Sedating, but lacking in anticholinergic properties. May cause priapism in a small number of men.
Dosage: 100–600 mg daily in divided doses.

Nefazadone
Has serotonin reuptake inhibition properties but is also a potent 5-HT$_2$ antagonist. This latter feature allows it to be free of some of the troublesome side effects of SSRIs. Its advantages include minimal ill effects on sexual function and sleep architecture (it does not suppress REM activity).
Dosage: 100 mg b.d., and increasing to 200 mg b.d. after 5–7 days; maximum dose is 300 mg b.d.

Side effects

- **GI tract:** dry mouth, nausea and constipation
- **Cardiac:** syncope (only rarely) and postural hypotension (uncommon)
- **Neuropsychiatric:** ataxia, confusion and dizziness
- **Ophthalmic:** ambylopia and other minor visual disturbances.

Other physical treatments for depression include:

- Electroconvulsive therapy (ECT)
- Psychosurgery
- Light therapy
- Alternative therapies.

For details see pp. 191–199.

Management of treatment-resistant depression

With the **first antidepressant**, try to maintain the therapeutic dosage or serum level for at least 4 weeks

↓

If **no response**, reassess diagnosis and/or clarify the subcategory of depression

↓

Then discontinue first antidepressant and begin the second (see section on switching antidepressant), preferably one with a different serotonin/noradrenaline profile (maintain therapeutic dosage or serum level for 4 weeks)

If **still no response**, consider

↓

- MAO inhibitor – irreversible or RIMA *or*
- **Augmentation strategies**, such as the addition of:
  — Lithium 600–900 mg/daily (60% of non-responders may show positive benefits; allow 3 weeks for a positive response, which may occur within 48 hours)
  — Thyroxine (T_3) 25–50 μg/daily (allow 3 weeks for a positive response, which may happen in 60% of non-responders)
  — Carbamazepine 400 mg/daily
  — Buspirone 30 mg/daily
  — Fluoxetine, sertraline or paroxetine to a tricyclic (however, monitor for the possibility of serotonin syndrome)
- ECT.

MANAGEMENT OF PERSONALITY DISORDERS

The management of personality disorders is usually fraught with difficulties and will vary with the particular type of disorder, its severity, the presence of other comorbid psychiatric conditions and social factors.

You should explore the following:

- A careful assessment must be carried out and all relevant sources of information used (see Chapter 3).
- The primary medical conditions that may lead to a personality change should be excluded. A frontal lobe tumour can easily present as personality change, as can a serious unrecognized head injury.
- The presence of comorbid psychiatric disorders: a high percentage of people with personality disorders have other psychiatric disorders. For example, as many as 40% of psychiatric inpatients have comorbid personality disorders. The recognition of other psychiatric disorders may facilitate management, as they can be actively treated.
- Abuse of alcohol and illicit drugs, which is particularly high in certain personality disorders such as borderline personality disorder.

| Note | Personality disorders are frequently overlooked in the elderly, and personality traits and disorders tend to become exaggerated and more fixed with dementia. |

Despite difficulties in management and the negative emotions these patients may evoke in health-care workers, attempts using a fresh and positive outlook should be made to help them.

Management strategies encompass:

- Psychosocial interventions, which include:
  — use of various psychotherapies
  — use of special psychiatric units
  — use of therapeutic communities (e.g. Henderson Hospital)
- Pharmacotherapeutic measures (see under specific personality disorders, as outlined below).

SPECIFIC PERSONALITY DISORDERS

PARANOID PERSONALITY DISORDER

This particular disorder is difficult to manage and paranoia may even be directed against the staff.

PSYCHOSOCIAL MANAGEMENT

A clear and straightforward explanation should be given for the reasoning behind history taking, tests and other therapeutic procedures.

Give an explanation and warn about possible side effects of the treatment, both verbally and in writing if at all possible.

Psychotherapies found to be useful include:

- Individual supportive therapy by an experienced therapist
- Behavioural therapy to improve social skills and reduce suspiciousness.

PHARMACOTHERAPY

Low-dose antipsychotics such as thioridazine, haloperidol, olanazapine or risperidone may be given for short periods.

SCHIZOID PERSONALITY DISORDER

Schizophrenia and schizotypal personality disorders should be excluded (unlike those with schizoid personality disorder, these patients may have affected relatives).

PSYCHOSOCIAL MANAGEMENT

- Individual supportive therapy
- Group therapy, usually after some progress in treatment has been made.

PHARMACOTHERAPY

- Low-dose antipsychotics
- Antidepressants have also been found to be useful in some cases.

DISSOCIAL (ANTISOCIAL) PERSONALITY DISORDER

These patients are more likely to be seen in a forensic setting (e.g. local and regional secure units, special hospitals); comorbid substance abuse is common and will need to be managed appropriately.

PSYCHOSOCIAL MANAGEMENT

These individuals are difficult to contain; however, when possible, individual or group psychotherapy, or self-help groups can be tried.

- Avoid being manipulated or made to feel guilty.
- Keep clear and firm boundaries, and inform the individual of the legal consequences of their antisocial behaviour.
- Severe cases may need to be managed in special units or therapeutic communities.

PHARMACOTHERAPY

- Low-dose antipsychotics
- Mood stabilizers/antiaggression drugs, e.g. carbamazepine or lithium
- Antidepressants (SSRIs) in some cases.

BORDERLINE PERSONALITY DISORDER

You are more than likely to meet this category in a general psychiatric setting. Individuals with borderline personality disorder are extremely difficult to manage and may even cause friction among staff owing to their use of the defence mechanism called **splitting**.

PSYCHOSOCIAL MANAGEMENT

- There should be clear communication between all staff involved, with an agreed management strategy.
- A senior member of staff (usually the consultant) should be in charge.
- Maintain clear, firm and, if at all possible, consistent boundaries.
- Avoid being blackmailed.
- Therapeutic goals should be realistic.

Some of the psychotherapies used include individual supportive therapy and group therapy.

PHARMACOTHERAPY (Table 4.18)

This is usually aimed at the psychiatric symptomatology (e.g. mood instability, aggressiveness, impulsive and episodic depressive and psychotic symptoms) or the presence of comorbid psychiatric disorders.

- Avoid using medications that may be dangerous in overdose (e.g. TCAs).
- Consider and provide appropriate management for the abuse of alcohol and illicit drugs, especially before prescribing medications.
- Clarify and discuss compliance issues.

TABLE 4.18 Pharmacotherapeutic targeting of symptoms in borderline personality disorder

Symptoms	Drugs of choice
Depression	SSRIs, SNRIs, nefazadone moclobemide
Mood lability	Lithium
Impulsivity/behavioural dyscontrol	Carbamazepine (follow the same guidelines as in manic disorders)
Anger/rage episodes	Low-dose antipsychotics, carbamazepine, lithium and β-blockers
Paranoia and brief psychotic episodes	Antipsychotics
Bulimia	SSRIs in relatively high doses

HISTRIONIC PERSONALITY DISORDER

It is often difficult to differentiate this condition from borderline personality disorder. You should also consider somatization disorder (Briquet's syndrome), psychotic disorders and dissociative disorder, which may coexist.

PSYCHOSOCIAL MANAGEMENT

Explore and clarify the patient's real feelings, which are often suppressed. Psychoanalytic psychotherapy has been found to be useful.

PHARMACOTHERAPY

This may be considered and is targeted towards the symptomatology.

- Antidepressants for depressive symptoms
- Anxiolytics for anxiety symptoms
- Antipsychotics for the derealization and delusions.

ANANKASTIC (OBSESSIVE–COMPULSIVE) PERSONALITY DISORDER

You should distinguish this from obsessive–compulsive traits and obsessive–compulsive disorder. Delusional and depressive disorders may also coexist.

PSYCHOSOCIAL MANAGEMENT

Individuals with this disorder often want minute details of their treatment. A balanced approach should be taken by giving appropriate amounts of information. Support groups, group therapy and cognitive behaviour therapy (CBT) have been found to be beneficial. Help should also be provided in improving the person's social interactions.

PHARMACOTHERAPY

Clomipramine and SSRIs (fluoxetine or paroxetine) in relatively high doses have been found to be beneficial where there are obsessive–compulsive features.

ANXIOUS (AVOIDANT) PERSONALITY DISORDER

These individuals may be difficult to help because of their extreme shyness and their sensitivity to the interviewer or the therapist.

PSYCHOSOCIAL MANAGEMENT

A trusting alliance with the therapist, who discourages dependence, is helpful. Individual, supportive, and group therapies and assertiveness training have been found to be useful.

PHARMACOTHERAPY

This is used to manage anxiety and depressive symptoms; drugs used include:

- Anxiolytics, e.g. buspirone
- Antidepressants, e.g. paroxetine
- β-Blockers, e.g. atenolol.

DEPENDENT PERSONALITY DISORDER

A number of management approaches can be tried to help those with this disorder. The overall goal is to encourage the patient to become more independent, assertive and self-reliant.

PSYCHOSOCIAL MANAGEMENT

Assertiveness training, individual, supportive, family, group and behaviour therapies have all been found to be useful.

PHARMACOTHERAPY

Drugs, when used, are to deal with the symptoms of anxiety and depression, which are common in this disorder. They include:

- TCAs: imipramine
- SSRIs: paroxetine and fluoxetine.

SCHIZOPHRENIA AND OTHER PSYCHOTIC DISORDERS

PSYCHOSIS

A patient is said to be suffering from psychosis if he or she exhibits symptoms such as delusions, hallucinations and disorganized patterns of thought and speech. However, not all of these symptoms may be present and it is important to assess their impact on the patient's life.

While carrying out a psychiatric evaluation you must exclude the presence of psychotic symptoms so that a serious psychotic disorder such as schizophrenia is diagnosed and treated early, thereby improving the prognosis.

Schizophrenia is one of the most common psychotic disorders and you must learn to recognize and treat this devastating illness.

MANAGEMENT

- Clarification of psychotic symptoms
- Exploring underlying medical causes, including drugs (prescribed and illicit)
- Clarification of the appropriate psychiatric diagnostic category
- Exploration of psychosocial and cultural issues
- Provision of a treatment package for specific disorders, which should include:
  — psychosocial treatments
  — drug treatments
  — other treatments such as ECT, if required.

Clarification of psychotic symptoms
The following points should be noted:

- Avoid putting words into the patient's mouth: it is usually better for the patient to reveal the psychotic symptoms voluntarily. However, many patients may not volunteer psychotic symptoms without specific questioning. If you suspect caginess from the patient, this should be recorded in the case notes.

- When the patient is being uncooperative observation of his or her non-verbal behaviour and collateral history may also be helpful.

Delusions A delusion can be described as a false belief that is firmly held despite evidence to the contrary, and which is out of keeping with the person's educational, cultural and social norms. A variety of delusions are described (see section on psychopathology).

When clarifying delusional beliefs, it is important to note the features of a particular delusion.

- A delusion which is described as **mood congruent** (i.e. appropriate to the mood of the patient) is more likely to occur in depression, whereas **mood-incongruent** delusions tend to be found in schizophrenia.
- Other qualities of a delusion that may point to a schizophrenic illness include **bizarreness** and whether the delusion is considered **primary**.
- In addition, the **delusion of being controlled** (the passivity phenomenon; a schneiderian first-rank symptom) is also more likely to be described in a patient suffering from schizophrenia.

> ⚠ **It is essential that you consider whether the alleged event is actually taking place or has taken place before labelling someone delusional.**

Some examples of delusions include (see also psychopathology):

- **Primary delusions:** An example is the **delusional perception** (a schneiderian first-rank symptom), where a delusional meaning is attached to a normally perceived object.
- **Paranoid (and persecutory) delusions:** The patient believes that he or she is being followed, persecuted, poisoned, or in some way picked out; this can occur in schizophrenics (where they tend to be more bizarre), as the result of drugs (e.g. amphetamines) and in psychotic depression (especially in the elderly).
- **Somatic delusions:** The content of these delusion refers to the patient's appearance and bodily functioning. They are more common in psychotic depression, especially in the elderly.
- **Grandiose delusions:** These refer to the patient's belief in his inflated self-worth, identity, power, knowledge, or special relationship with some important person or even with God. They are common in manic patients, but the more bizarre grandiose delusions tend to occur in schizophrenia.

Hallucinations A hallucination is defined as a false sensory perception which appears realistic to the patient in the absence of a real external stimulus. Hallucinations can occur in a number of modalities, including auditory, visual, olfactory and tactile (see Chapter 6).

- **Auditory hallucinations:** Generally the **second-person auditory hallucination** is more common in psychotic depression, whereas, **third-person auditory hallucinations** (schneiderian first-rank symptom) tend to occur in schizophrenic illness.
- **Visual hallucinations:** These usually occur in delirium, most commonly secondary to an organic medical disorder. The non-verbal behaviour of the patient may point to the likelihood of the presence of the visual hallucinations.
- **Olfactory hallucinations:** These classically occur when there is an abnormality of the temporal lobe, such as in **temporal lobe epilepsy**. When olfactory hallucinations occur in depressed or schizophrenic patients they are generally bizarre.
- **Tactile hallucinations:** These may occur during drug intoxication, for example with cocaine (e.g. cocaine bug).

Disorganization of behaviour, speech or thinking A psychotic patient may exhibit grossly disordered or even bizarre behaviour. The speech may be disordered (unintelligible), as may be his or her thinking (abnormalities of content and form of thoughts). See Appendix for details.

Once again, the more bizarre the behaviour, speech and thoughts, the more likely it is that the patient is suffering from schizophrenic illness.

Exploring the underlying medical causes
Medical disorders and drugs (both prescribed an illicit) can both cause psychotic symptomatology.

It is therefore essential that you exclude psychiatric causes for an apparently psychotic behaviour, because the removal of the causative factors may relieve the psychotic symptoms without the need for antipsychotic drugs.

Some of the clues for a possible medical aetiology for psychotic symptoms include sudden onset of the symptoms, a history of medical illness, and a lack of personal and family psychiatric history.

Medical disorders and drugs that can cause psychotic symptoms	
Disorder/drug	**Symptoms**
Amphetamine	Paranoid delusions
Procyclidine	Visual hallucinations
Delirium	Visual hallucinations
Delirium tremens	Hallucinations
CVA affecting language area	Bizarre speech
Temporal lobe epilepsy	Delusions and hallucinations

Clarification of appropriate psychiatric diagnostic category
Once you have established the presence of psychotic symptoms and excluded possible medical causes, the next task is to try and establish possible psychiatric diagnostic category(ies), as many psychiatric disorders feature psychotic symptoms.

Psychiatric disorders featuring psychotic symptoms:

- Bipolar affective disorder (mania)
- Brief reactive psychosis/acute and transient psychotic disorders
- Delusional disorders
- Personality disorder (borderline personality disorder)
- Psychotic depression
- Schizophrenia
- Schizoaffective disorders
- Schizotypal disorder.

Exploration of psychosocial and cultural issues
When assessing a patient with psychotic symptoms it is essential that you also explore the psychosocial and cultural issues, for these have both diagnostic and prognostic implications. Many beliefs which may appear delusional may be sanctioned by an individual's religion or culture.

Persistent suffering from discrimination, of whatever type, may lead to beliefs that appear paranoid.

Finally from the prognostic point of view it has been shown that a schizophrenic patient living in a family where high expressed emotions are prevalent is likely have a poor prognosis.

Provision of a treatment package
This should include:

- Psychosocial treatments
- Drug treatments
- Other treatments such as ECT, if required.

SPECIFIC DISORDERS WITH PSYCHOTIC SYMPTOMS

BIPOLAR AFFECTIVE DISORDER (MANIA)

See p. 139.

PERSONALITY DISORDER (BORDERLINE PERSONALITY DISORDER)

See p. 167.

PSYCHOTIC DEPRESSION

See p. 170.

BRIEF REACTIVE PSYCHOSIS/ACUTE AND TRANSIENT PSYCHOTIC DISORDERS

The psychotic symptoms usually appear within 2 weeks of some traumatic/stressful event.

These typically include bereavement, unexpected loss of partner or job, divorce, or other forms of psychotrauma. Recovery usually occurs within 2–3 months, and often within a few weeks or even days.

MANAGEMENT

This is targeted towards the cause and usually involves **psychosocial management**, such as supportive measures, reassurance and observation; it is very rare to resort to the use of antipsychotics.

DELUSIONAL DISORDERS

These include a number of disorders (for example delusional disorder and late paraphrenia) in which long-standing, unusually isolated delusional beliefs are present.

MANAGEMENT

Many respond to antipsychotic medications and, if possible, **psychosocial measures**.

SCHIZOPHRENIA

See Chapter 3 (p. 99).

MANAGEMENT

The management of schizophrenic disorders needs to be tailored to the individual.

Factors that need to be taken into consideration include:

- Whether the presentation is acute or chronic
- The symptomatology, e.g. the presence of positive or negative symptoms or both; its severity, and its implications for the patient and others (e.g. safety issues)
- The risk of suicide or homicide
- The presence of comorbid psychiatric disorders (such as depression, personality disorders and substance abuse)
- Compliance with treatment by the patient
- If the patient can be treated voluntarily or involuntarily (i.e. use of the Mental Health Act)

- Previous exposures (and response) to antipsychotics
- Any evidence of previous treatment failure or resistance
- The social support available for the patient.

PSYCHOSOCIAL TREATMENTS/INTERVENTIONS

These are easily neglected (especially during an acute presentation) but must not be forgotten.

Supportive psychotherapy and counselling are important for both the patient and the family as well as carers. Cognitive behavioural techniques are increasingly being used to help patients cope with persistent delusions and hallucinations, and for modifying behaviour to be more acceptable. Some of the of the operant techniques can also be used in patients with socially embarrassing or withdrawn behaviours.

Rehabilitation measures are an important part of the overall management strategy, along with drug therapy. Rehabilitation usually includes occupational therapy (commonly at the day hospital), counselling and supportive therapy. Many non-medical members of the multidisciplinary team (MDT) play an important part in rehabilitation. Social workers can help with accommodation problems, financial difficulties and various claims (e.g. application for social security, travel passes and disability living allowance). The patient may attend the day hospital (on an inpatient or an outpatient basis), where various therapies and social skills training are provided. Some patients are then encouraged to attend classes for training in certain skills and possible future employment.

Rehabilitation can continue well after discharge from the hospital: where appropriate, patients should be helped to attend the day hospital, sheltered workshops and/or a day centre. This helps to ensure that they continue with appropriate activities and recreation, as well as gaining work experience. It may also permit monitoring of their mental state and compliance with medication regimens.

In the UK psychiatric patient are part of the **care programme approach** (CPA) which, by using a key or case worker for the individual patient and regular CPA meetings, is designed to ensure that the above should occur as smoothly as possible.

Many patients who are considered to be a danger to themselves or others may be placed on the **supervision register**, usually under the direction of their consultant psychiatrist.

It is also important to teach the relatives or carers that both under- and overstimulation (i.e. **high expressed emotions**) should be avoided, as this has been shown to increase the likelihood of relapse.

DRUG TREATMENTS

An increasing numbers of antipsychotics are available. The choice is usually dictated by the clinical profile of the patient, familiarity with the particular drug, and its availability (unfortunately this is sometimes dictated by the costs).

The following may help in choosing an appropriate antipsychotic:

- Use the general prescribing guidelines described earlier
- It is best to carry out baseline investigations (e.g. FBC) in those who have never been exposed to antipsychotics
- Clarify any previous successful or unsuccessful use of a particular antipsychotic, even in first-degree relatives
- Give the drug a good trial – at least 3–4 weeks – before considering changing to another
- A change of drugs because of intolerable side effects should be documented in the case notes
- Abrupt stoppage of drugs with a shorter half-life may lead to withdrawal symptoms and should be avoided
- Switching to another class of drug within 24 hours is possible following the use of a drug with a shorter half-life. However, avoid (or exercise caution) following the use of depot preparations.

When prescribing a particular antipsychotic consider the following:

Drug factors

- The side-effect profile (e.g. sedating or non-sedating, troublesome parkinsonian effects)
- Choice between typical (conventional) and atypical (novel) drugs
- Pharmacological parameters such as dosage, half-life, drug interactions etc.
- Cost: generic drugs are cheaper, but this should be balanced by factors such as side-effect profile (atypical antipsychotics are in general better tolerated than the typical ones and may help with compliance, indirectly improving the prognosis) and indirect savings made by keeping patients out of hospital.

Patient and illness factors

- Age, sex, special situations (e.g. pregnancy) and disease status
- Compliance, previous use
- Suicide risk from overdose
- Presentation, whether acute or chronic
- Psychotic symptoms (positive or negative) to be targeted: atypical antipsychotics appear to be more suitable when there are negative symptoms.

Figure 4.1 is an algorithm for the drug treatment of schizophrenia.

TREATMENT RESISTANCE

For those who fail to respond to two classes of antipsychotics a revision of diagnosis should be considered, and a second opinion may be needed; you should also consider:

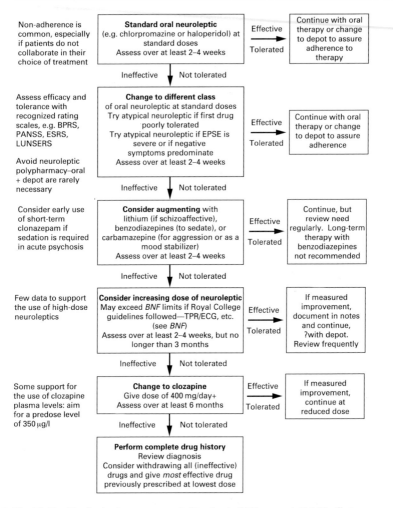

Fig. 4.1 Algorithm for the drug treatm,ent of schizophrenia. (EPSE, extrapyrimidal side effects; BPRS, brief psychiatric rating scale; PANSS, positive and negative symptom scale; ESRS, extrapyrimidal side effects rating scale; LUNSERS, Liverpool University side effect rating scale; BNF, British National Formulary; TPR, temperature, pulse, respiration; ECG, electrocardiogram.)

Reproduced with permission from David Goldberg, 1997. The Maudsley Handbook of Practical Psychiatry, 3rd edn (fig 10.1, pages 182–183), Oxford University Press.

- Is the patient compliant with therapy?
- Has the patient received an adequate dose of antipsychotic for a sufficient period?
- Concurrent abuse of illicit drugs and alcohol.

Treatment-resistant (i.e. with refractory positive symptoms) patients may be helped by:

- Clozapine or other atypical antipsychotics
- Augmentation with drugs such as:
  — **Anticonvulsants;** (carbamazepine and valproate), **but note** that carbamazepine can reduce antipsychotic plasma levels and **should not be combined with clozapine**
  — **Lithium** (plasma levels 0.9–1.2 mmol/l)
  — **Benzodiazepines**, but improvement may be modest and short-lived
- ECT may be beneficial, especially if catatonic or affective symptoms are present.

ECT – INDICATIONS IN SCHIZOPHRENIA

ECT should be considered for catatonic schizophrenics and in cases where there is severe behavioural disturbance refractory to traditional management. It should also be considered in patients with severe depressive symptoms that overwhelm the schizophrenic symptoms and there is a risk of suicide requiring urgent treatment. Similarly, where extreme manic symptoms overwhelm the schizophrenic symptoms ECT should also be considered.

For refractory negative symptoms the following antipsychotics may be helpful:

- **Clozapine** or other **atypical antipsychotics,** as suggested above
- **Dopamine agonists:** L-dopa at a dose of 300–2000 mg/day, but the response may not be evident for 7–8 weeks
- **Antidepressants:** TCAs, SSRIs and MAOIs may help to reduce negative symptoms and poor social or work functioning in some patients
- **Benzodiazepines:** alprazolam has been a reported to be useful in those with predominant anxiety and negative symptoms
- **Selegiline:** at a dose of 5 mg b.d. has been reported to improve negative, depressive and extrapyramidal symptoms.

Antipsychotics

Typical or 'conventional' antipsychotics (neuroleptics)

Class	Drug
Butyrophenones	Haloperidol, droperidol
Dibenzoxazepines	Loxapine
Diphenylbutylpiperidines	Pimozide, fluspirilene
Phenothiazines	

Antipsychotics (contd)

Aliphatic	Chlorpromazine, promozine
Piperidines	Thioridazine (considered atypical)
Piperazines	Fluphenazine, trifluperazine
Thioxanthenes	Flupenthixol, zuclopenthixol

Atypical or 'novel' antipsychotics

Class	Drug
Benzisoxazoles	Risperidone
Dibenzodiazepines	Clozapine
Dibenzothiazepines	Quetiapine
Thienobenzodiazepines	Olanzapine
Imidazolidinones	Sertindol

Other antipsychotics (also considered atypical)

Class	Drug
Substituted benzamides	Sulpiride
Benzamides	Amisulpiride

Note: At the time of writing many newer antipsychotics are in development and close to their introduction into clinical practice. Furthermore, some of the anticonvulsants (e.g. vagabatrin) are being introduced as antipsychotics.

Antipsychotics play an important role in the management of psychiatric disorders when psychotic symptoms are present. Occasionally they are also used in conditions such as obsessive–compulsive disorder (as augmenting agents), mental handicap and Gilles de la Tourette's syndrome.

Clinical indications	Comments
Schizophrenia	Treatment of psychotic symptoms both in the acute and the chronic phase; prophylaxis of schizophrenia; **Note:** atypical antipsychotics are favoured in situations where negative symptoms and increased vulnerability to extrapyramidal symptoms are prominent.
Schizoaffective disorders	Antidepressant may be added
Acute/brief psychosis	For example as a result of drugs, medical disorders, or in brief reactive psychosis
Delusional disorders	Sometimes resistant to antipsychotics
Bipolar affective disorder	Especially during the manic phase; also useful as augmenting agents with lithium
Psychotic depression	In addition to antidepressants
Personality disorders	Examples include paranoid, schizoid, schizotypal and borderline personality disorders
Psychosis in dementia	Small-dose, low-potency drugs such as thioridazine (25 mg) clozapine (6.25–50 mg/day)

Antipsychotics (contd)	
Obsessive–compulsive disorder	As augmenting agents to SSRIs
Mental handicap	To control behaviour even in the absence of psychotic symptoms
Gilles de la Tourette's syndrome	Haloperidol (0.2 mg/kg/day) and pimozide have been used
Anti depressants	Low-dose fluphenthixol (0.5–4. 5 mg) has been used for this purpose
Antiemetic	Prochlorperazine
Antipruritic	
Anaesthetic	As an adjunct to anaesthesia

Despite their troublesome side effects **typical antipsychotics** continue to play an important role in the management of schizophrenia and other psychoses; **atypical** drugs, although still relatively expensive, are increasingly being prescribed. Their advantages over typical antipsychotics lie in the fact that they have fewer, if any, extrapyramidal side effects, and are consequently better tolerated.

It is also thought that they may play some role in preventing cognitive decline in schizophrenia.

The exact mechanism of action of antipsychotics is unknown. Traditionally the antipsychotic effect has been attributed to the dopamine D_2 receptors, but it seems increasingly likely that their effect may also involve other dopamine receptors (e.g. D_3 or D_4), and that other neurotransmitters (e.g. serotonin, glutamate) also have a role.

These drugs appear to control the symptoms of schizophrenia, such as hallucinations, paranoid delusions, passivity phenomena and thought disorder, whereas in mania they reduce euphoria, excitement, irritability and expansive behaviour. Generally, the negative symptoms such as anhedonia, amotivation, poverty of speech and thought and cognitive impairment are thought to respond better to atypical antipsychotics.

Dosage

The D_2 receptor-binding studies suggest that lower doses (i.e. haloperidol 2–10 mg daily or equivalent) are sufficient for the antipsychotic effect. In practice, however, schizophrenic patients with acute presentations require higher doses than do chronic patients and manic patients may also need higher doses. Lower doses should be used in the elderly, in patients with delusional disorder and in those presenting with the first episode of schizophrenia. In normal clinical practice plasma levels are not checked. Table 4.19 gives the appropriate doses for specific antipsychotics.

TABLE 4.19   Antipsychotic doses

Atypical antipsychotics	Starting dose (mg)	Daily range for psychosis (schizophrenia)	Elimination half-life (h)
Benzisoxazole Resperidone	1–2	1 mg bid. to start and increase gradually Usual daily dose: 4–8 mg daily Doses above 16 mg/day not recommended	20–24
Dibenzodiazepine Clozapine	12.5–25	Daily to start, increase gradually up to 300–450 mg daily Doses should not exceed 900 mg daily	5–16
Dibenzothiazepine Quetiapine	50	25 mg bid. to start; increase 25–50 mg bid. as tolerated, to a target dose of 300 mg/day (given bid.) within 4–7 days Usual daily dose: 300–600 mg in divided doses. Doses above 800 mg/day not recommended	6–7
Thienobenzodiazepine Olanzapine	5–10	5–10 mg daily to start; usual dose of 10 mg Further dose increases should occur at intervals of not less than 1 week Doses above 20 mg/day not recommended	21–54
Imidazolidinones Sertindol	12	12–24 In UK ECG monitoring required	
Substituted Benzamides Sulpiride	200–600	200 mg–2.4 g daily in divided dose Hyperprolactinaemia is a problem	
Benzamides Amisulpiride	600	400 mg–1.2 g daily in divided dose Fewer problems with hyperprolactinaemia than with sulpiride	
Butyrophenone Haloperidol	6	2–100 mg daily	12–36
Dibenzoxazepine Loxapine	20	60–200 mg daily; higher than 250 mg is not recommended	8–30

TABLE 4.19   Antipsychotic doses (contd)

Atypical antipsychotics	Starting dose (mg)	Daily range for psychosis (schizophrenia)	Elimination half-life (h)
Diphenyibutylpiperidine			
Pimozide	2	2–20 mg daily; average dose: 6 mg/day Doses above 20 mg/day not recommended	29–55
Phenothiazines – Aliphatic			
Chlorpromazine	100	Usual dose: Oral 75–1000 mg daily. i.m.: 30 to 150 mg daily For severe psychosis, doses up to 1 g or more daily, in divided doses Usual dose: 60 mg i.m. up to a maximum of 150 mg/day	16–30
Piperazine			
Fluphenazine HCl	2.5–10	Up to 20 mg daily	13–58
Trifluoperazine	5	Up to 40 mg daily; doses up to 80 mg daily used rarely	13
Piperidine			
Thioridazine	100	Usual dose: up to 400 mg daily; 200–800 mg daily in hospitalized patient	9–30
Thioxanthenes			
Flupenthixol	10	3–6 mg daily as maintenance dose; up to 12 mg daily used in some patients	26–36
Zuclopenthixol	10	10–50 mg to start; increase by 10–20 mg every 2–3 days; usual daily dose: 20–60 mg; doses >150 mg daily not recommended	12–28

The above doses are approximations, and are applied to the management of acute schizophrenia. Variations in dose required for clinical effectiveness will occur because of number of factors. Doses are usually lower in chronic schizophrenia or the elderly.

TESTS PRIOR TO COMMENCING ANTIPSYCHOTICS

Exercise caution in antipsychotic-naive patients. It is useful to take blood for baseline FBC.

Where cardiac disease or epilepsy is suspected an ECG or EEG should be carried out.

TESTS DURING ANTIPSYCHOTIC TREATMENT

It is prudent to monitor patients with laboratory tests (e.g. FBC, ECG) at appropriate intervals, and other investigations relating to the clinical picture and on presentation of significant side effects. **Note:** Clozapine has its own special monitoring procedures (see later).

Side effects of typical antipsychotics (neuroleptics)

Anticholinergic	These result from antimuscarinic effects (Ach) and vary between antipsychotics; they include dry mucous membranes, blurred vision (check for glaucoma), constipation and urinary retention
CNS	
Cognitive	Sedation, confusion, disturbance in concentration and orientation; possibly negative-like symptoms and worsening of cognitive problems
Neurological	Extrapyramidal

Early (hours/days):
Akathisia in 40% (restlessness)
Dyskinesia (abnormal muscle movements)
Dystonia or abnormal muscle tone, such as torticollis (neck rotation), oculogyric crises (eye turning upwards), opisthtonus (back arching), lingual and laryngeal (very rare)

Middle (days/weeks):
Akinesia (often mistaken for depression), parkinsonian tremor, facies, rigidity

Late (weeks/months):
Tardive dyskinesia
Tardive dystonia
Rabbit syndrome
Pisa syndrome
Choreoathetosis of extremities; clonic jerking of fingers, toes
Loss of gag reflex
Lowering of seizure threshold

Cardiovascular	Due to antagonism of α_1-adrenergic and muscarinic receptors, hypertension, tachycardia, non-specific ECG changes and, in rare cases, arrhythmias (especially with pimozide and thioridazine)
Endocrine	Prolactin levels raised by many (such as sulpiride) and this leads to sexual side effects and gynaecomastia in males, menstrual irregularities, false-positive pregnancy test and changes in libido. Hypoglycaemia or hyperglycaemia may also occur. Tardive hypothalamic syndrome (polydipsia and polyuria of SIADH) is known to occur rarely
Gastrointestinal	Increased appetite and weight gain are common; rarely, anorexia, dyspepsia, dysphagia, diarrhoea and vomiting. Constipation is regularly complained of
Genitourinary/sexual	Decreased libido, erectile difficulties, impotence, inhibition of ejaculation, retrograde ejaculation (thioridazine) and, rarely, priapism (thioridazine, chlorpromazine)

Side effects of atypical antipsychotics (contd)

Ocular	With long-term use lenticular pigmentation (chlorpromazine), retinitis pigmentosa/*blindness* (chronic use of thioridazine >800 mg daily)
Hypersensitivity/others	Agranulocytosis (>0.1%)
	Choleostatic jaundice, transient elevation of liver enzymes
	Photosensitivity, photoallergy and skin reactions
	Neuroleptic malignant syndrome (NMS)
Withdrawal symptoms	See p. 108, withdrawal of antipsychotics
Toxicity (see later)	

Side effects of atypical antipsychotics
CNS

Cognitive	Sedation, usually first 2 weeks (mainly with clozapine) Headache (risperidone, olanzapine and quetiapine), confusion, disturbance in concentration and orientation at higher doses in the elderly; agitation and insomnia reported with olanzapine and risperidone. Negative-like symptoms and cognitive problems **less likely**
Neurological	Extrapyramidal side effects **less likely** (clozapine has the lowest risk) but may occur at higher doses (risperidone) Lowered seizure threshold (especially with clozapine)
Cardiovascular	Owing to antagonism of α_1-adrenergic and muscarinic receptors, hypotension (risperidone and clozapine dosing needs to be increased gradually), tachycardia, non-specific ECG changes and, in rare cases, arrhythmias. Rare reports of cardiomyopathy with clozapine
Endocrine	Prolactin levels may be raised (least likely with clozapine), leading to sexual side effects and gynaecomastia in males, menstrual irregularities, false-positive pregnancy test and changes in libido Hypoglycaemia or hyperglycaemia may also occur (clozapine) Tardive hypothalamic syndrome (polydipsia and polyuria of SIADH) is known to occur rarely
Gastrointestinal	As with typical antipsychotics, increased appetite and weight gain are common and, rarely, anorexia, dyspepsia, dysphagia, diarrhoea and vomiting. Constipation is regularly complained of (especially clozapine)
Genitourinary/sexual	Decreased libido, erectile difficulties, impotence, inhibition of ejaculation, retrograde ejaculation (risperidone) and anorgasmia
Ocular	Lens changes with chronic use of quetiapine can occur
Hypersensitivity/others	Agranulocytosis in 1–2% of patients on clozapine; eosinophilia and transient leucocytosis (clozapine)

Side effects of atypical antipsychotics (contd)

Choleostatic jaundice (>0.1%), transient elevation of liver enzymes
Photosensitivity, photoallergy and skin reactions (risperidone)
Neuroleptic malignant syndrome (NMS) much rarer than in typical antipsychotics
Rhinitis (risperidone, olanzapine and clozapine)

MANAGEMENT OF SIDE EFFECTS OF ANTIPSYCHOTICS
(see Table 4.20)

TABLE 4.20   Some suggestions for the management of antipsychotic side effects

Side effect	Management
Dry mouth, blurred vision, constipation other anticholinergic effects	Fluid intake (non-sugar) should be encouraged; use of sugarless gum; high-fibre diet and/or stool softener for constipation; use of bethanechol for peripheral anticholinergic side effects; switch to more potent agent if other strategies unsuccessful
Extrapyramidal symptoms	Reduce dose of antipsychotic if possible; add anticholinergic (Procyclidine, Benzhexol); for akathisia add β-blocker (propranolol 10 mg t.i.d. or atenolol 50 mg b.i.d.); for refractory EPS amantadine 100 mg b.i.d. (but may worsen psychosis in some patients); benzodiazepines sometimes helpful
Dizziness and hypotension	Instruct patient to dangle legs, rise slowly from bed; reduce dose of antipsychotic and/or divide into smaller amounts (e.g. 100 mg b.i.d. and 200 mg thioridazine rather than 400 mg); increase salt intake (e.g. salt tablets); use of support stockings; in difficult cases, use fludrocortisone
Sexual side effects	Reduce dose of antipsychotic if possible; switch to more potent agent (avoid aliphatic piperidine phenothiazines); add small amount of cyproheptadine (or ?yohimbine); bethanechol

Adapted with permission from R.W. Pies, 1998. Handbook of Essential Psychopharmacology. American Psychiatric Press, Washington, D.C.

Clozapine (clozaril)

This drug is mainly used in treatment-resistant schizophrenia: between one-third and two-thirds of patients will respond positively over a period of 2 years. It blocks $5-HT_{2a}$, $5-HT_{2c}$, D_1, D_4, α-adrenergic histamine and D_2 receptors. Its unusual receptor profile may be responsible for its effectiveness and the lack of extrapyramidal side effects. The major difficulty is that there is a small risk of agranulocytosis, which unfortunately can be fatal and requires special monitoring.

In the UK it is usually prescribed in hospital (at least initially, i.e. the first year) and all patients must be registered with the clozapine patient monitoring service (CPMS), details of which can be obtained from:

The Clozaril Patient Monitoring Service Manager
Novaritus Pharmaceuticals UK Ltd
Frimley Business Park
Camberley
Surrey GU16 5S J
Tel: 01276 692255

Current guidelines (UK) for initiating treatment with clozapine include:
Prior to commencement:

- The patient should be in the hospital.
- The patient should be registered with CPMS.
- WBC should be greater than $3.5 \times 10^9/l$.
- FBC and differential should be normal.

After commencement:

- Monitor FBC weekly for first 18 weeks.
- 2-weekly thereafter for 1 year.
- Then 4-weekly if there have been no concerns regarding WBC.

Dosage

- Usual **starting** dose is 12.5 mg nocte, day 1
- 12.5 mg b.d., day 2
- Increasing in 12.5 mg increments daily
- **Maximum** dose 900 mg/daily.

Contraindications

- History of agranulocytosis/neutropenia
- Severe cardiac, renal and hepatic impairment
- Alcohol/drug intoxication
- Epilepsy
- Pregnancy and breastfeeding
- History of poor compliance with monitoring.

Side effects

See under side effects for atypical antipsychotics.

- Least likely to cause extrapyramidal side effects
- Potentially fatal agranulocytosis and neutropenia
- Lowering of the seizure threshold
- Headache and dizziness
- Hyperglycaemia
- Hypersalivation
- Hypotension
- Fever (first 3 weeks).

Antipsychotic depot injections (usual doses and frequencies)

Drug	Trade name	Test dose (mg)	Dose range (mg/weeks)	Dosing interval (weeks)	Clinical effects
Flupenthixol decanoate	Depixol	20	12.5–400	2–4	Mood elevating; or may worsen agitation
Fluphenazine decanoate	Modecate	12.5	6.25–50	2–5	Depression High EPSE
Haloperidol decanoate	Haldol	25*	12.5–75	4	Low incidence of sedation High EPSE
Pipothiazine palmitate	Piportil	25	12.5–50	4	Lower incidence of EPSE
Zuelopenthixol decanoate	Clopixol	100	100–600	2–4	Useful in agitation and aggression

Notes

The elderly should be given 25 or 50% of the stated doses.

After the test dose, wait 4–10 days before starting titration to maintenance therapy.

Dose range is given in mg/week for convenience only: avoid using shorter dose intervals than those recommended, except in exceptional circumstances, e.g. a long interval necessitates a high-volume (> 3–4 ml) injection.
EPSE = extrapyramidal side effects.
*Test dose not stated by manufacturer.

The **pharmacokinetics** vary with individual drugs. In general peak plasma levels are reached 1–4 hours after **oral** administration. Most are highly bound to plasma proteins and many phenothiazines and thioxanthenes have active metabolites. With i.m.. administration plasma levels are reached sooner and bioavailability is greater.

Recently injectable atypical antipsychotics, Risperidone (long-acting) and Olanzapine (short-acting) have become available in clinical practice.

DEPOT PREPARATIONS: TYPICAL CONVENTIONAL ANTIPSYCHOTICS (NEUROLEPTICS)

Depot antipsychotics have an important role in the management of psychotic patients where there are problems of compliance with oral intake. They are given (mostly by nursing staff) via deep intramuscular injection, usually at intervals of 1–4 weeks. Patients should first be given a small test dose, and the usual preantipsychotic cautions apply. Injections must be given correctly (e.g. use of the z-track technique). Avoid giving more than 2–3 ml of an oily injection at any one site, which should be regularly varied.

TABLE 4.21   Dose equivalents for some common antipsychotics

Drug	Approximate mg equivalent to 100mg chlorpromazine
Clozapine	100
Fluphenazine	2
Haloperidol	2
Olanzapine	3.5
Risperidone	1.5
Thioridazine	100
Thiothixene	4
Trifluoperazine	5

The above equivalents are only approximate as they vary from patient to patient.

Adapted with permission from R.W. Pies, 1998. Handbook of Essential Psychopharmacology. American Psychiatric Press, Washington, D.C.

SWITCHING DRUGS (see p. 111)

ANTIPSYCHOTICS DOSAGE: *BNF* UPPER LIMITS (ROYAL COLLEGE OF PSYCHIATRISTS ADVICE)

Unless otherwise stated, doses in the *BNF* are licensed doses: any higher dose is therefore **unlicensed**.

● Consider alternative approaches, including adjuvant therapy and newer or atypical antipsychotics such as clozapine.
● Bear in mind the risk factors, including obesity; particular caution is indicated in older patients, especially those over 70.
● Consider the potential for drug interactions (published in an appendix to the *BNF*).
● Carry out ECG to exclude untoward abnormalities such as a prolonged QT interval; repeat ECG periodically and reduced the dose if a prolonged QT interval or other adverse abnormality develops.
● Increase the dose slowly, and not more often than once weekly.
● Carry out regular pulse, blood pressure and temperature checks; ensure that the patient maintains an adequate fluid intake.
● Consider high-dose therapy for a limited period, and review it regularly; abandon it if there is no improvement after 3 months (return to standard dosage).

Note	When prescribing an antipsychotic for emergency administration it must be borne in mind that the intramuscular dose should be *lower* than the corresponding oral dose (because of the absence of a first-pass effect), particularly if the patient is very active (increased blood flow to muscle considerably increases the rate of absorption). The prescription should specify the dose in the context of *each route* and should *not* imply that the same dose can be given by mouth or intramuscularly. The dose should be reviewed *daily*.

> ⚠ **The main dangers of high-dose antipsychotics are:**
> ● **Sudden cardiac-related death**
> ● **CNS toxicity.**

ANTIPARKINSONIAN DRUGS

In psychiatric practice these drugs are used to counteract the neurological side effects induced by antipsychotics. There is no clear evidence for the superiority of one drug over another. Individual patients may respond better to, or tolerate, one drug rather than another.

There is some controversy over whether these drugs should be given prophylactically to patients being treated with neuroleptics, or only when extrapyramidal side effects (EPS) develop.

Akathisia appears to respond to anticholinergic drugs only when symptoms of parkisonism are also present.

Indications

● Acute dystonias and dyskinesias
● Akathisia
● Akinesia
● Parkinsonism.

Dosage (see Table 4.22 for specific drugs)

Contraindications
For antimuscarinic drugs:

● Closed-angle glaucoma
● Urinary retention
● Gastrointestinal obstruction.

Side effects

● **Anticholinergic:** dry mouth and eyes, blurred vision, constipation and urinary retention
● **CNS:** usually in elderly and at high doses, stimulation ('high', euphoria, and therefore potential for addiction), confusion, disorientation, hallucinations and cognitive impairment (memory disturbance)
● **Cardiac:** palpitation, tachycardia, arrhythmias (high doses)
● **Gastrointestinal:** nausea, vomiting.

TABLE 4.22   Comparison of some antiparkinsonian drugs

Drug	Usual dose (mg)	Clinical effects	Adverse effects	Dose
Amantadine	100	Useful for akinesia, rigidity, acute dystonia, parkinsonism Tolerance to a particular dose may develop after 1–8 weeks Useful in treating neuroleptic and SSRI-induced sexual dysfunction Useful in treating weight gain caused by neuroleptics	**Common:** indigestion, excitement, difficulty in concentration, dizziness **Less common:** peripheral or oedema, skin rash, tremors, slurred speech, ataxia, depression, insomnia and lethargy (these are dose related and disappear on drug withdrawal) Less anticholinergic than other drugs; safe to use low doses in glaucoma	Orally: 100–400 mg daily
Orphenadrine	50	Some alteration of rigidity Modest effect on sialorrhoea Mild stimulant Beneficial effects tend to wear off in 2–6 months	Some dryness of mouth, sedation, mild central excitation	Orally: 50 mg t.i.d. up to 400 mg/day
β-Blockers Propranolol	10	Useful for akathisia and tremor	Monitor pulse and blood pressure; do not stop high dose abruptly because of rebound tachycardia. Avoid in asthmatics	Orally: 10 mg t.i.d. to 120 mg daily
Benzodiazepines Diazepam	5	Helpful for akathisia and acute dystonia Muscle relaxant	Drowsiness, lethargy	i.v.: 10 mg for acute dystonia by slow direct i.v.
Lorazepam	2	Helpful for akathisia Excellent for acute dyskinesia (sublingual works quickest)	Drowsiness, lethargy	Orally: 0.5–2 mg t.i.d. i.m.: 1–2 mg for dystonia; Orally: up to 2 mg q.i.d.
Benztropine	2	Helpful for rigidity Relieves sialorrhoea and drooling Powerful muscle relaxant; sedative action Cumulative and long-acting; once-daily dosing can be used i.m./i.v.: dramatic effect on dystonic symptoms	Dry mouth, blurred vision, urinary retention, constipation Increases intraocular pressure Psychosis may result with abuse	Orally: 1–2 mg b.i.d. up to 6 mg b.i.d. if required i.m./i.v.: 1–2 mg; may repeat in 30 min
Biperiden	4	Helps rigidity and akinesia	Less likely to cause peripheral anticholinergic effects May cause euphoria and increased tremor	Orally: 2–8 mg daily; up to 40 mg tolerated in younger patients

TABLE 4.22 Comparison of some antiparkinsonian drugs (contd)

Drug	Usual dose (mg)	Clinical effects	Adverse effects	Dose
Procyclidine	5	Commonly prescribed Useful to use in combination when muscle rigidity is severe	Slight blurring of vision Stimulation and giddiness in some patients Has potential for abuse	Starting oral dose: 2.5 mg b.i.d. May need up to 30 mg/day
Trihexyphenidyl Benzhexol	5	Mild to moderate effect against rigidity and spasm (occasionally get dramatic results) Stimulating – can be used during the day for sluggish, lethargic and akinetic patients	Dry mouth, blurred vision, GI distress Less sedating potential Severe and persistent mental confusion may occur, esp. in the elderly Toxic doses may cause restlessness, delirium, hallucinations; these disappear when the drug is discontinued	Orally: 4–15 mg daily, up to 30 mg tolerated in younger patients

Adapted with permission from K. Bezchlibnyk-Butler and J. J. Jeffries (eds), 1998. Clinical Handbook of Psychotropic Drugs, 8th edn. Hogrefe & Huber Publishers, Göttingen.

OTHER PHYSICAL TREATMENTS

- Electroconvulsive therapy (ECT)
- Psychosurgery
- Light therapy
- Alternative therapies.

ELECTROCONVULSIVE THERAPY (ECT)

Despite its poor image and the lack of clear scientific understanding with regard to its therapeutic mode of action, ECT remains an important treatment option in psychiatric practice. It is a medical procedure in which a brief electrical stimulus is given to the brain to induce a seizure under controlled conditions, with the aim of treating certain major psychiatric disorders.

The patient is anaesthetized and given a muscle relaxant before the procedure.

Overall the procedure, is safe with an associated mortality of approximately 2 per 100 000 treatments.

There is little doubt that it is effective in selected psychiatric disorders, but with rare exceptions it is not considered a first-line treatment.

In the UK ECT is usually given by trainees, therefore it is essential that you receive adequate training and supervision.

INDICATIONS

- **Major depressive illness (commonest indication)** It should be considered in the patient who fails trials of medications, cannot tolerate the risks or side effects, and in whom there is a need for an immediate response (e.g. severe suicide risk, or anorexia due to depression). Elderly patients and those with severe psychomotar retardation also benefit from this treatment.
- **Mania** It is especially useful in manic bipolar patients who are resistant to drug treatment.
- **Acute schizophrenia** ECT is usually reserved for acutely ill schizophrenic patients, especially those with prominent affective or catatonic symptoms. It is not effective for negative symptoms or the chronic phase of the illness. It has also been used in schizoaffective disorder.
- **Puerperal depression/psychosis** Here ECT is a reasonably safe and an effective option.
- **Other disorders**
  — Delirium
  — Severe organic psychosis
  — Refractory epilepsy
  — Parkinson's disease
  — Neuroleptic malignant syndrome

CONTRAINDICATIONS

Absolute

- Where there is **raised intracranial pressure** (check the fundus), a space-occupying lesion, cerebral aneurysm or cerebral haemorrhage
- **Glaucoma**, as the intraocular pressure may rise during treatment
- **Serious anaesthetic risk**.

Relative

- Recent myocardial infarction (MI) or cerebrovascular accident (CVA); it is usual to wait 3 months before giving ECT treatment
- Severe hypertension, bleeding, valvular and vascular abnormalities, ventricular arrhythmias
- Phaeochromocytoma
- Retinal detachment
- Other less serious anaesthetic problems, such as obstructive airways disease.

   Caution should be exercised with certain drugs (see interaction with ECT below).
   Note: Pregnancy (ECT can be used in all trimesters; consult obstetrician) and **old age** are **not** contraindications.

SIDE EFFECTS

Common side effects, which are usually short-lived, include headache, memory impairment and confusion; the elderly are particularly vulnerable to the latter two.

- **Cognitive:** confusion, headache; short-term memory impairment; acquisition and retention of new memories and the longer term memory are *not* impaired. The chance of cognitive impairment is increased in the elderly, with bilateral electrode placement, higher stimulus intensity, more frequent treatments and concomitant use of psychotropic medications
- **Cerebrovascular:** a brief, but marked rise in intracranial pressure
- **Cardiovascular:** the majority of deaths attributed to ECT relate to cardiac complications, most of which (hypertension, hypotension, bradycardia tachycardia) are transient
- **Intraocular:** there is a rise in intraocular pressure (avoid in glaucoma)
- **Intragastric:** there is a rise in intragastric pressure which may lead to regurgitation or pulmonary aspiration (caution needed in patients with hiatus hernia)
- **Neurological:** prolonged seizure (should be terminated after 3 minutes' duration)
- **Anaesthesia related** laryngospasm, tooth damage

DRUG INTERACTIONS WITH ECT (see Table 4.23)

PREPARATIONS FOR ECT

Consent/legal issues (England and Wales)

- Informed consent is required prior to the treatment, unless the Mental Health Act or the common law (in an emergency) is used.
- The patient should be given a full explanation of the procedure and informed about the possible side effects as well as the alternatives; this should be both verbally and in writing.
- ECT can proceed following valid consent if the patient is informal.
- For a patient detained under a treatment order (e.g. section 3) and giving valid consent, form 38 (section 58(3)(a)) will need to be completed.
- Where the patient refuses and ECT is deemed to be urgent:
  — For an informal patient ECT can be given under common law
  — If the patient is under a treatment order, ECT should be given under section 62 and a second opinion should be sought through the MHAC (section 58(3)(b) and 58(4)).
- Where the patient is incapable of giving informed consent and is detained:
  — If the patient is refusing ECT a second opinion should be sought from the MHAC.

TABLE 4.23   Drug interactions with ECT

Class of drug	Example	Interaction effects
Anticonvulsants	Carbamazepine, valproate	Increased seizure threshold with potential adverse effects of subconvulsive stimuli; Increased electrical stimulation can override above effect
Antidepressants Irreversible MAOI		Avoid this combination because pressor drugs may be required for resuscitation
Cyclic	Trazodone	Prolonged seizures reported
SSRI	Fluoxetine	Prolonged seizures reported. Clinical significance unknown. But concurrent administration not contraindicated
Antihypertensives	β-blockers, e.g. propranolol	May worsen bradycardia and hypotensive with subconvulsive stimuli Reports of confusion
Benzodiazepines	Lorazepam, diazepam	Increased seizure threshold with potential adverse effects
Caffeine		Increased seizure duration Hypertension, tachycardia, and cardiac dysrhythmia have been reported
Clozapine		Spontaneous (tardive) seizures have been reported following ECT Delirium reported with concurrent, or shortly following, clozapine treatment; But many case reports of uncomplicated concurrent use exist
Lithium		Lithium toxicity may occur: decrease or discontinue lithium and monitor patient. Concurrent administration not contraindicated
L-tryptophan		Increased seizure duration
Theophylline		Increased seizure duration, status epilepticus

EXAMINATION AND INVESTIGATIONS

- You should discuss the patient with the anaesthetist involved.
- The appropriateness of ECT should be confirmed by a thorough medical and psychiatric history, MSE and physical examination. Particular attention should be paid to cardiovascular and respiratory problems.
- Check for current medications (with regard to interactions with ECT and anaesthesia) and note any previous anaesthetic problems.

Investigations

- FBC, urea and electrolytes, blood glucose (especially diabetics)
- ECG (cardiac problems, age over 45)
- Chest X-ray and spine X-ray if indicated
- Sickle-cell status in Afro-Caribbean, Middle Eastern patients
- Coagulation screen for those on anticoagulants.

Instructions for nursing staff

- Patient should be kept nil by mouth for 8 hours prior to ECT.
- Some important medications may be given prior to ECT with small sips of water.
- Reassurance and support for patient should be available.

ECT procedures

As stated earlier, you should ensure that you have received adequate training and continue to be given supervision as necessary. In the UK an instruction manual and video are available from the Royal College of Psychiatrists, and many hospitals have their own training programmes.

Many psychiatric units have an ECT rota: you should make sure of your duties. Before you give your first treatment you should make sure that you have performed ECT under direct supervision until you are comfortable enough to carry out the procedure on your own.

You will need to become familiar with:

- The ECT suite (or the theatre where it is given)
- Local procedures
- The ECT machine
- The placement of electrodes
- Whether to give a unilateral or bilateral treatment
- Frequency and the dosage to be given
- Recognition of fit/seizure
- What to record
- Resuscitation procedures.

ECT machine

Make sure that you become familiar with your local machine. Modern machines have brief pulse stimuli and allow dose titration according to the needs of the patient (i.e. production of an adequate seizure). You should also be able to select the required amount of current and the duration of its application. Be guided by previous responses, and patient and treatment factors (see below).

Electrode placement (Fig. 4.2)

Once the patient is anaesthetized place the electrodes on the scalp, either bitemporally (for bilateral treatment) or unilaterally. Make sure that the area is clean and free from grease. After establishing contact, press the button on the electrode and check for the seizure response.

Unilateral or bilateral

Bilateral ECT is considered to be more potent, inducing a faster recovery; however, it has greater side effects. Unilateral non-dominant ECT should be considered in patients who suffered cognitive side effects (memory impairment) during previous ECT treatments, and in the elderly.

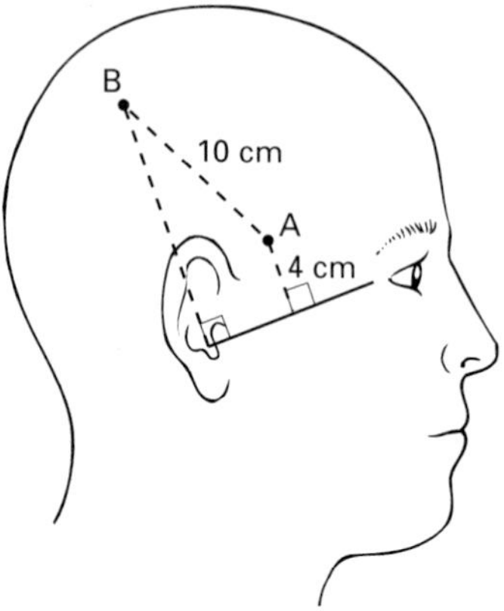

Fig. 4.2 Positioning of electrodes for ECT. Point A is 4 cm perpendicular to the mid-point of the line joining the angle of the orbit and the external auditory meatus. Point B is 10 cm from A. The electrode is usually placed over point A.

Frequency and the dosage

In the UK ECT is usually given twice weekly and in most cases 4–8 treatments are given. Some will receive 10–12 treatments or even more. In the USA it is given thrice weekly and nine treatments appear to be the norm. With regard to the actual current dosage you are advised to consult local guidelines. You will need to establish the seizure threshold for the individual patient. This refers to the minimum setting required on the ECT machine to induce a generalized seizure.

Seizure threshold is affected by many factors, including patient age, sex, weight and medical status, drugs, and whether ECT is given bilaterally or unilaterally.

The seizure threshold usually increases during the course of treatment and the length of seizure may decrease as a reflection of this. If the seizure length drops below 15 seconds in two consecutive treatments, the dosage should be increased for the next session.

Drugs that *raise* seizure threshold	Drugs that *lower* seizure threshold
Anaesthetic drugs	Alcohol
Anticonvulsants	Antipsychotics (clozapine)
Benzodiazepines	Antidepressants (TCAs, SSRIs)

The patient should be reviewed after treatment regarding their response and continued need for ECT.

Recognition of fit/seizure

Many modern ECT machines have an EEG monitor, which allows generalized seizures to be recognized. A generalized seizure usually has both tonic and clonic phases. A seizure lasting 15–20 seconds is considered the minimum, and if it continues for 3 minutes it should be terminated.

What to record

It is essential that you record ECT procedures accurately in the case notes and on special sheets provided. At a minimum the information should include the number of treatments (1/2), bilateral/unilateral, dosage (current setting) and the production/failure of seizure. Comments concerning the patient's recovery should also be recorded.

Resuscitation procedures

Ensure that you have received training in resuscitation procedures.

PSYCHOSURGERY

Psychosurgery, though controversial, is still used in rare circumstances when the patient has intractable symptomatology and all other treatment methods have failed. It is carried out in special units where neurosurgeons and psychiatrists work closely together. In the UK approximately 20–30 operations are carried out annually, and all data concerning them are recorded and monitored prospectively.

The procedure involves making lesions in specific brain regions (e.g. lobotomies and cingulotomies) or their connecting tracts (e.g. tractomies and leukotomies).

Modern techniques involve the use of stereotactic neurosurgical equipment, allowing the neurosurgeon to place discrete lesions in the brain. The actual lesions are made using various tools, including:-

- Cryoprobes
- Electrical coagulation
- Proton beams
- Radioactive implants
- Ultrasound waves.

INDICATIONS

- The presence of debilitating chronic psychiatric disorders
- When most other treatment methods have failed
- The disorder is diagnostically clear and has been present for 5 years
- The presence of vegetative symptoms and masked anxiety seems to improve the likelihood of a successful outcome.

Disorders usually considered for psychosurgery include:

- Chronic intractable major depression
- Chronic intractable obsessive–compulsive disorder (OCD).

SIDE EFFECTS

- Postoperative seizures (>1%), which are controlled using phenytoin
- Undesirable changes in personality (very rare nowadays).

OUTCOME FOLLOWING CAREFUL SELECTION PROCEDURES

- 50–70% improve significantly.
- >3% become worse.
- Interestingly, many become more responsive to traditional psychiatric treatments (drugs and psychological treatments).
- Improvements in IQ and cognitive ability have also been noted.

LIGHT THERAPY

Also known as phototherapy, this is used to treat major depression with a seasonal pattern such as seasonal affective disorder (SAD). Its mechanism of action is uncertain, but one theory suggests that the exposure to bright artificial light in the morning leads to a phase advance in biological rhythms which effectively treats the delayed circadian rhythms associated with SAD. Commonly the patient is exposed to a bright light (2500 Lux) for 2 hours in the morning, usually before dawn; in some cases it is also given in the evening. The treatment is given daily during the affected period or season.

INDICATIONS

- **Seasonal affective disorder (SAD):** symptoms include seasonal (i.e. during winter months) symptoms of depression, carbohydrate craving, fatigue, hyperphagia and hypersomnia
- **Mild depression** with subsyndromal symptoms of mood disorder with a seasonal pattern.

OUTCOME

- Response seems to occur within 2–4 days of treatment.
- Relapse occurs 2–4 days after stoppage of treatment.

Adverse effects include:

- Headache
- Eyestrain
- Irritability.

These adverse effects can be reduced by reducing the length of exposure to light.

SLEEP DEPRIVATION

Approximately 60% of patients with depressive disorder show a dramatic reduction in depressive symptoms following one night of sleep deprivation; however, the beneficial effects last only 1 day. In contrast, for some patients the beneficial effects last longer (about 1 week) if they go to bed early and rise early (this is known as phase-advancing the sleep cycle). It has also been reported that preventing rapid eye movement (REM) sleep has the same beneficial effects as total sleep deprivation.

In some cases sleep deprivation methods have been used as an adjunct to antidepressant drug treatment.

ALTERNATIVE THERAPIES

These include:

- Psychological treatments such as meditation and yoga
- Acupuncture
- Herbal treatments, e.g. Chinese, Greek and Indian
- Extract of *Hypericum perforatum* (St John's Wort), widely used in Germany, has been shown to be an effective treatment of mild to moderate depressive disorder. The usual dosage is 300 mg t.d.s.

FUTURE TREATMENT METHODS IN PSYCHIATRY

TRANSCRANIAL MAGNETIC STIMULATION (TMS) AND REPETITIVE TRANSCRANIAL MAGNETIC STIMULATION (rTMS)

At the time of writing these interesting procedures are being investigated for their application in psychiatric disorders, for both diagnosis and treatment.

TMS is a procedure whereby electrical activity in the brain is influenced by a pulsed magnetic field, which is generated by passing current pulses through a conducting coil held close to the scalp; the field is focused in the cortex and passes painlessly through the skull. Magnetic induction dictates that the changing field acts on charges in the neurons through which it passes, causing small local currents to flow. The dramatic effects of TMS are easily demonstrated by the contractions seen in hand muscles when the corresponding area in the motor cortex is stimulated. The stimulation can be delivered in form of a brief (0.5 ms) single pulse, described as TMS, or at higher frequencies (up to 50 Hz), called repetitive TMS, or rTMS.

Researchers around the world are using TMS to study the pathophysiological basis of neuropsychiatric disorders such as depression, OCD, schizophrenia and chronic fatigue syndrome.

There have also been recent published studies where TMS (given daily for 2 weeks) applied to the dorsolateral prefrontal cortex of severely depressed patients has resulted in a significant improvement. Others have demonstrated the beneficial effects of rTMS in mania and OCD.

It is being suggested that rTMS could become a safer and cheaper alternative to ECT, as it is painless and does not require anaesthesia; however it is too early to be sure of its full potential.

GENE THERAPY

The field of genetic research is moving at a tremendous pace and there will undoubtedly be the potential to apply gene therapy to many neuropsychiatric disorders (e.g. Huntington's chorea).

CHAPTER 5

PSYCHOLOGICAL
TREATMENTS

**Assessment for
psychotherapy** 202

Counselling 203

The holistic view 204

Cognitive therapy 205

**Behavioural
psychotherapy** 206

Other therapies 208

**Psychological treatments
for alcohol-related addiction/
dependence disorders** 211

Psychological treatments encompass a broad range of therapies using psychological approaches and play an important part in the management of a number of psychiatric disorders. They are given either alone or in conjunction with physical treatments.

As in most cases treatments are given by non-medically qualified professionals, the patients are often referred to as clients. Whoever gives the treatment, empathic communication is essential. The basic components of psychotherapy are listening, talking, empathy, emotional expression, interpretation and advice. All these occur to varying degrees in different forms of therapy. Interpretation is likely to play a significant form in psychodynamic/analytic therapy, whereas advice is more likely to be more prominent in cognitive therapy.

ASSESSMENT FOR PSYCHOTHERAPY

The decision to refer patients for psychological treatment will depend on a number of factors.

Patient factors

- Their wishes/co-operation/demand for psychological treatment
- Their particular psychiatric disorder
- Overtly psychotic disordered patients may not initially be amenable to psychological interaction
- Their ability (verbal competence, education, culture) to deal with/benefit from psychological intervention.

Service provision/availability of resources

- The availability of and waiting time for a specialized therapist will influence referral policies.
- You will need to know which therapies are available (CBT, CAT, dynamic etc.).

What model of psychotherapy?

Psychotherapy is dependent on the relationship between the patient and the psychotherapist; beyond that is the question of which psychotherapy to choose:

- Individual psychotherapy (with further subdivisions)
- Family therapy
- Group psychotherapy.

It is possible to move the patient from one form to another. This will depend on the patient's need and the overall management plan of the therapist.

Where to carry out psychotherapy?

Psychotherapy may be carried out in any of the following places:

- In hospital
- Outpatient clinics
- Day services/day hospital
- In the community.

The decision depends on the risks posed by the patient, and a detailed assessment is required. Psychotherapy at the patient's home is *not* recommended.

The following factors should also be decided:

- Overall duration of psychotherapy
- Duration of the session
- Frequency with which the patient will be seen.

Sessions may be short in duration: about 30–50 minutes, but some can last up to one and a half hours. The duration should be decided from the outset. There may also be ultrabrief sessions. The overall duration of therapy may vary, depending on the need, but generally brief therapy lasts for weeks whereas others may last longer.

- **Brief therapy:** 20 sessions lasting up to 6 months
- **Long-term therapy:** for example in interpretative psychotherapy, may last up to 3 or even 5 years.

The various **psychotherapeutic techniques** are as follows:

- Supportive: this includes advice, reassurance, limit setting, lending ego and praise
- Directive:
  — Cognitive
  — Cognitive behavioural
  — Rational emotive
  — Cognitive analytical
  — Goal directed/problem focused
  — Feedback
  — Reality
  — Desensitization therapies.

COUNSELLING

This form of 'talk therapy' is cheap, readily available and non-intense. It is not there to cure or treat, but to provide a feeling of being listened to and empathized with.

Like all therapies it is non-judgemental, non-directive and supportive. Patients are able to express their feelings, encouraged to look at other aspects of problems, and to discuss their social or personal concerns. The purpose is to provide emotional support so that an individual can deal with his or her crises more effectively, without feeling isolated and abandoned.

Individuals facing imminent crises (of any nature) and those with long-term problems may benefit from counselling. The aim is to facilitate a better adaptive response by the patient to the crisis at hand. Support is provided to encourage, enable, guide and facilitate resolution of the crisis. Some people who are going through an episode of grief, bereavement, trauma and loss are able to seek solace and support from a counsellor.

By its nature counselling is not intended to deal with long-lasting and serious mental health issues. For some **personality-disordered individuals** it may be **contraindicated**.

Counsellors are usually registered with the British Association of Counselling.

Counselling may be carried out by:

- Counsellors employed by GP surgeries
- Social workers
- Nurses
- Private counsellors
- Volunteer counsellors
- Charity-employed counsellors.

THE HOLISTIC VIEW

SOCIAL, ECONOMIC AND SPIRITUAL NEEDS

Psychiatric interventions and psychological treatments have limitations. Unless patient/client needs are understood in their holistic context, there can be no solution to the problems experienced by the individual.

'Holistic' means that whole is bigger than the sum total of its components. It means that human beings are bigger than their genetic, biochemical, organic and psychological components.

To facilitate a better life for a patient who has been acutely psychiatrically ill, prescribing of psychotropics may not be enough: the individual's social circumstances should also be considered. Economic pressures and worries should also be thought about and spiritual needs taken into consideration.

For some, unemployment may be a socioeconomic need resulting in severe emotional and psychological distress, culminating in psychiatric symptomatology. A narrow, isolated approach would be unsatisfactory.

Psychotropic medication cannot, by itself, overcome unhappiness: it can help a person to view life in a positive light, but if there are serious problems then social and other interventions may help.

It is a first principle of psychiatry that if someone is not responding to treatment, socioeconomic factors must be taken into account. Social factors exert a strong influence in perpetuating psychiatric syndromes; the social environment determines the nature of the disorder and its expression, in many cases. These factors also influence the final outcome of clinical management.

A homeless, unemployed person may not respond readily to antidepressants unless these needs are met. Meeting these needs is, in itself, a successful therapeutic intervention, enabling the person to maintain him or herself in the community.

COGNITIVE THERAPY

This is based on the work of Aaron Beck in the USA and is closely linked with Albert Ellis' independently developed **rational emotive therapy**.

These therapies are:

- Time limited
- Directive
- Structured.

They also alleviate symptoms by dealing with distorted cognitions.

Cognitive therapy (also known as cognitive behavioural therapy, CBT) is effective in the following conditions:

Disorder	Methods used
- Depressive disorders (mild to moderate)	Relaxation, social skills, assertiveness, cognitive challenge
- Panic disorder	Exposure, relaxation, cognitive challenge
- Phobic disorder	Exposure, relaxation modelling, cognitive challenge
- Generalized anxiety disorder	Above
- Obsessive–compulsive disorder	Exposure, response prevention, modelling, thought stopping

- Perceptual and delusional symptoms in psychotic patients
- Dementia
- Eating disorders
- Bereavement reactions
- Post-traumatic stress disorder
- Somatization disorder
- Addictions
- Sexual dysfunction
- Personality disorders
- Childhood behavioural problems.

Cognitive therapy is based on the **cognitive triad of distortions**, which include:

- Negative view of self

- Negative view of the world
- Negative view of the future.

Cognitive distortions include:

- All or nothing thinking
- Overgeneralization
- Arbitrary inference or jumping to conclusions
- Catastrophizing
- Minimization and magnification
- Disregarding the positive
- Selective abstraction
- Labelling or mislabelling
- Personalization
- 'Should' statements or masturbatory thinking [Ellis].

UNDERLYING ASSUMPTIONS

Every person has a set of beliefs according to which he or she behaves. These assumptions give rise to cognitive distortions and undesirable behaviours. Therapists examine the underlying assumptions and try to treat the cognitive distortions. This leads to a change in both the cognitive distortions and the underlying beliefs.

BEHAVIOURAL PSYCHOTHERAPY

As mentioned above behavioural therapy is used mostly in conjunction with cognitive therapy, and these may be considered as two parts of cognitive behaviour therapy.

Behaviour therapy is based on two learning theories:

- Pavlov's theory, based on the work of the famous Russian neurologist Ivan Pavlov
- Skinner's theory.

Pavlov described **classical conditioning** and **Skinner**, **operant conditioning**. These were brought together in the **double learning theory**. This is reflected by the following sequence of events:

An unconditioned stimulus gives rise to a response; a condition stimulus also gives rise to a response. This response varies in avoidance, which will result in the reduction of fear, which itself will be the reward.

The treatment involves **a**, **b** and **c**:

- **a:** Antecedent of behaviours
- **b:** Behaviour (actual)
- **c:** Consequences of behaviour.

The emphasis is on symptoms, whether these are actions or consequences, not the underlying causes. It is time limited, with clear targets.

It is effective in:

- Phobias
- Obsessive–compulsive disorder
- Obsessional traits
- Sexual problems
- Rehabilitation of chronic psychotic patients
- People with learning disability
- Childhood neurotic symptoms.

Commonly used behaviour treatments:

- **Systematic desensitization:** This stems from the principle of reciprocal inhibition, which states that anxiety will be extinguished if relaxation is elicited. It is achieved through:
  — Hierarchy construction: during this a hierarchy of anxiety-provoking situations is constructed, scoring from 0 to 100
  — Relaxation training: the patient is trained to relax, usually through tensing and relaxing all muscle groups systematically. Other methods may be used, for example mild tranquillizers, relaxation tapes and hypnosis
  — Desensitization proper: after achieving relaxation the patient is gradually exposed to the anxiety-provoking stimulus in imagination, followed by exposure to the real stimulus; for that the patient has to be in a total state of relaxation during the preparatory stages
- **Aversive therapy:** an example of this is the use of disulfuram (Antabuse). This causes vomiting when a person suffering from alcohol dependence syndrome ingests alcohol. To avoid vomiting, the patient has to refrain from alcohol. In this way there is an effective, aversive stimulus which stops unwanted behaviour. This has been proved of value in alcohol and substance misuse, smoking, sexual offending, binge eating and self-destructive behaviours which need acute management
- **Token economy:** this was originally tried on chronic, long-term institutionalized psychotic patients. They were encouraged to perform activities conducive to more adaptive and positive functioning which earned them certain tokens, which could be exchanged for things they desired, e.g. cigarettes, social outings, pub meals etc.
- **Modelling:** this is based on the theory that observational learning encourages adaptive behaviour. This is done gradually, especially in the treatment of phobias, where the model gradually approaches and becomes familiar with the anxiety-provoking object. During this process the model encourages and helps the patient
- **Flooding/implosion:** these are exposure therapies during which, instead of systematic desensitization, the patient is exposed to the feared object immediately, or flooded with the anxiety-provoking stimulus. The patient

is put in anxiety-provoking situations for long enough without negative consequences, and the anxiety is gradually overcome. An example is jumping off a diving board for the first time: once the person overcomes his or her fear by being helped or gently pushed off the diving board for the first time he or she is subsequently able to do it alone.

OTHER THERAPIES

Experiential psychotherapies:

- Existential therapy
- Art therapy
- Psychodrama
- Gestalt psychotherapy
- Client-centred psychotherapy.

Exploratory/interpretative psychotherapies:

- Psychodynamic psychotherapy
- Psychoanalysis
- Analytical psychotherapy
- Hypnoanalysis
- Eidetic psychotherapy.

SUPPORTIVE THERAPY

The purpose of this psychotherapy is:

- To increase the patient's ability to face reality
- To develop their confidence and encourage them to deal with life's challenges
- To provide advice about coping mechanisms when faced with the reality of life.

This depends on:

- The patient's baseline ability to cope with life challenges, i.e. decision making
- The patient's detailed activities
- The patient's relationship with family, friends and the community at large.

The role of the therapist is that of a supportive observer by:

- Educating the patient to deal with the various problems he or she encounters
- Providing advice, reassurance, and appreciation of their already present or newly acquired coping skills.

PSYCHODYNAMIC PSYCHOTHERAPY

Here emphasis is placed on the resolution of unconscious conflicts as a way of changing undesirable thoughts and feelings. The relationship between the therapist and the patient plays a very important role in bringing about this change.

This form of therapy is usually appropriate for patients with the following characteristics:

- Fairly intelligent
- Good verbal communication skills
- Aware of psychotherapy and believes in its value
- Able to think abstractly
- Able to make long-term commitments
- Will adhere to the psychotherapy programme
- Desirous of alleviating the problem through psychotherapy
- Able to show patience and able to resist immediate gratification of desires
- Able to tolerate different points of view.

RELATIVE CONTRAINDICATIONS

Interpretative psychotherapies are not indicated in people suffering from:

- Major depressive disorders
- Antisocial personality disorder
- Organic brain disease
- Acute psychotic disorders

There are also difficulties with obsessive–compulsive disorder, but some have advocated this form of therapy for all the above patient types.

In interpretative psychotherapy, especially psychoanalysis, the techniques used for treatment are free association, dream work/dream interpretation and parapraxes.

- **Free association** means the free and uninterrupted flow of words and thoughts.
- **Dreams** are interpreted according to the theories of psychoanalysis.
- **Parapraxes** mean omissions in a person's description or in daily life which may have a significant symbolic value. These forms of therapies also deal with the ego defence mechanisms.
- **Transference** is the emotional attitude and attachment of the patient towards the therapist, which develops during the phase of treatment.
- **Countertransference** is the therapist's emotional and psychological attitude towards the patient.
- **Therapeutic alliance** is the relationship that develops during psychotherapy, which is then gradually interpreted over the duration of treatment.
- **Working through** is the resolution and understanding of repeated conflicts, which may occur while resolving transference.
- **Defence mechanisms** (e.g. denial, projection, splitting) are also explored.

GROUP PSYCHOTHERAPY

This helps to develop patients through self-awareness, sensitivity and social skills. In a psychiatric setting, community meetings, ward meetings, day hospital/services groups/day centre groups are all based on group therapy. It facilitates interaction between members to encourage their self-confidence and self-awareness.

Such groups could be:

- **Homogeneous**, i.e. same sex, same age group, etc.
- **Heterogeneous**.

Homogeneous groups could be:

- **Open:** membership is open and people come and go as required and as needed, depending on circumstances
- **Closed:** membership is fixed and once a member leaves no other member is taken in.

They can be:

- **Ongoing** groups, which go on indefinitely
- **Time limited**.

There is no particular group size, but most have between 6 and 12 members, except for large ward and community meetings.

Groups can be:

- **Supported**, in which people with similar problems help each other, for example Alcoholics Anonymous, Narcotics Anonymous, CRUSE, social clubs, etc.
- **Analytic**, which are for interpretative treatment of members through 'analysis of the group' and by 'analysis in the group'.

Curative factors in group therapy are:

- Interpersonal learning
- Catharsis
- Group cohesiveness
- Insight
- Development of socializing techniques
- Imitative behaviour
- Guidance
- Corrective recapitulation of family group
- Altruism
- Instillation of hope
- Universality
- Existential awareness.

THERAPEUTIC COMMUNITIES

These are residential communities based on the principles of group therapy, in which people with personality disorders or severe problems with substance misuse, alcoholism and sometimes neurotic disorders, live for long periods of time.

There are two types of therapeutic communities, **democratic** and **hierarchical**.

The basic features of a democratic therapeutic community are:

- **Communalism**, which means that everybody has an equal share in the community
- **Permissiveness**, in that people in the community will tolerate disturbed behaviours in its members
- **Democratization:** there will be no hierarchy
- **Reality confrontation**, in which other members of the community give feedback to the individual on the effects of his or her behaviour.

IS PSYCHOTHERAPY FOR EVERY PATIENT?

In some cases psychotherapy may not be beneficial to a person's mental health. It is essential to bear in mind that not everyone will respond positively to psychotherapy, and do not consider it as a method of treatment if inappropriate.

There is no bar to using medication competently with any form of psychotherapy.

PSYCHOTHERAPY IN THE NHS (UK)

In the current functioning of the NHS trainee psychiatrists cannot offer psychotherapy unless they are attached to a psychotherapy department for training.

However, many trainees take on at least one psychotherapy patient under supervision. It is essential not to offer psychotherapy, nor to practise it without competent and adequate supervision, because of the potential dangers.

PSYCHOLOGICAL TREATMENTS FOR ALCOHOL-RELATED ADDICTION/ DEPENDENCE DISORDERS

There are two aspects of dependence/addiction:

- Psychological
- Physical.

Psychological addiction is much more refractory to treatment than physical. Detoxification is possible but it is not easy to overcome the psychological dependence: this may require long-term or intermittent therapy.

Education is the first step in dealing with addiction. One must be aware of the dynamics, effects, consequences and results, of one's habits, e.g. the physical, psychological, familial and social consequences.

All forms of psychotherapy are effective in the treatment of alcohol-related dependence disorders. Whether interpretative or behavioral, all have been known to have some impact on the motivated.

Motivation is the key: if the patient is motivated then any form of therapy will have an impact; if not, then nothing will have any benefit.

If the patient is motivated some therapies are more effective than others. Those that have been found especially valuable are:

- Supportive therapy
- Support groups
- AA 12 Steps
- Cognitive behavioral therapy
- Therapeutic communities
- Community reinforcement therapy
- Group therapy
- Family therapy.

Alcoholics Anonymous 12 Steps is a stepwise therapy where recovering dependents help the motivated patient find his or her way to recovery. Every step is thoroughly discussed and the person evaluated before he or she graduates to the next step.

It takes a long time and participants should not be time-limited. The support system works to reject the culture of branding and provide support in the community for those who have been shunned by those around them.

Interpretative therapies are effective for this problem but they take a long time and may not be available on the NHS.

Behavioural therapies are short-term, symptom-focused therapies.

Cognitive therapies are also time-limited focused therapies that deal with symptoms and relate to thoughts about the habit.

All this should be part of the overall *detoxification programme*, which involves:

- Reducing drinking
- Harm minimization
- Gradual abstinence
- Detoxification using medication.

This may be carried out either in the hospital or on an outpatient basis.

CHAPTER 6

PSYCHIATRIC EMERGENCIES AND THEIR MANAGEMENT

Emergency assessment and admission 216

Dealing with psychiatric emergencies 217

Specific psychiatric emergencies 220

Drug-related (including alcohol) psychiatric emergencies 249

Substance withdrawal 259

Lithium toxicity 262

Serotonin syndrome 264

Hypertensive crisis due to MAOIs 264

Antidopaminergics: acute side effects 265

Neuroleptic malignant syndrome 267

Other possible medical problems on psychiatric wards 270

While caring for psychiatric patients you may also face some purely medical problems and your management strategies are likely to vary with your particular experience/expertise and the resources available (investigative equipment, particular drugs, i.v. fluids and suitably qualified nurses).

You will be expected to have at least some basic knowledge of investigations and management strategies.

It is essential that you think of and try and exclude life-threatening disorders, as well as involving or referring to the relevant experts at the earliest movement: it is always better to err on the side of caution.

Many psychiatric units run regular courses in cardiopulmonary resuscitation: you are strongly advised to attend these and continue to refresh your basic medical training.

A variety of situations can be described as psychiatric emergencies and there will be occasions when what seems an emergency to a patient, his or her carer or even other staff, is not quite what the duty psychiatrist would consider an emergency. However, in this position you will need to decide upon the urgency of a particular situation, whether it requires immediate attention, or if it can be dealt with later.

- Familiarize yourself with the layout of the casualty area/emergency room and your wards.
- If at all possible, shadowing a relatively experienced trainee may be very helpful before you start your own duty.
- When on duty be contactable and respond quickly and politely. Know your rota, bleep number and other relevant contact numbers (e.g. security, bleep holder/nursing officer, relevant wards).
- Find out about the bed state (i.e. beds available for admission), local policies regarding patient transfers and extracontractual referrals (ECR).
- Know about the catchment area and the division of consultant responsibilities.
- Obtain as much information as you can before dealing with an emergency, but do not take too long.
- Communicate by telephone if you cannot attend straight away.
- It is difficult, if not impossible, to carry out a mental state examination over the telephone.
- The switchboard should not put a patient directly through to the duty psychiatrist, but on occasions this may happen. Avoid a telephone consultation: tell the patient that it is not appropriate for you to do an assessment over the telephone and that they should either contact their own GP or attend the emergency department.
- It is almost impossible to do a proper psychiatric assessment on an intoxicated person, but this does not mean that any patient who has taken alcohol or drugs should be flatly refused. Assess each situation carefully and offer psychiatric input when appropriate.

- Prioritizing of tasks is important and can be achieved by acquiring a theoretical knowledge of potential emergencies as well as by gaining suitable experience.
- When approaching an emergency, plan your response. Thinking about diagnostic possibilities and their management may help to focus your attention.
- Take a calm approach; this will also help to calm others, including the patient. Remember that **calmness can be as infectious as laughter**.
- Act as a psychiatrist and not as a policeman.
- The overall long-term plan should have some influence on the immediate management.
- Seek advice from senior colleagues when you are unsure. It may help to rehearse how you will to present the information, which ought to be relevant, clear and concise.
- Record all the relevant information as accurately as possible. The management plan should be clearly recorded, as well as conveyed to the persons involved without ambiguity.
- Remember that information may be biased: be objective and use your medical and psychiatric skills fully when dealing with the emergency.
- Having completed the emergency presentation, formally hand the patient over to those who will be responsible for his or her future care.
- Communicate with the patient's GP/psychiatrist and other involved agencies as regards your assessment and treatment.
- Debriefing at the end of the emergency may be helpful, especially if it provoked considerable anxiety.
- Learn the relevant parts of the Mental Health Act (MHA) that may be used in an emergency.
- Avoid taking or being seen to be taking sides: management decisions should be in the best interest of the patient, not to make life comfortable for others. Decisions regarding a particular emergency should take into account all the factors that can interact.
- On occasions there may be disagreement with the patient, relatives or even the staff involved. Little is gained by unhelpful confrontation and it may be useful to seek advice from a more senior colleague. It is usually best to listen actively to all those involved and try to defuse any possible confrontational problems.

EMERGENCY ASSESSMENT AND ADMISSION

ASSESSMENT IN A&E

Assessment in A&E is usually limited by time and often by the inappropriateness of the setting. It is important to be flexible with the history taking and examination, tailoring it to the urgency of the situation. However, you should ensure that comprehensive and accurate notes are recorded and that the assessment findings and treatment plans are communicated to the relevant agencies, including the patient's GP.

PHYSICAL ASSESSMENT

All patients should be physically examined although on occasions this may be impossible.

It is especially useful in the A&E setting as urgent medical or surgical assessments can be requested and are usually easily obtained.

INVESTIGATIONS IN CASUALTY

Certain investigations are especially useful:

- Urine tests for glucose, drugs, infection
- Blood tests for FBC, glucose, U&E
- Breathalyser if intoxication is suspected.

LEGAL CONSIDERATIONS

INTERACTION WITH THE POLICE

An acutely disturbed individual thought to be mentally ill may be removed from a public place by the police and brought in under Section 136 of the Mental Health Act. Some psychiatric units have a designated 136 room, but in many the assessment is carried out in A&E. The assessment is made by an approved social worker (ASW) and the psychiatrist on duty. Some hospitals require that the SR/SpR/consultant (usually Section 12 approved) on duty carry out the initial assessment, whereas in the others the duty SHO is usually the first doctor involved.

The police should be asked to wait until the assessment is completed, in case the patient is found not to be suffering from a mental disorder and therefore technically their responsibility.

If admission is required it may be on an informal basis or formally under an appropriate section of the Mental Health Act. Patients should not normally be transferred to the admitting hospital under Section 136.

ADMISSION PROCEDURES

These vary from hospital to hospital and may be informal (voluntary) or formal (requiring the use of the Mental Health Act).

If the patient is from outside the catchment area transfers may need to be arranged. You should contact the duty doctor from the relevant area and the bleep holder/nursing officer. The senior psychiatrist on call (consultant/SpR) may also need to be informed.

Difficulties may arise if the patient is amnesic or mute, or there are difficulties with the transfer (e.g. late at night). In these situations transfer may be postponed, and it may be safer and kinder to admit the patient overnight.

Admission is usually required when the patient is:

- Suicidal
- Homicidal
- Acutely psychotic (especially the first presentation) with disturbing delusions or hallucinations (e.g. command hallucinations)
- Behaviourally disturbed, with a psychiatric history
- Agitated or excited
- With psychiatric symptoms related to psychotropic drugs
- Lacking social support.

The following alternatives to admission should be considered:

- Discharge back to GP
- Further assessment in A&E or an emergency psychiatric clinic
- Outpatient referral (psychiatrist)
- Referral to other members of the MDT (CPN, SW)
- Referral to the day hospital
- Referral to a substance misuse or other specialized clinic
- Referral to other agencies (AA, drop-in centres, ethnic groups, hostels).

DEALING WITH PSYCHIATRIC EMERGENCIES

The framework outlined below may be used for collecting information, making an assessment and devising a management plan.

HISTORY/INFORMATION GATHERING

This should take account of the following:

- Medical and surgical diagnosis
- Psychiatric diagnosis (especially any history of suicidal/homicidal episodes)

- Head injuries
- Drugs, both prescribed and/or illicit
- 'Dirt' (infections)

TARGET SYMPTOMS

These should be elucidated from the history and MSE; clarify whether the patient is:

- Mute
- Delirious/incoherent
- Agitated
- Behaving in a bizarre manner
- Suicidal
- Homicidal/violent
- Delusional
- Hallucinating.

PHYSICAL EXAMINATION

- General impression: is the patient well or not?
- Signs of head trauma
- Meningeal signs
- Autonomic signs: temperature, heart rate, respiratory rate, blood pressure
- Cranial nerve abnormalities
- Motor abnormalities.

PRELIMINARY DIAGNOSIS

- **Organic/medical:** alcohol and drugs related, delirium tremens etc.
- **Psychiatric:** schizophrenia/affective psychosis (bipolar, unipolar), neurotic (acute anxiety)
- **Personality disorders:** borderline personality disorders etc.

MANAGEMENT

Some issues to be considered:

- Safety/security (for both patients and staff, including yourself)
- Appropriate levels of observations in a suitable setting (e.g. appropriate ward), as well as the level of observations needed initially
- Medical treatment required
- Psychiatric treatments required (pharmacological or non-pharmacological, or both)
- Further monitoring/instruction to the nursing staff (e.g. levels of observations needed: level 1, 2, etc.)
- Who will be responsible for care when the emergency situation is over
- Formal handover to medical/nursing colleagues.

RISK ASSESSMENT AND ITS MANAGEMENT

When carrying out a psychiatric evaluation you should also carry out a risk assessment. The aim of this should be not only to reduce the risk of harm to self or others, but also to decide upon the level of risk that is acceptable. The risk assessment should also consider future reviews of the risk.

Factors that increase the likelihood of risk include:

- History of harm (to self or others)
- Threats of harm (to self or others)
- Access to or possession of weapons
- Use/withdrawal of alcohol or drugs (illicit or prescribed)
- Medical disorders (e.g. head injury, cranial infections, brain tumours, dementia)
- Psychiatric disorders (e.g. psychosis, schizophrenia, mania, depression, psychopathic personality disorder, borderline personality disorder)
- Demographic factors (young men, lower intelligence)
- Social factors (recent major stressors or losses, criminal record)
- Mental state abnormalities (e.g. thoughts of self-harm or violence to others, paranoid thoughts, command hallucinations, disturbance of mood).

It is also important to clearly document and communicate to others the risk assessment, as well as the subsequent management plan.

MANAGEMENT

Having carried out a risk assessment you will have to decide on:

- The potential for harm to self or others
- The probability of harm to self or others
- Whether the risk is imminent, short-term or long-lasting
- How to reduce or eliminate the risk.

The following should be considered as part of the management strategy.

Immediate interventions:

- Removal from the risky setting and access to the tools of self-harm
- Arrest and removal by the police
- Admission with close observations or seclusion (use of Mental Health Act if necessary)
- Pharmacological intervention (sedation with benzodiazepines, antipsychotics)
- Non-pharmacological intervention (calming or talking down, diffusion of tension)
- Making associated individuals aware of the risk (e.g. partner of an individual with pathological jealousy).

Longer-term interventions:

- Treatment of psychiatric disorder and provision for longer-term care
- Help with psychosocial difficulties
- Teaching of certain skills, such as anger management, enrolment in self-harm groups
- Use of care programme approach (CPA), supervision orders, community orders.

SPECIFIC PSYCHIATRIC EMERGENCIES

Psychiatric emergencies in general do not come neatly packaged, but for simplicity we have grouped them into **behavioural**, **drugs-related** and **other**.

Specific emergencies may of course overlap, so the following should be regarded as guiding principles only.

Good theoretical knowledge and a build-up of clinical experience will help you manage emergencies effectively. In many cases the diagnosis will not be clear and the patient may present with many features that could be called 'psychiatric problems'.

BEHAVIOURAL

SUICIDE/DELIBERATE SELF-HARM (DSH)

Dealing with suicide attempts is routine for the duty psychiatrist, but their management may be fraught with uncertainty. As a psychiatric trainee you will be expected to assess a suicidal person by asking questions and gathering relevant information (these should be documented in the notes), allowing some judgement to be made about the degree of risk. If you are unsure or relatively inexperienced, seek a second opinion from a senior colleague. Try to involve as many relevant persons as possible in the management plan.

Note	Remember, simply asking about suicidal intent does not put ideas into a patient's head.

⚠ **ALL PATIENTS BEING EVALUATED PSYCHIATRICALLY SHOULD BE ASSESSED FOR SUICIDE (AND INDEED HOMICIDE) RISK.**

Completed suicide is a major contributing factor to psychiatric disorder-related mortality.

COMMON PRESENTATIONS

- In A&E following an overdose or other forms of attempted self-harm
- Referral from A&E or other medics; referral from non-psychiatric wards (patient expressing suicidal ideation)
- In emergency psychiatric clinics
- Psychiatric outpatient department
- From GP and other health workers, for example social worker, community psychiatric nurse (CPN), psychologist
- Telephone calls from suicidal patients, or even their relatives. It is usually rare for a suicidal patient to be put through directly to the duty psychiatrist: such calls are often taken by nursing staff or the casualty officer.

EPIDEMIOLOGY

Suicide accounts for approximately 1% of all deaths in the UK: approximately 6000 suicides a year are recorded, which is probably less than the true incidence. The rate varies from country to country and there may be a number of factors responsible for this.

RISK FACTORS

- **Previous attempts:** 1% of those who have attempted suicide die from suicide within 1 year. In the year following a suicide attempt the repetition rate is 100 times greater than that in the general population. Between 12 and 20% repeat an attempt during the first year.
- **Suicidal ideation** (communicated by 60% of those attempting suicide)
- **Presence of psychiatric disorders:**
  — *Depression:* 15% of patients eventually kill themselves
  — *Schizophrenia:* this may be related to depressive symptoms if they coexist, or to the presence of command hallucinations (10%)
  — *Alcohol and drug-related disorders:* (20%)
  — *Personality disorders,* especially borderline personality disorder (5–25%)
- **Chronic physical/medical illness:**
  — *Cancer patients* have a suicide risk approximately twice as high as the general population, and it is also significantly elevated among AIDS patients
  — *Poor sleep*
  — *Chronic pain:* retired, separated, widowed or divorced
  — Approximately 50% of those who commit suicide **had seen a doctor** in the previous month
- **Demographic and social factors:**
  — age over 40, but rising in younger men
  — male sex.

> **Note**   Demographic factors appear to be changing: young males are increasingly presenting with suicide attempts.

— more females attempt suicide, but a greater number of males succeed
— single/unmarried/divorced
— occupation (doctors, especially psychiatrists and anaesthetists, pharmacists, farmers)
— unemployed
— recent life crises.

EVALUATION OF SUICIDAL INTENT

The clinical evaluation of a suicidal patient is not an exact science. However, an evaluation is more likely to be successful if a through approach (i.e. taking account of all the risk factors) is supplemented with acquired clinical experience. **If in doubt, consult your seniors**.

● Use graded questions. Start with some general (open) questions and gradually home in with specific (closed) questions relating to the intent (see Box).
● Suicidal ideas ought to be explored, i.e. whether present or not, how often, and is there a specific plan.
● Enquire about the means, e.g. violent methods rather than sleeping tablets, for example (guns usually imply a greater risk).
● Enquire about any previous history of suicide, and the number of attempts.
● Enquire about the most recent attempt and the precipitating factors, e.g. concurrent use of drugs and alcohol; the methods used; was it planned; any suicide note; what active attempts were made to avoid being discovered; how was he or she discovered; and how brought to medical attention.
● Look for evidence of mental illness, especially depression.
● One should also ask what would stop a person attempting suicide, e.g. religious or social beliefs, responsibilities, any children?
● Explore excessive guilt and loss of self-esteem (some suggest this leads to inward aggression, i.e. self-harm)
● What social support is there, and who will take over the responsibility of looking after the patient should they be discharged home?

Useful questions in assessing suicide risk

● How do you feel about the future?
● Does life seem worth living?
● Do you have thoughts of hurting or harming yourself?
● Have you ever thought of ending it all?
● Have you made any plans?
● What would you use to carry out your suicide plan?
● What might prevent you from carrying out your plan?

MANAGEMENT

If a patient presents with a significant suicide risk:

- Do not allow the patient to leave the interview without an appropriate treatment plan.
- Admit voluntarily and treat any medical/psychiatric illness.
- Admit involuntarily under the Mental Health Act (e.g. if refusing to comply with treatment).
- Remove the means to commit suicide, e.g. potentially toxic substances (including medications). If admitted, recommend the appropriate level of observation to the nursing staff, and ensure these instructions are written in the case notes.
- If admission is not warranted and responsible supervision can be arranged, inform all those who may be involved, e.g. family, friends and/or professionals, and ensure they have clear guidelines regarding what to do in an emergency.
- It may help to form a 'no suicide pact' with the patient (contract for safety), which may be especially helpful for those with a lower level of risk and where some form of supervision/support is available in the community. The pact implies that the patient agrees not to attempt suicide for a specified period, e.g. a fortnight, while you both explore all aspects of the situation, including alternatives to dying.
- Those admitted should be reviewed daily, so that appropriate level observation (see below) can continue and cease when appropriate.
- If a patient requires emergency ECT for severe suicidal intent, **remember the riskiest time is near the end of the course of ECT, when the patient begins to feel better**.
- Those discharged home should also be reviewed, for example by visits from psychiatrists, community psychiatric nurses, social workers or other care workers. Alternatively they may be asked to come to the psychiatric clinic for review.

CRITERIA FOR ADMISSION

The decision whether to admit a suicidal patient or not is difficult, especially for a new trainee. Unfortunately, even the most experienced psychiatrists do not always get it right.

The decision usually rests upon the balance of all the factors that apply to the patient and how the risk can be minimized. It can never be eliminated, and therefore the decision to discharge depends upon the level of risk that most psychiatrists would consider acceptable.

During the early part of the training you are advised to discuss the management of suicidal patients with your seniors, especially if admission is not considered.

Admission should be considered:

- When there are serious/significant risk factors not countered by any protective factors
- When a serious attempt has been made (e.g. hanging, use of firearms)
- When an effort was made to conceal the attempt, or a note was left
- For those with a significant psychiatric disorder (e.g. depression, schizophrenia)
- For those with chronic physical/medical illness (e.g. cancer, chronic pain).

Non-admission may be considered:

- For those who make a minor attempt at suicide (e.g. superficial cuts on wrist, swallowing a handful of relatively safe drugs – but remember that swallowing more than 10 paracetamol tablets poses some medical risk, which should be evaluated)
- In 'cry for help' type attempts
- In the absence of a significant psychiatric disorder/substance abuse
- In situational crises (e.g. a young girl breaking up with her boyfriend)
- In personality disorder (e.g. patient with borderline personality disorder but no other comorbid psychiatric disorders); some argue that admission is detrimental for these individuals
- For those who have a reasonably low risk and good and reliable social support/supervision
- For those with whom a 'no suicide pact' is possible.

Interviewing a suicidal patient

Preparation
Discuss with referrer, check that patient is sufficiently alert but avoid long delays that allow the patient to put up defences. Check medical notes.

Rapport establishment
Introduce by name and explain purpose of interview. History taking: problem oriented, helping patient to take an active role. *Style:* conversational, active listening, minimal note taking. Setting: quiet without interruptions. Do not hurry, take non-judgemental approach. Permit ventilation and communication.

Clarifying and understanding the attempt
Detailed account of 48 hours preceding the attempt. When, where, how, presentation. What is meaning of action (wanted to die, blot out distress, escape problems, communicate distress, express anger, elicit guilt, manipulate situation). Whether alcohol taken, who was present. Previous attempts.

Exploring intent at time of attempt
Planning; premeditation; precautions taken against discovery; actions taken to get help; last acts (will made, pet arrangements, note); lethality of method (subjective and objective)

Clarification of medical/psychiatric/social factors
Psychological and physical problems; relationship with partner, family, children; work (unemployment, threatened); friend/isolation; loss/bereavment (also job, money, status); alcohol/drugs; financial; legal/criminal; housing

Interviewing a suicidal patient (contd)

Relevant family and personal factors
Coping strategies
Current resources (e.g. friends, social, GP, CPN, samaritans, church, NSF)
Previous ways of coping/personality and strengths
Current mental state
Level of consciousness; rapport depression/agitation/hopelessness; psychosis;
current intent (regret or pleased at recovery – is it genuine?); understanding of
problems and solutions
Management
Decide
  Presence of psychiatric disorder
  Is psychiatric disorder present and under effective treatment?
  Current risk
  Is there ongoing risk of suicide (1-2% in next year) or DSH (15% in next year)
  To admit
  Not to admit
  Make contract or no-suicide pact. Agree problem solving plan: clarify
  problems and steps needed to achieve goals; provide information and advice;
  offer referral or treatment with limits set; explore preventative measures and
  identify sources of help in further crisis; e.g. 'medication – can you cope
  having tablets around?', 'do you feel safe between now and the next
  meeting?', 'what would you do if the old feeling's came back?'
Communication
  With colleagues, relatives, written notes.

SUPERVISION FOR SUICIDAL INPATIENTS

- **Close observation:** the patient remains continuously within the sight of
  the designated supervising nurse. This is usually appropriate for an
  acutely suicidal patient.
- **Continuous observation:** the patient is always within reach of a nurse.
  This is used in situations when the patient is exhibiting self-destructive
  behaviour.
- **Routine observation:** normal observations when the suicide risk has
  diminished significantly.

Many hospitals use terms such as level I, level II, level III observations.
You should ensure that all involved (including yourself) understand the exact
meaning/implications of the particular term used. The observation level should
also be written in the case notes, reviewed, and discussed regularly with nursing
and medical colleagues.

REPEATED SUICIDE ATTEMPTS

The chronically suicidal patient, for example suffering from borderline
personality disorder, features quite heavily in this category. Such patients are

often angry and manipulative, and commonly use a defence mechanism called splitting, all of which makes management decisions quite difficult. They have a high risk (up to 25%) of eventual suicide. Hospitalization is not always suitable, but the decision not to hospitalize should only be taken after consultation with a more senior colleague and those previously involved in the patient's care. If not hospitalised, a documented, alternative outpatient treatment plan should be made. If there is any concurrent diagnosis, such as depression, psychosis or drug and alcohol-related disorders, a brief hospital admission may be needed to treat these conditions.

PROCEDURES FOLLOWING COMPLETED SUICIDE/SUSPECTED SUICIDE

- Be guided by local protocols.
- The family should be informed early by appropriate staff (usually the senior staff involved with the patient). Clear communication and support should be available to involved staff (including yourself).
- Those who may have witnessed the event (staff, other patients or relatives) may need counselling/debriefing.

The following should be notified:

- Next of kin
- RMO/consultant, GP
- Other involved staff (nursing, medical, paramedical)
- Hospital managers
- Police and the coroner.

You should avoid contact with the media, which is best dealt with by senior management.

VIOLENT/HOMICIDAL

All too often health workers come face to face with aggressive patients, and psychiatric practice is no exception.

- Be aware of the risk factors that predispose to violence:
  — individual medical factors
  — certain mental illness and use of drugs (prescribed and illicit)
  — settings/environment.
- Learn about verbal methods of diffusing violence and physical methods of restraint
- Seek out the reasons behind the aggression and try to treat the underlying disorders, whether medical, psychiatric or psychological.
- Avoid responding with drugs in a knee-jerk manner.
- When using drugs take into account the situation/setting, your own knowledge of specific drugs, and the safety issues.

PRESENTATIONS

Violent or homicidal patients may present in a number of ways:

- They may be brought in by the police to a designated place of safety (such as a Section 136 room, either in A&E or in a psychiatric unit).
- The patient may present in A&E, or be brought by relatives or friends.
- An inpatient may become violent or homicidal, either in a psychiatric ward or elsewhere.

RISK FACTORS FOR VIOLENCE

- Young male
- Previous/recent history of violence
- Psychopathic personality traits or disorder
- Brain impairment, which may be associated with disinhibition and impulsiveness. These include head injury, frontal lobe damage, and any medical condition (e.g. meningitis, encephalitis, epilepsy, diabetes) affecting the brain; intoxication with drugs (especially stimulants) and alcohol, as well as withdrawal from these
- Use of drugs and alcohol
- Psychiatric disorder: schizophrenia, especially with positive symptoms such as hallucinations, paranoid delusions and command hallucinations; mania, depression (e.g. postnatal), borderline and severe personality disorder, dementia
- Inability to reason and deal with frustration. This can occur in those with learning disability as well as those described above.

ASSESSMENT

Seek as much information as possible before dealing with a potentially violent patient. **The personal safety of all those involved is of the utmost importance**. Avoid assessing alone. Both the patient and the doctor should have easy access to the exit.

Warning signs of impending violence

Recent/previous history of violence
Patient grievance
Threats being made
Possession of an object that could be used as a weapon
Signs of extreme anger or irritability
Patient making interviewer fearful
History/presence of psychiatric symptoms
Intoxication/withdrawal state

Mental State Examination (MSE)

As with suicide evaluation a series of questions, initially general and open-ended but progressing to more specific (closed) ones, can be used to evaluate the risk of violence (see Box). However, do not forget that the situation may be quite urgent and that a long-winded assessment may prove dangerous. Indeed, a formalized MSE may be difficult and even counterproductive.

Helpful questions to assess a homicidal/violent patient

- Are you upset with anyone?
- Do you have thoughts of hurting anyone?
- Have you made plans to harm someone?
- You appear to be angry with this particular person.
- You mention you want to hurt this particular person. How would you do that? e.g. What method would you use?

Note Homicidal ideation planning can have a spectrum of responses, from the non-specific, e.g. 'I feel so mad that I could kill someone', to a more specific description of a plan, e.g. 'When I get there I am going to stab him with a knife'.

Assessing **non-verbal behaviour** is quite useful. Features to look out for include:

- Aggressive eye contact
- Aggressive stance
- Clenched fists
- Body posture
- Lack of personal space.

Never forget that the patient may be in possession of an object that could be used as a weapon. The presence of **disinhibition**, as well as delirium or a delirious state, which may impair impulse control and judgement, is also important.

Verbal threats should always be taken seriously.

- **Angry mood** and **irritability** increase the risk of violent behaviour.
- **Paranoia** is a significant symptom, especially if focused on some individual.
- **Pathological jealousy**, whatever the cause, should be excluded.
- The presence of **command hallucinations** should also be assessed, as these are potentially very dangerous symptoms.
- **Cognitive impairment** and **lack of insight** can be significant factors with regard to aggression.

DIAGNOSTIC POSSIBILITIES

- **Intoxication and withdrawal states**: *alcohol:* impulsiveness, disinhibition (release of aggression); *drugs* (amphetamine, cocaine, especially 'crack'): associated with unpredictable violence

- **Organic brain impairment**: any organic brain disorder may lead to unpredictable violence; prescribed drugs may also contribute
- **Psychosis**: violence associated with psychosis may be bizarre. A schizophrenic may commit acts of violence as a result of hallucinations (especially command hallucinations) or paranoid delusions. In chronic patients general excitability, frustration and confusion may also contribute to the violence
- **Manic patients** may also become embroiled in acts of violence
- **Morbid jealousy**: this is an important cause of domestic violence and has a number of causes. It may lead to violence against the person to whom the jealousy is directed, or against others associated with that person
- **Personality disorder**: individuals with antisocial personality disorder show acts of violence without remorse. Those with borderline personality disorder exhibit repeated acts of aggression which may be against themselves, others or both.

MANAGEMENT

Familiarize yourself with local rules, guidelines and procedures for dealing with violence. It also helps to be familiar with the geographical area where the assessment is being made, i.e., the best escape routes. Where there is physical violence, involve the police or security staff to disarm and isolate the offender. Try to avoid the 'knee-jerk' use of drugs, although there are circumstances when their urgent use may be necessary. Be cautious, but give a sufficient amount at a time.

There are a number of approaches (see below) that may be applied individually or in combination, depending on the degree of threat, the perceived level of threat or the actual level of violence.

The main options are:

- **Behavioural approach:**
  — verbal, i.e. talking down
  — physical restraint, by either staff or police
  — use of seclusion rooms

Adopt a calm, confident approach, avoiding encroaching an personal space and avoid physical contact; try to listen and acknowledge the patient's fear, distress and anger, even if delusional. Refrain from argument.

- **Use of drugs**:

  Rapid tranquillization. The aim is to rapidly load medications to decrease behavioural disturbance.
  — *With benzodiazepines:* the most commonly used drug is lorazepam 0.5–2 mg i.m. every 1–2 hours until behaviour is well controlled, but **remember**:
  contraindications of respiratory depression in CO_2 retainers and those on narcotics

cautions and risks of psychomotor impairment, excessive sedation and disinhibition.

— *With antipsychotics:*

5 mg haloperidol i.m. every 30–60 minutes until the patient is calm

doubling of the above dose every 30–60 minutes until the patient is calm

oral preparations such as droperidol (favoured by many as sedating), haloperidol and chlorpromazine

Zuclopenthixol acetate 50–150 mg (for the elderly 50–100 mg) injection to the gluteal muscles or lateral thigh can also be used for short-term management of aggression/agitation. The injection may be repeated a day later, with a maximum cumulative dose of 400 mg per course (maximum of four injections).

If drug treatment is used it must be monitored for possible side effects and complications. Once you are in a position to assess the nature of violence, the next step is to try and assess whether or not it is due to mental illness.

LEGAL ASPECTS

- Common law allows emergency involuntary treatment.
- The Mental Health Act (MHA) may be invoked if there is likely to be a continuing need for compulsory assessment and treatment.

Aggression may be formally assessed using an overt aggression scale (Yodofsky):
- Verbal aggression
- Physical aggression against objects
- Physical aggression against self
- Physical aggression against other people

If appropriate, the police should be involved in violent incidents and the patient should be informed that having a psychiatric disorder does not necessarily protect him from the consequences of his violence and the procedures of the law. At the end of a violent episode debriefing of all the people involved is useful, as it allows them to vent their feelings and provides mutual support and reassurance.

DOCUMENTATION

Nursing staff will require the duty psychiatrist to sign an 'incident form' in which accurate details of the incident should be recorded, as in the case notes.

An audit of violent incidents is also needed for the Mental Health Commission, managers/purchasers, to deal with for future needs, and for research purposes.

There will be occasions when a psychiatrically ill, violent patient may need to be transferred to a specialist unit (e.g. a psychiatric intensive care unit, local secure unit, regional secure unit or even a special hospital). It is useful to obtain local guidelines regarding this, and of course the transfer decision is likely to be made by your seniors.

FURTHER PHARMACOTHERAPY FOR AGGRESSIVE PATIENTS (ACUTE AND CHRONIC)

Anticonvulsants: these tend to be used when the aggressive behaviour is more pervasive, i.e. not during an acute presentation, and their mood-stabilizing qualities may make them more effective.
— *Carbamazepine*:
  - Starting dose of 200 mg daily. The usual range is 400–800 mg daily
  - Because of the possibility of blood dyscrasia it will be necessary to do a full blood count, most importantly in the first 3 months
  - Although serum level monitoring has been called into question, it can still be useful for checking toxicity levels and compliance.
— *Clonazepam*: useful in those showing agitation, and may simply work through its anxiolytic effects.
  - A starting dose of 1 mg (500 µg in the elderly) and gradually increasing by 1 mg every 3 days until the benefits are noticeable. The usual range is 4–8 mg daily
  - Serum levels used for antiepileptic effects do not appear to correlate with antiaggressive properties.
— *Sodium valproate (valproic acid)*: mainly used in mania with agitation.
  - Starting dose of 600 mg daily, in divided doses, increasing by 200 mg daily at 3-day intervals until the benefits are noticeable. The usual range is 800–1600 mg
  - Liver function tests (LFTs) should be carried out every month, especially during the first 6 months, to monitor hepatotoxicity.
Antimanic:
— *Lithium*: although lithium is the drug of choice for bipolar manic patients it has also been used in a variety of other disorders, especially in impulsive aggressive outbursts, as may be the case with borderline personality disorder. It is also very useful in anger outbursts among patients with learning disabilities.
  - The same pretreatment laboratory work-up should be used as in the case of bipolar manic disorder.
  - The starting dose is 300 mg daily, but the maintenance dose tends to be lower than that used in bipolar manic disorder.
  - The scientific evidence for its use in the control of aggression, and its correlation with the serum levels, is limited.
  - The usual monitoring procedures should be carried out, which is also useful for checking on compliance and the development of toxicity.

Anxiolytics:
— *Benzodiazepines* are useful in the short-term acute management of, for example, episodic aggressive behaviour.
  - Be on the alert for paradoxical agitation/disinhibition in some patients.
  - Avoid long-term use in cases of abuse or addiction.
  - An example of the drugs used includes lorazepam 1–4 mg daily in divided doses.

Others:
— *β-Adrenergic blockers:* Propranolol is occasionally used for aggressive agitated behaviour.
  - Watch out for **side effects** of hypotension, bradycardia and **contraindications** of asthma and heart failure.
  - The starting dose is 40 mg b.d., gradually increasing by 20 mg every 4 days until behaviour improves.
  - Medical status and side effects need to be kept under constant review.

Some other drugs occasionally used in special cases include:

- Cyproterone
- Oestrogens
- Phenytoin
- Primidone
- SSRIs (in those with learning disabilities).

MANIA

PRESENTATION

Mania may present in a number of ways and can easily be confused with other diagnostic entities, such as schizophrenia. It may also be secondary to a medical disorder such as thyrotoxicosis, or as a result of illicit or prescribed drugs.

Eliciting a history from a manic patient may not be easy and his train of thought may be difficult to follow. Occasionally the patient may attempt to interview you, tempting you to smile or even laugh; try to keep your composure. Always attempt to obtain a collateral history and obtain any previous psychiatric history either from the case notes or from the established staff, who may know the patient from previous contacts.

A known bipolar (manic–depressive) patient can have a relapse of the manic episode (e.g. following stoppage of lithium) and may be brought to the hospital by the police (usually under Section 136) or by relatives/friends.

ASSESSMENT

There is usually marked overactivity, distractibility, irritability and agitation. The personal appearance may be flamboyant and showy, with clothing favoured by younger people, rather provocative and with strong colours; there may also be impulsiveness and sometimes violent behaviour. There may be overspending and indiscriminate sexual behaviour. Classically **speech** may be emphatic, with pressure, and there may be a **flight of ideas**.

The patient may also describe having **racing thoughts** and **psychotic** symptoms may be present.

Note	20% of manic patients have schneiderian first-rank symptoms

The **cognitive assessment** may reveal attention deficit as well as impairment of judgement, and there may be **lack of insight**.

The presence of comorbid substance misuse may cloud the picture further.

DIFFERENTIAL DIAGNOSIS

Organic causes:

- **Infection**: this may include HIV, syphilis, encephalitis and endocrine (hyperthyroidism)
- **Tumours**: these may include gliomas, meningiomas and brain metastases
- **Connective tissue disease**: sarcoidosis and various forms of arthritis
- **Neurological**: epilepsy, especially temporal lobe epilepsy (TLE); hamartoma; multiple sclerosis; strokes; Wilson's disease
- **Drugs**: alcohol (intake or withdrawal); antidepressants; amphetamines; alprazolam; antihypertensives; (captopril; β-blockers; anticholinergics (procyclidine) and steroids; hallucinogens; antituberculous medication such as isoniazid; and other antibiotics
- **Others**: alcoholism, anaemia, haemolysis.

The most common organic causes include alcohol, drugs (prescribed and illicit) and hyperthyroidism.

Psychiatric causes:

- Bipolar affective disorder (manic phase)
- Schizophrenia (NB: 20% of manic patients have schneiderian first-rank symptoms)
- Brief reactive psychosis related to experiencing a stressful event
- Adult attention deficit/hyperactivity disorder (ADHD)
- Bereavement or other significant life events.

MANAGEMENT

Use the guidelines for dealing with psychiatric emergencies, i.e. gather as much relevant information as possible and try to exclude treatable causes.

A number of management options are available and their use will largely depend on the severity of the manic behaviour, possible diagnostic causes and current circumstances. They include:

- Talking down
- Restraining
- Medication.

Talking down

Approach the patient in a confident, open and neutral way. Try to confront him or her about their behaviour, explaining that you wish to help and that they may be unwell. Avoid arguing and shouting.

Restraining

This may be required in emergencies when a patient is likely to harm themselves or others. For safe and effective restraint of an intensely agitated patient who cannot be talked down it is important for the staff to have had both training and experience in restraint techniques.

When restraint is required consider the following:

- Use it only if no other safe alternatives are available
- Call the security staff to assist
- Have a sufficient number of staff — at least five
- Use of specific medications and the details should be clearly documented
- Tell the patient calmly and clearly what is happening
- The need for restraint should be re-evaluated as soon as possible.

Medication

Rapid tranquillization The aim is to rapidly load medications to decrease behavioural disturbance.

- With **benzodiazepines**: the most commonly used drug is lorazepam 0.5–2 mg i.m. every 1–2 hours until behaviour is well controlled, but remember:
  - **contraindications** of respiratory depression in CO_2 retainers and those on narcotics
  - **risks** of psychomotor impairment, excessive sedation and disinhibition
- With **antipsychotics**: some approaches include:
  - 5 mg haloperidol i.m. every 30–60 minutes until the patient is calm
  - double the above dose every 30–60 minutes until the patient is calm.

Droperidol (favoured by many as sedating) or haloperidol or chlorpromazine may also be used orally. However, in those who refuse they may have to be injected. If the situation is urgent the patient should be admitted and given the required dosage every 30–60 minutes until calm.

Injectable preparations such as zuclopenthixol acetate (clopixol acuphase) 50–150 mg can also be used, but with extreme caution in those who are antipsychotic naïve.

This is an effective way of beginning antipsychotic treatment, but the disadvantages include possible side effects such as dystonia, akathisia, parkinsonism and, occasionally at a later stage, neuroleptic malignant syndrome (NMS).

If drug treatment is used it must be monitored for possible side effects and complications. Once you are in a position to assess the nature of the violence, the next step is to try and assess whether it is due to mental illness or not.

> ⚠ **Constant review and evaluation are essential throughout. You should also be guided by the drug formularies and senior staff with regard to the maximum dose allowed.**

LEGAL ASPECTS

- **Common law** allows emergency involuntary treatment.
- The appropriate section of the Mental Health Act (MHA) may need to be applied if there is likely to be a continuing need for compulsory assessment and treatment.

USE OF LITHIUM AND OTHER MOOD STABILIZERS

Lithium is usually the drug of choice in the treatment of mania but its use in emergency management is limited. Nevertheless, unless contraindicated, it should be commenced as soon as possible. Make sure the patient has been screened for the use of lithium, which should include checking urea and electrolytes, kidney and thyroid status (see Chapter 4 on drug treatment).

Other alternative drugs used in the treatment of mania (bipolar affective disorder) include carbamazepine, sodium valproate (especially useful for rapidly cycling bipolar affective disorder) and clonazepam.

Some patients with a history of mania may already be on lithium. The levels should be checked and the dosage altered accordingly. The addition of an antipsychotic may also be needed. At a later stage those thought to be treatment resistant may be helped by augmentation strategies (see Chapter 4 on drug treatments).

HALLUCINATING

Hallucinations are defined as perceptions in the absence of a real stimulus and may occur in any modality, such as auditory, visual or olfactory, and occasionally in more than one.

It is important to assess a hallucinating patient carefully and to try and ascertain the possible underlying disorder. Care should also be taken to differentiate true hallucinations from distortion of perception, illusions and pseudohallucinations. Some hallucinations, such as hypnapompic and hypnagogic are not considered abnormal and some cultures may accept certain hallucinations, not considering them to be a sign of illness and having a different explanation for their presence.

Distortion of perception may include hyperacusis, micropsia, macropsia, xanthopsia, and dysmegalopsia.
Illusions can be described as a misinterpretation of real external sensory stimuli, e.g. seeing snakes in an open fire.
Pseudohallucinations can be described as imagery located in the mind and not in the external space. They lack the substantiality of a normal perception and cannot be consciously manipulated. Unlike true hallucinations, pseudohallucinations are usually egosyntonic.

The underlying reasons for hallucinations can be grouped as follows:

- **Organic:** medical disorders including infections such as meningitis, encephalitis and HIV; brain tumours, including metastases; dementia, metabolic disorders, hepatic and renal failure; neurological disorders such as TLE and ophthalmic and auditory disorders of the senses; post surgery and head injury.
- **Alcohol and drugs** (prescribed or illicit) can also cause hallucinations. Examples include steroid psychosis, amphetamine psychosis, delirium tremens and hallucinations due to solvent abuse. Some of the drugs implicated include amphetamines (speed), cannabis, cocaine, LSD, PCP, prescribed drugs such as tricyclic antidepressants and procyclidine.
- **Functional**: schizophrenia, schizoaffective disorder, paranoid psychoses and brief psychoses; bipolar affective disorder; unipolar depression and puerperal psychosis
- **Neurotic disorders**: during times of extreme stress and when experiencing strong emotions such as bereavement: these are usually referred to as pseudohallucinations
- **Dissociative disorders and personality disorder**: individuals with borderline personality disorder may experience brief periods of hallucination.

PRESENTATIONS

- A&E
  — Patient with a psychiatric history, such as a schizophrenic who may present with a relapse

— Secondary to medical illness such as infection, head injury, brain
tumours, metastasis, TLE
— Secondary to prescribed drugs during treatment and as a result of an
overdose
— Patients who are intoxicated either by drugs or alcohol or who are
withdrawing from intoxicants
● Medical/surgical ward
— As above.
● Psychiatric Wards
— Relapse of illness
— Iatrogenic owing to tricyclic antidepressants or anticholinergics such as
procyclidine
— Overdoses and use of illicit drugs (**Remember that illicit drugs are
surprisingly easily available in many psychiatric wards and hospitals**)
● Community
— Referral by the GP
— Referral by other health workers, such as CPN, social worker, care worker

ASSESSMENT

The hallucinatory experience should be carefully assessed and an attempt
made to elucidate the possible underlying disorder/illness. Try also to clarify
the nature of the hallucinations (see Box).

The **modality** of hallucination should be clarified, and whether they are
occurring in more than one modality.

Note	Sometimes delusions are mistaken for hallucinations, e.g. thought broadcasting.

Ask yourself, 'Is the patient likely to act on these hallucinations?'
A detailed mental state examination should also be carried out to look for
other psychiatric symptomatology, and a detailed medical and psychiatric
history taken if practical.

The **past psychiatric history** is especially important and the presenting
hallucinatory symptoms should be assessed in that context. The patient's
educational, social, linguistic and cultural background should also be
clarified, as many sociocultural groups accept certain hallucinatory
experiences and do not consider them a sign of illness.

COMMON HALLUCINATIONS

● **AUDITORY**: When assessing a patient with auditory hallucinations, look
for distractibility, apparent listening posture, holding of a conversation with
the voice(s), and muttering or whispering. Check that the hallucination is

congruent with the mood (usually in mania and depression) or **incongruent** (likely in schizophrenia). Note the blunting of affect regardless of the content of the hallucination (likely in schizophrenia). Clarify whether the hallucination is in the second person, i.e. 'You should do this' (likely in depression), or the third person: 'He should do this' (likely in schizophrenia). Explore whether the voices are commanding, and whether patient is likely to act upon them. An **opening question** may be: *Do you hear sounds or voices when there is nobody around?* If the answer is positive this can be followed up with further questions to establish the nature of the hallucinatory experience. However, try not to put words into the patient's mouth and avoid closed questions, especially at the outset.

- **VISUAL:** These are especially common in organic disorders, as described above. The patient may have a number of manifestations of the particular organic disorder (e.g. delirium) he is suffering from. So far as visual hallucinations are concerned, the patient may complain of seeing objects, people and faces. He may look into the corners of the room and display an affective response to the hallucinations, such as pleasure, fear or terror. An **opening question** may be: *Do you have visions or see things that others cannot see?*

  Again, a positive reply should be followed by further exploration of the hallucinatory experience.

For other specific hallucinations see Appendices.

MANAGEMENT

The overall aim is to elucidate possible underlying disorders (organic/psychiatric) and to alleviate the hallucinatory experience.

- Hallucinations may be acknowledged but not agreed with, i.e. try to reassure the patient by saying that what he is experiencing, though not real, may appear real to him.
- Attempts should be made to keep patients in contact with reality.
- The assessment should take place in a calm and quiet setting, with appropriate reassurance.
- If there is overwhelming anxiety, agitation and disturbance, benzodiazepines (if not contraindicated) may be used to calm/sedate the patient.
- Where the underlying disorder is reasonably clear and there are no contraindications, use neuroleptics such as haloperidol 2–10 mg (oral/i.m./i.v.) or an atypical antipsychotic.

> ⚠ **CAUTION IS REQUIRED WITH NEUROLEPTIC-NAÏVE PATIENTS AND IT IS ADVISABLE TO TAKE BLOOD FOR HAEMATOLOGY AND BIOCHEMISTRY IF AT ALL POSSIBLE, BEFORE COMMENCING NEUROLEPTIC TREATMENT.**

- Where the presentation is new or atypical, diagnostic possibilities are unclear and social support is unavailable, admit the patient for further observation prior to the use of medications (benzodiazepines or neuroleptics).
- It is not always necessary to admit hallucinating patients and, where the diagnosis is clear (e.g. schizophrenia) and acceptable care is available in the community, they may be treated on an outpatient basis with the help of neuroleptics.
- Formal admission (i.e. use of Mental Health Act) may be required if there are sufficient grounds, such as risk to the patient or to others. Such situations may occur particularly with dangerous command hallucinations and patients having a previous history of having acted upon them.

DELIRIUM

A patient can be said to be suffering from delirium if there is a fluctuating level of consciousness (which may be noted as confusion) alternating with periods of lucidity. The speech may be described as mumbling, normal or shouting, and the thought process may appear incoherent, rambling or disorganized. Anxiety, irritability and perceptual abnormalities may also be present.

PRESENTATION

- In A&E
- In psychiatric wards (as a result of drugs or medical disorders)
- Referral from medical/surgical wards (possibly erroneously thought to be suffering from a psychiatric disorder).

MANAGEMENT

A thorough medical and psychiatric evaluation will need to be carried out to exclude underlying disorders.

Investigations

- **Urine**: screen for drugs, glucose and infection
- **Blood**: FBC, U&Es, creatinine, glucose, LFTs, TFTs, blood cultures (if appropriate)
- **Depending on clinical findings, other investigations include**: chest X-ray, skull X-ray, lumbar puncture, syphilis serology, HIV test, arterial blood gases, serum toxicology (drug screen), CT/MRI scans.

Immediate management

This will depend upon the clinical state of the patient and presence of a life-threatening disorder.

Nursing management

- Provide a calm and reassuring environment.
- Lighting should be optimal.
- All procedures should be explained to the patient, in order to reassure them and reduce the effects of disorientation and perceptual abnormalities.
- An adequate fluid and electrolyte balance should also be maintained.

Use of medications

This should be kept to a minimum, especially while the underlying disorder is being investigated. Haloperidol and lorazepam may be used cautiously where there is a need to treat agitation and paranoia. Physical restraints should be avoided unless absolutely necessary.

MUTISM OR UNRESPONSIVENESS

Mute or unresponsive patients are usually difficult to deal with. They are particularly challenging and may cause frustration on the part of the examiner, especially if a careful, logical and patient approach is not taken during the assessment.

PRESENTATION

The underlying cause may be organic (medical), psychiatric or even psychosocial.

- **Organic**: a number of medical disorders can lead to muteness/unresponsiveness. These include delirium (for whatever reason), dementia, drugs, intoxication, head injury, metabolic disorders and neurological disorders (such as convulsion, meningitis, encephalitis and HIV infection). These organic disorders may have been overlooked or misdiagnosed. All these can present in any setting.

> **Note** Among organic disorders, one should also consider akinetic mutism, which is a stupor (usually due to lesions of the midbrain or the third ventricle) in which the patient appears to be quite asleep, with relaxed breathing. He may be awakened but very rapidly falls asleep again, and sometimes may fall asleep while talking. On recovery there is usually total amnesia for the event.

- **Psychiatric**: these patients may also present in any of the settings described above.

The pointers towards a psychiatric aetiology may include a previous psychiatric history, a lack of physical abnormalities and bizarre presentation.

The diagnostic possibilities include:

— *schizophrenia*, especially the catatonic type; complications of neuroleptic treatment, such as parkinsonian state, neuroleptic malignant syndrome and dystonia

— *affective psychosis*, psychomotor retardation, and stupor in both manic and depressive states

— *dissociative states* include fugue, psychogenic amnesia, and hysterical mutism. The patient often shows characteristic *belle indifférence*. Elective mutism may also occur in a patient with a personality disorder.

● **Psychosocial**: Psychosocial reasons for mutism/unresponsiveness include, those who may be transiently overwhelmed by emotional stress (e.g. severe grief reaction); malingering (the possibility of secondary gain should be considered); and Munchausen's syndrome.

ASSESSMENT

The *history* (especially from a reliable informant) is of paramount importance. Attempts should be made to communicate with the patient, both verbally and non-verbally. Show tact and courtesy, and assume that the patient can hear and understand you. Assess the *degree of mutism* and decide whether it is selective, partial or complete. Attempt to carry out a *mental state examination*, as well as the *mini mental state examination* (MMSE), which in reality is likely to be only partly complete. The *physical examination* should exclude obvious signs of injury, such as to the head. (**Note:** members of certain vulnerable groups, e.g. alcoholics, children, the elderly, and those with personality disorder and schizophrenia, are more prone to head injuries.)

Vital signs including the temperature, should be recorded and, if appropriate, a *Glasgow Coma Scale* may be used to score the degree of impairment of consciousness.

A *neurological screening* can be carried out using minimal observations such as:

● Facial asymmetry
● Pupillary abnormalities
● Eye movements
● Limb movements.

This may be followed by a full neurological examination, if possible. The investigations should be guided by history and the examination, and it is also useful to carry out screening tests of urine and blood. Further investigations (if clinically indicated, and at appropriate times) include chest and skull X-ray, ECG, EEG, CT and MRI.

MANAGEMENT

The aim should be first to exclude life-threatening brain pathology, which will need urgent referral to appropriate medical/surgical specialists.

> When taking blood for screening it is always worth making an urgent check of glucose level. If there is any hint of an organic problem, do not hesitate to involve medical/surgical colleagues. Minor organic problems may be dealt in a psychiatric setting with advice from medical colleagues. The effective management will depend on the accuracy of assessment and investigations. Often, provided there are no life-threatening disorders, the most effective initial management is to provide an appropriate environment for further assessment/observation.

Catatonic schizophrenia

The patient may show marked psychomotor disturbances (excitement or stupor) which may lead to fatal exhaustion. This may be treated with rapid tranquillization using an antipsychotic such as haloperidol or droperidol (i.m./i.v.). Failing this, ECT may be used. It is important to monitor vital signs and to ensure that the patient is adequately hydrated, and that medical complications are not overlooked.

Remember catatonic stupor may also be caused by organic disorders, which should be excluded.

Acute dystonia

This is usually caused by neuroleptic drugs and can be effectively treated using i.m. anticholinergics such as procyclidine 5–10 mg.

Neuroleptic malignant syndrome (NMS)

See section on NMS for management.

Affective psychosis leading to psychomotor retardation

This may be life-threatening, especially where oral intake of fluids is minimal. Ensure adequate hydration (i.v. fluids, if required), and emergency ECT treatment may be required. No consent is required in such a situation and common law may be used. Manic or depressive stupor may also be treated with rapid tranquillization, as described above.

Dissociative states

Psychogenic mutism or stupor may occur as a part of hysterical reaction. Catatonic symptoms are rare and the patient is usually responsive, with the exception of aphonia. Reassurance and support may be sufficient. However, on occasions admission may be necessary and abreaction (amytal interview) and hypnosis should be considered. If unable to exclude affective psychosis or catatonic schizophrenia, consider emergency ECT.

Note	Consent is not needed if common law (UK) is invoked during an emergency. However, it is sensible to inform the patient and his or her carers.

ANXIETY

The main features of anxiety include a feeling of fear, usually accompanied by autonomic symptoms such as rapid breathing/sweating. It is important to distinguish between normal and pathological anxiety states. Pathological anxiety differs from normal in terms of the response to a given stimulus (usually inappropriate) and the intensity or duration of the symptoms.

Severe anxiety should be taken seriously as it is associated with significant morbidity (psychiatric and medical) and may in some cases lead to death (owing to association with poor judgement and suicidal behaviour). It is also important to distinguish primary anxiety from the anxiety secondary to non-psychiatric causes (medical diseases, drugs and alcohol, etc.).

PRESENTATION

- A&E — self referral
- GP referral
- Psychiatric wards
- Medical/surgical wards.

Signs and symptoms of anxiety

Respiratory	**Cardiovascular**	**Autonomic**
Chest pressure	Tachycardia	Dry mouth
Choking	Palpitations	Sweating
Sighing	Chest pain	Headaches
Dyspnoea	Faintness	Hot flushes
Hyperventilation		
Musculoskeletal	**Genitourinary**	**Gastrointestinal**
Aches/pains	Frequency	Swallowing difficulty
Twitching	Urgency	Abdominal pain
Stiffness	Sexual dysfunction	Nausea
Fatigue	Menstrual problems	Irritable bowel
		Diarrhoea
Neurological	**Psychological**	**Appearance**
Dizziness	Apprehension	Strained
Numbness/tingling	Avoidance	Furrowed forehead
Visual disturbance	Irritability	Pale
Weakness	Restlessness	Sweaty
Tremor	Fear, startle response, hypervigilance	
Headache	Worrying thoughts, rumination	
Paraesthesia		

ASSESSMENT

The clarification and request for further information need to be tailored to the requester. The request is more likely to be from the nursing staff if the patient is from your own ward, whereas medical staff may contact you if the patient is in A&E or on a non-psychiatric ward.

From the requester, clarify:

- The urgency of the request
- The main presenting symptoms and vital signs
- Medical/surgical illness
- Prescribed drugs
- History of illicit drugs and alcohol use/abuse
- History of psychiatric disorder.

Depending on the information obtained, inform the requester:

- Your likely time of arrival
- What further observations/investigations you would like carried out.

The urgency of your attendance will depend upon:

- The severity of the patient's symptomatology
- Involvement of the cardiovascular and respiratory systems
- Vital signs pointing to a life-threatening situation
- Knowledge/experience, expertise and competence of the requester.

DIFFERENTIAL DIAGNOSIS

Medical

- Drugs-related (Table 6.1)
- Other (Table 6.2).

Psychiatric

- Adjustment reaction
- Acute reaction to stress
- Depression
- Generalized anxiety disorder (GAD)
- Mania
- Obsessive–compulsive disorder (OCD)
- Panic disorder
- Phobic disorder
- Post-traumatic stress disorder (PTSD)
- Schizophrenia.

TABLE 6.1   Drugs that may cause anxiety

Drugs with anticholinergic affects	Dopaminergics/Antidopaminergics
Benzhexol	Amantadine
Benztropine mesylate	Bromocriptine
Oxybutynin	Levodopa (L-dopa)
Tricyclics	Levodopa-carbidopa (Sinemet)
Procyclidine	Metoclopramide
	Neuroleptics
Drug Withdrawal	**Stimulants**
Barbiturates	Amphetamines
Benzodiazepines	Aminophylline
Narcotics	Caffeine
Alcohol	Cocaine
Sedatives	Methylphenidate
	Theophylline
Sympathomimetics	**Miscellaneous**
Adrenaline	Baclofen
Ephedrine	Cycloserine
Phenylpropanolamine	Hallucinogens
Pseudoephedrine	Indomethacin

TABLE 6.2   Medical causes of anxiety-like symptoms

Type of Cause	Specific Cause
Cardiovascular	Angina pectoris, arrhythmias, congestive heart failure, hypertension, hypovolaemia, myocardial infarction, syncope (multiple causes), valvular disease, vascular collapse (shock)
Dietary	Caffeine, monosodium glutamate ('Chinese restaurant syndrome'), vitamin deficiency diseases
Drug related	Akathisia (secondary to antipsychotic drugs), anticholinergic toxicity, digitalis toxicity, hallucinogens, hypotensive agents, stimulants (amphetamines, cocaine, related drugs), withdrawal syndromes (alcohol, sedative–hypnotics), bronchodilators (theophylline, sympathomimetics)
Haematological	Anaemias
Immunological	Anaphylaxis, systemic lupus erythematosus
Metabolic	Hyperadrenalism (Cushing's disease), hyperkalaemia, hyperthermia, hyperthyroidism, hypocalcaemia, hypoglycaemia, hyponatraemia, hypothyroidism, menopause, porphyria (acute intermittent)
Neurological	Delirium, encephalopathies (infectious, metabolic, toxic), essential tremor, intracranial mass lesions, post-concussive syndrome, seizure disorders (especially of the temporal lobe), vertigo
Respiratory	Asthma, chronic obstructive pulmonary disease, pneumonia, pneumothorax, pulmonary oedema, pulmonary embolism
Secreting tumours	Carcinoid, insulinoma, phaeochromocytoma

Psychosocial

- Psychological response to social upheaval/events, e.g. assault (robbery/theft/rape etc.) or bereavement
- Other losses, - e.g. jobs/house/possessions.

MANAGEMENT

- **Short-term**: medical/psychosocial
- **Long-term**: Referral to colleagues; outpatient arrangements; drug treatment (antidepressants, buspirone).

Short-term

When dealing with acutely anxious patients the following should be considered:

- Exclude treatable acute medical conditions causing anxiety and involve other specialties if appropriate.
- Exclude drugs/alcohol (prescribed or illicit) as a cause.
- Look and remain calm.
- Calm and reassure the patient appropriately (remember, calmness can be infectious as laughter).
- Take the patient seriously and provide a safe, secure environment, with the help of colleagues.
- Seek the help of a senior experienced nursing colleague/senior psychiatrist (if necessary).

Medical Having made sure of the above, if drugs are still required use anxiolytics (mostly benzodiazepines; see Table 6.3). However, first consider the contraindications, interactions and side effects, and dependency/abuse issues. With **benzodiazepines** you should be aware of the following:

- Addiction (addicts may want it) and withdrawal symptoms are possibilities.
- Behaviour disinhibition may occur.
- Children and the elderly are especially sensitive.
- Metabolism of some benzodiazepines (least likely with lorazepam, temazepam and oxazepam) may be reduced by liver dysfunction and other drugs.
- Synergism with other CNS depressants, such as alcohol, barbiturates and narcotics, is possible.
- Side effects include:
  — cognitive/psychomotor impairment
  — confusion
  — depressive symptoms
  — disorientation, drowsiness.

TABLE 6.3	Benzodiazepines (BDZ)			
Specefic BDZ	Oral dosage equivalence (mg)	Onset after oral dose	Distribution half-life	Elimination half-life (h)
Alprazolam	0.5	Intermediate	Intermediate	6–20
Chlordiazepoxide	10.0	Intermediate	Slow	30–100
Clonazepam	0.25	Intermediate	Intermediate	18–50
Clorzepate	7.5	Rapid	Rapid	30–100
Diazepam	5.0	Rapid	Rapid	30–100
Flurazepam	30.0	Rapid-intermediate	Rapid	50–160
Lorazepam	1.0	Intermediate	Intermediate	10–20
Midazolam	—	Intermediate	Rapid	2–3
Oxazepam	15.0	Intermediate-slow	Intermediate	8–12
Temazepam	30.0	Intermediate	Rapid	8–20
Triazolam	0.25	Intermediate	Rapid	1.5–5

The elimination half-life encompasses the total for all metabolites; the elderly usually have the longer half-lives in the range reported. Chlordiazepoxide, clorazepate and diazepam have desmethyldiazepam as a long-lived active metabolite.

Lorazepam is usually preferred for emergency use. It is well absorbed and can be administered i.m. or i.v. (slowly). Give 1–2 mg p.o./i.m./i.v. and repeat every 30 minutes until a clinical response is achieved.

It is useful to use a particular benzodiazepine to which the patient has previously shown a good response. When prescribing PRN do not write '1–2 mg p.o./i.m., but specify separately, i.e. 1–2 mg p.o.; 1–2 mg i.m.

> ⚠ **Do not send the patient home with benzodiazepines (or having been just given some) without warning about and discussing the side effects and the potential dangers (e.g. while driving or using machinery). Ideally a responsible and informed person should accompany the patient home.**
> **In general, following the administration of benzodiazepines the patient should be monitored for a few hours before being sent home.**

Psychosocial

● If the patient is overbreathing/hyperventilating teach him to rebreathe into a paper bag for short periods.
● Show him how to breathe more regularly and deeply if there is evidence of a deteriorating pattern of breathing, e.g. shallow.
● If there is time and appropriately trained staff are available, consider teaching progressive muscle relaxation or relaxation muscle response.

Long-term

This should always be considered and appropriate measures taken, including:

Drugs:

- **Neuroleptics** (e.g. thioridazine) where there is agitation and some psychotic symptoms and if benzodiazepines cannot be used
- **β-Blockers** where there are peripheral manifestations of anxiety, such as tremor or performance anxiety, but *not* if there is a history of asthma, heart failure or hypoglycaemia
- **Azapirones** (e.g. buspirone), especially in generalized anxiety disorder
- **SSRIs** (e.g. paroxetine) for panic disorder or anxiety related to agoraphobia or obsessive–compulsive disorder
- **Other** Antihistamines are occasionally used. They are sedative and have no specific anxiolytic properties.

Non-drug/psychosocial:

Refer to anxiety management classes, which are usually run by day hospital services, or advise the patient to seek private instruction (e.g. information from libraries and Citizens' Advice Bureau).

FACTITIOUS DISORDER (MUNCHAUSEN'S SYNDROME, 'HOSPITAL HOPPER' SYNDROME)

This is a curious disorder in which physical or psychological signs and symptoms are intentionally feigned. The motivation is to assume a sick role in the absence of obvious gains/benefits (e.g. economic gain, or avoiding legal responsibility). It is not quite the same as malingering.

Where the complaints relate to physical signs and symptoms it is often called Munchausen's syndrome (after an 18th century German storyteller, Baron von Munchausen), whereas in others psychiatric symptoms are feigned, and these usually include depression, hallucinations, dissociative and conversion symptoms with bizarre behaviour. Factitious disorder with both physical and psychiatric features may also occur. In such cases the individual often has personality problems (e.g. borderline personality disorder) and relationship difficulties. Munchausen's syndrome is usually easier to recognize than factitious disorders where psychiatric symptoms predominate. The former is more likely to be dealt with by a surgeon or physician, and many hospitals keep a register of individuals with this disorder. The latter may have received high doses of psychiatric drugs, or may have even undergone ECT because of a poor therapeutic response. In most cases management is problematic, owing to the difficulty of engaging the individual. Constant and close observation is helpful.

PRESENTATIONS

- A&E
- Medical/surgical wards
- Psychiatric wards/clinics.

As a trainee psychiatrist you are less likely to meet these individuals in an emergency setting (especially those with Munchausen's syndrome), and those with psychiatric symptoms may successfully gain admission unless they are well known and on the register.

MANAGEMENT

Be aware of this diagnostic possibility, paying special attention to various features common to this condition so that fruitless investigations/procedures are not carried out.

If suspicious:

- Check the special name register kept by the hospital.
- Contact other neighbouring hospitals to check their registers.
- Maintain professionalism: avoid feelings of resentment and hostility; remember that even though the illness is factitious, the patient is ill.
- The idea of confronting these individuals is controversial and should really be dealt with by more senior colleagues. Most individuals leave when confronted.
- Your job is more likely to be to help educate other colleagues in dealing with such individuals.
- In a few cases individual psychotherapy has been found helpful.
- It is better to inform and involve the patient's GP.

DRUGS-RELATED (INCLUDING ALCOHOL) PSYCHIATRIC EMERGENCIES

INTOXICATION

Intoxication, whether from drugs or alcohol, frequently leads to behavioural problems, and on many occasions psychiatric symptomatology is exhibited. Overall the incidence of drugs/alcohol abuse is higher in patients with a psychiatric history. It is therefore not surprising that the duty psychiatrist is often requested to evaluate an intoxicated patient with only the merest hint of psychiatric symptoms or history.

It is difficult to carry out an effective psychiatric evaluation on an intoxicated patient. Therefore, if a significantly intoxicated patient presents in A&E it is better to leave a detailed psychiatric evaluation until he or she is sufficiently sober.

You should explain your reasoning to A&E staff, but do not totally refuse to see anyone who is intoxicated, instead provide psychiatric input until it is appropriate to take over the care of the patient.

A&E staff should evaluate the intoxicated patient medically and perhaps admit him or her overnight for further observation, if clinically indicated.

It is often helpful to request that the patient be breathalysed in order to establish the actual level of intoxication.

Intoxicated patients can be divided into two groups:

● Lethargic, sedate or even in a coma (less likely to be referred to a psychiatrist).
  Intoxicants may include:
  — alcohol
  — sedative hypnotics: benzodiazepines, barbiturates, non-barbiturate sedatives
  — opiates: morphine, heroin, opium, methadone
● Restless and agitated (more likely to be referred to a psychiatrist).
  Intoxicants may include:
  — psychostimulants: amphetamines, 3,4-methylene-dioxymethamphetamine (MDMA, Ecstasy), cocaine
  — hallucinogens: lysergic acid diethylamide (LSD), phencyclidine hydrochloride (PCP, 'angel dust'), marijuana.

PRESENTATIONS
● A&E
● Medical/surgical wards
● Psychiatric wards
● Outpatient department/day hospital.

The following points should be clarified before offering advice or agreeing to a psychiatric evaluation:

● The patient's conscious state (e.g. Glasgow Coma Scale, if appropriate)
● The vital signs
● What intoxicant(s) used, how much and for how long
● The resulting behaviour and psychiatric symptoms.

Depending on the information obtained, advice may be offered over the telephone or in person, either immediately or later.

If you agree to an evaluation, inform the requester of your approximate time of arrival.

The decision to visit will depend on a number of factors. For A&E presentations this has been partially discussed above. The difficulty lies with the patient with a clear psychiatric history but who is only partially intoxicated, but little is gained by refusing to visit in such circumstances.

Consultation in a non-psychiatric setting may culminate in advice regarding further management, which should be clearly communicated to the relevant staff and documented.

Where psychiatric symptomatology is significant and there are no significant medical problems that might best be managed on a non-psychiatric ward, admission to a psychiatric ward may be considered.

Such situations include:

- Patients with a history of psychiatric disorder
- The presence of a serious suicide/homicide risk

In cases of intoxication on a psychiatric ward the medical responsibility lies with you. You will need to assess the patient further, but if there are significant medical complications the management may be shared with medical colleagues, or the patient may be transferred to an appropriate non-psychiatric ward.

MANAGEMENT

ASSESSMENT

Before you evaluate the patient certain observations by the nursing staff should have been undertaken. These include:

- Level of consciousness (e.g. Glasgow Coma Scale. **Note**: not all nursing staff will know about this, especially on psychiatric wards)
- Vital signs such as pulse rate, blood pressure, pupil size and reaction, respiratory rate and temperature
- Blood glucose: this is especially useful in serious alcohol intoxication, which may lead to serious hypoglycaemia
- Urine for drugs screening.

Consider:

- The type of drugs that may have been ingested
- A mixture of drugs may have been ingested together with alcohol
- Street drugs (surprisingly, it is often easier to obtain these in psychiatric hospitals) are often impure and can lead to a mixed intoxicated/withdrawal state.

Examination
Briefly assess:

- Appearance and behaviour/activity
- Level of consciousness
- Recheck vital signs.

Further history

- The length of history and time spent will need to take account of the clinical state of the patient and his location (i.e. in psychiatric ward etc.).
- Obtain as much information as possible regarding the identity of the substances taken, the amount and when taken, and if the use was acute or chronic. Involve friends and relatives of the patient in order to obtain further details.

A modified physical examination should include:

- Pupils: size, reaction, etc.
- Presence of tremor
- Signs of needle marks
- Neurological examination
- A modified form of mental state examination.

MANAGEMENT

The **acute management** will depend on the type of intoxicants taken (see below).

Further **long-term management** should include:

- Appropriate counselling/information for the patient, as well as friends and relatives
- Guidance advice for those taking over the care (i.e. medical staff)
- Referral to the appropriate agencies, especially where there is a history of drugs/alcohol dependency syndrome (e.g. drug dependency clinics/units).

SPECIFIC INTOXICANT-RELATED SYNDROMES AND THEIR MANAGEMENT

ALCOHOL

SIGNS AND SYMPTOMS

- Aggression
- Ataxia
- Coma
- Disinhibition
- Hypothermia
- Nystagmus
- Slurred speech
- Tachycardia.

Note: These are not listed in order of occurrence.

MANAGEMENT

- Evaluate the patient in a calm and quiet environment.
- Monitor vital signs.
- If the patient is agitated and violent treat with benzodiazepines, such as lorazepam 1–2 mg orally or i.m. every 4 hours.
- Involve medical colleagues early and hand over.
- Patients whom you suspect of using excessive alcohol should be given thiamine (100 mg i.m./i.v. then orally for 6 days) to prevent the onset of Wernicke's encephalopathy (note the CSM warning; see Chapter 4, p. 125). Folate 1 mg orally should also be given for 7 days. Patients with other B-vitamin deficiencies should be given appropriate supplements.

Serious intoxication

A person with a blood alcohol level of 0.1–0.15 mg/dl is considered legally intoxicated. A level of 0.3–0.4 mg/dl will cause a coma.

Management should be in a medical setting, and includes:

- Gastric lavage
- Thiamine 100 mg i.m./i.v. as prophylaxis for possible Wernicke's encephalopathy (note CSM warning)
- i.v. fluids
- 50 ml 50% glucose to prevent hypoglycaemia
- Intensive care monitoring
- Monitor for withdrawal symptoms (see Chapter 4, p. 121).

ANXIOLYTICS/BENZODIAZEPINES

SIGNS AND SYMPTOMS

- Ataxia
- Confusion
- Slurred speech

Note: Benzodiazepine overdose alone is rarely fatal, but mixture with other drugs, particularly alcohol, can cause fatal respiratory depression.

MANAGEMENT

This will depend on the severity of the overdose: a severe overdose should be treated in a medical setting.

- Monitor vital signs and support airway when needed.
- Flumazenil (a benzodiazepine antagonist) may be used to reverse the effects of an overdose. Make sure the airway is secured, then administer 0.2 mg i.v. over 30 seconds; after waiting a further 30 seconds repeat 0.2–0.5 mg over 30 seconds at 1-minute intervals until the patient

responds. Do not exceed 3 mg. Caution should be exercised if the patient has taken a concomitant tricyclic antidepressant or is benzodiazepine dependent, as flumazenil may precipitate seizures.

BARBITURATES (PHENOBARBITAL) AND NON-BARBITURATES (GLUTETHIMIDE, MEPROBAMATE)

SIGNS AND SYMPTOMS

- Ataxia
- Confusion
- Decreased level of consciousness
- Decreased respiration
- Hypotension
- Nystagmus
- Slurred speech.

Note: These are not listed in order of occurrence.

MANAGEMENT (MEDICAL)

- Admit under the care of medics, as overdose can be fatal.
- Monitor vital signs and support airway when needed.
- Keep awake the patient who is already awake.
- No specific antidote is available, but gastric lavage should be used if the drug was taken within the last 4–6 hours, to reduce further absorption.
- Forced diuresis and dialysis may need to be carried out.
- Monitor for withdrawal symptoms (see later).

PSYCHOSTIMULANTS (COCAINE, AMPHETAMINES, 3, 4-METHYLENE-DIOXYMETHAMPHETAMINE [MDMA, ECSTASY])

SIGNS AND SYMPTOMS

- Coma
- Cardiac arrhythmias, tachycardia
- Decreased appetite
- Dilated, reactive pupils
- Euphoria
- Fever
- Hypertension
- Psychosis, hallucinations
- Restlessness
- Seizures.

Note: These are not listed in order of occurrence.

The paranoia of the chronic high-dose cocaine abuser can mimic schizophrenia. Extremely high doses may lead to autonomic instability and hyperthermia, which may progress to seizures, strokes and death.

MANAGEMENT

- Assess in a calm, quiet environment.
- Reassure the patient with mild symptoms.
- For acute agitation use lorazepam 1–2 mg as often as every 1–2 hours (avoid exceeding 8 mg in a 24-hour period) until the patient has calmed down.
- Give neuroleptics such as haloperidol 5 mg every 30 minutes until the patient has calmed down, to severely paranoid or agitated patients.
- Exclude medical complications such as myocardial infarction, stroke and intracranial haemorrhage. Involve medical colleagues and hand over care if appropriate.
- Adrenergic reactions (diaphoresis, tachycardia, hyperpyrexia, hypertension) may be treated with β-blockers such as propranolol, 20–40 mg orally or 1–2 mg i.v. (but **avoid in asthmatics, diabetics** and patients with **cardiovascular disease**). Involve medical colleagues and hand over care if appropriate.
- Temperatures higher than 38°C should be investigated and treated aggressively. Involve medical colleagues and hand over care if appropriate.
- Treat seizures with i.v. diazepam 5–20 mg/min, repeated at 15-minute intervals as necessary. Involve medical colleagues and hand over care if appropriate.
- Consider hospitalization if the paranoid behaviour persists and may lead to harm. If not, then discharge to a responsible supervisor. An immediate follow-up appointment should be considered.
- To increase drug excretion acidify the urine with ascorbic acid (vitamin C) or ammonium chloride.

Serious cocaine intoxication
Serious complications may result from this which should really be managed in an ICU setting, i.e. hand over to medical colleagues.

Signs, symptoms and management

- Seizures: use benzodiazepine as previously described
- Hyperthermia: manage with a cooling blanket if > 38°C
- Tachycardia, arrhythmias: use supportive measures
- Monitor withdrawal symptoms (see Chapter 4, p. 108).

MARIJUANA (CANNABIS)

SIGNS AND SYMPTOMS

- Altered perceptions
- Euphoria, silliness, feeling of wellbeing
- Increased appetite, thirst
- Increased anxiety, paranoia
- Injected conjunctivae
- Lack of coordination
- Tachycardia.

   Note: These are not listed in order of occurrence.

MANAGEMENT

- Reassure the patient of the likelihood of effects subsiding.
- Manage acute anxiety with lorazepam 1–2 mg orally every 1–2 hours as needed (avoid exceeding 8 mg in a 24-hour period).

HALLUCINOGENS

These include lysergic acid diethylamide (LSD), psilocybin (mushrooms), dimethoxymethylamphetamine (STP or DOM), dimethyltryptamine (DMT) and methylene dioxyamphetamine (MDA, MDMA).

SIGNS AND SYMPTOMS

- Extreme or labile affect
- Alternating periods of lucidity and hallucinations
- Diaphoresis
- Dilated pupils
- Hypertension
- Hyperthermia
- Perceptual distortions, including hallucinations and synaesthesia, in which, for example, sound is perceived as colour
- Piloerection
- Tachycardia, palpitations
- Tremor, incoordination.

   Note: These are not listed in order of occurrence.

   These effects mostly occur over 6–12 hours, but may last up to several days. Presentations may vary from an acute panic reaction to a brief psychotic state. The patient may describe feelings of helplessness, fear of losing control, fear of going crazy, and paranoia. They may also exhibit signs of intense anxiety, depression and hallucinations (mostly visual). Flashbacks may occur suddenly with chronic LSD use, and last from several minutes to several hours.

MANAGEMENT

- Reassure and talk down.
- Do not leave the patient alone, as behaviour can become dangerous and consequences may be fatal.
- Treat with lorazepam 1–2 mg orally or i.m. every 1–2 hours until the patient has calmed down.
- Use an antidopaminergic (e.g. haloperidol) in conjunction with lorazepam especially if hallucinations persist following removal of the hallucinogen.
- Hospitalize if the reaction lasts longer than 24 hours despite medical treatment.
- Discharge should be into the care of responsible friends or family and with appropriate follow-up.
- Monitor for withdrawal symptoms (see later).

PHENCYCLIDINE (PCP, ANGEL DUST)

SIGNS AND SYMPTOMS

- Decreased sensitivity to pain
- Disorientation, memory impairment
- Hallucinations, synaesthesia
- Hyperreflexia, numbness
- Hypertension
- Nystagmus, ataxia, dysarthria
- Rigidity
- Stupor, coma, death
- Tachycardia.

MANAGEMENT

This should be in a medical setting.

- Hospitalization, as overdose can be fatal
- Minimization of sensory stimulation
- Treatment of psychosis with haloperidol 2–5 mg orally or i.m. every hour until the patient is calm
- Treatment of anxiety or agitation with lorazepam, 1–2 mg orally or i.m. every 30–60 minutes until the patient is calm
- Acidification of urine with ascorbic acid or ammonium chloride
- Close monitoring of vital signs, especially if large amount is ingested, because of the possibility of coma and death; support for pulmonary and cardiovascular functioning, when necessary.

INHALANTS

SIGNS AND SYMPTOMS

- Altered states of consciousness, ranging from euphoria to clouding
- Chest pain
- Dizziness, syncope
- Nausea, vomiting, epigastric distress
- Odour of the breath
- Organ damage (brain, liver, kidney, heart)
- Psychosis.

   Note: These are not listed in order of occurrence.

> **Note** Acute intoxication can last from 15 to 45 minutes, whereas drowsiness and stupor may last for hours.

MANAGEMENT

This should involve medical colleagues, who should take over the management with psychiatric input from yourself.

- Give oxygen, which should resolve symptoms within minutes.
- Try to identify the solvent. Leaded petrol may require the use of a chelating agent.
- Treat acute psychosis with haloperidol 2–5 mg orally or i.m.

OPIOIDS

These include opium, morphine, heroin, meperidine, methadone, pentazocine and propoxyphene.

SIGNS AND SYMPTOMS

- Bradycardia
- Depressed respiration and consciousness level
- Hypothermia
- Pinpoint pupils unresponsive to light, except for meperidine, which may produce dilated pupils
- Pulmonary oedema.

   Note: These are not listed in order of occurrence.

   Overdose can cause pulmonary oedema and respiratory depression, which should be treated in the intensive care unit.

MANAGEMENT (MEDICAL)

- Make sure the airway is supported.
- Treat with naloxone 0.4–2.0 mg i.v. every 2–3 minutes until respiration is stable. However, after 10 mg consider other causes for the symptoms.

- As the half-life of naloxone is much shorter than that of most opioids (approximately 1 hour), you will need to observe closely for the re-emergence of symptoms (e.g. coma) and re-treat with naloxone.

SUBSTANCE WITHDRAWAL

Like intoxicated patients those suffering from substance (drugs/alcohol) withdrawal may also be referred to you, as they may exhibit psychiatric symptomatology and behavioural problems. The patient presenting with substance withdrawal may:

- Have taken these drugs for the first time, either deliberately (e.g. as part of a suicide attempt) or inadvertently
- Be an established abuser who, when unable to obtain drugs, may feign symptoms in order to obtain a further supply
- Be known to other services, such as a drug treatment clinic, which may provide vital information for effective immediate management.

The patient's presentation may be bewildering, and therefore it is essential that you seek relevant information (details regarding specific drugs taken as well as when taken) and guidance from experts.

Many presentations will be mild and self-limiting, requiring no specific measures. However, some may progress to life-threatening conditions such as delirium tremens (DTs). Remember that DTs is a medical emergency with a high mortality rate and should be managed in a medical setting (usually a medical ward).

PRESENTATION

- A&E
- Medical/surgical wards
- Psychiatric wards, day hospital or clinics (e.g. emergency psychiatric clinic)
- Detoxification clinic associated with the hospital.

Clarify from the referrer:

- Physical state of the patient:
  — level of consciousness (Glasgow Coma Scale, if appropriate)
  — vital signs
- Signs of withdrawal:
  — anxiety, agitation, vomiting, diarrhoea
  — state of pupils (dilatation), lacrimation
  — piloerection, rhinorrhoea.
- What, how much and when taken, and other prescribed medication the patient may be taking
- Whether the patient is suicidal or violent, and the objective level of distress exhibited.

Before you visit:

- Inform the requester of your likely time of your arrival.
- Ask for any of the above, e.g. vital signs.
- Ensure that lorazepam (2 mg) or haloperidol (5 mg) for i.m. injections is available.
- While on your way try to put together a picture of the likely drugs involved and a possible management plan (see effects of specific drugs for withdrawal below).

Do not forget:

- Withdrawal from a combination of drugs may complicate the picture (especially alcohol and other CNS drugs).
- The presence of a concomitant psychiatric diagnosis. Could the symptoms be better accounted for by a medical or psychiatric disorder?
- Withdrawal syndrome can be life-threatening.
- Possibility of medical complications, e.g. endocarditis, HIV.
- Individuals may feign symptoms in order to obtain medications, or to avoid the law enforcement agencies.

EXAMINATION

Physical/general

- Is the patient well/unwell?
- State of airway; also rule out stigmata characteristic of substance abuser, such as needle marks and poor state of nutrition
- Piloerection, rhinorrhoea, muscle twitching, post-seizure incontinence
- Vital signs: be aware of changes such as raised or lowered blood pressure and pulse rate
- Neurological: signs of agitation, confusion, size of pupil, sixth cranial nerve palsy, reflexes and gait.

Mental state examination:

This is may have to be relatively brief. However, you should explore the presence of psychomotor abnormalities, thought disturbance (including paranoia), perceptual abnormalities, affective lability, suicidal and homocidal ideation and relevant cognitive impairment.

MANAGEMENT

General (see also above)

It is of the utmost importance to carry out a thorough medical evaluation to rule out life-threatening situations. Depending on the clinical findings, this should include the following:

- Urine analysis (drug screen)
- Full blood count, blood biochemistry (urea and electrolytes, liver function tests, calcium, thyroid function tests)
- B_{12} and folate
- ECG
- EEG
- CT, if required to rule out subdural haematoma, which is fairly common among substance abusers.

You should also involve other specialists, or ask them to take over the care of the patient if clinically indicated.

Note	Remember that drug abusers have a high mortality. Do not be judgemental and value-laden when it comes to providing medical care. Many drug abusers recover and go on to become valuable members of society.

Specific substance withdrawal

Alcohol (see Chapter 4, p. 121)

Delirium tremens (see Chapter 4, p. 127)

Antidepressants (see Chapter 4, pp. 150–165)

Antipsychotics (see Chapter 4, p. 175)

Anxiolytics/sedatives (see Chapter 4, p. 110)

Opiates Opiate withdrawal may appear dramatic but is not usually life-threatening. You should try to manage the objective physical findings (autonomic disturbance, including hypertension, piloerection, rhinorrhoea, and sweating) with supportive measures. The patient's subjective complaints are usually less reliable: he or she should be reassured and told to expect some discomfort.

> ⚠️ **With heroin and morphine (short-acting) withdrawal symptoms appear within 6–24 hours of the last dose, peaking at 48–72 hours, and may last as long as 7–10 days. With methadone (longer–acting) symptoms may take as long as 36–72 hours to appear.**

Symptoms

- Anxiety, irritability, craving, yawning
- Autonomic disturbance (hypertension, tachycardia, tachypnoea, pupillary dilatation)

- Lacrimation, rhinorrhoea, diarrhoea ('discharge from all the orifices')
- Nausea, vomiting
- Insomnia, dysphoric mood
- Muscle twitching, increased sensitivity to pain.

Management
General management is as described above.

Drug treatment

- **Methadone**: (5–10 mg i.m. initially with most) is used as a replacement drug because of its long half-life. The above dose may be repeated every 4–6 hours until symptoms subside. In most cases it is best to avoid exceeding 40 mg of methadone in a day.
- **Clonidine** (α-agonist antihypertensive): 0.1–0.3 mg orally t.d.s./q.d.s. (avoid exceeding 0.8 mg/day) for 2 weeks as an adjunct to methadone. It helps alleviate nausea, vomiting, diarrhoea, craving, restlessness and insomnia. Discontinue gradually (to avoid rebound hypertension); its main side effects include hypotension and sedation.

Stimulants (cocaine, amphetamine) There is a strong risk of suicide in those experiencing withdrawal from both cocaine and amphetamine. This should be managed appropriately.

Symptoms

- Anxiety
- Drug craving
- Severely depressed mood, psychomotor retardation or agitation
- Sleep disturbance, disturbing dreams
- Paranoid ideation/delusions
- Increased appetite
- Fatigue.

Management

- **Lorazepam** (1–2 mg orally/i.m.) can be used to control agitation, anxiety and disruptive behaviour.
- **Antipsychotics** such as haloperidol (5–10 mg orally/i.m.) may be used for paranoid ideation/delusions.

LITHIUM TOXICITY (see also Chapter 4)

The main indication for lithium use is in the treatment of bipolar illness, such as manic depression, both acutely and prophylactically. Because this drug has a narrow-range therapeutic index it is essential to carry out regular blood level monitoring.

The preferred blood levels for lithium are:

- In acute treatment of mania, 0.8–1.2 mmol/l
- In prophylactic treatment, 0.6–1.0 mmol/l
- Lower levels (0.4–0.6 mmol/l) are sufficient in the treatment of the elderly, those with impaired renal or CNS function, and in cases where augmentation (an antidepressant) is needed.

> ⚠ **Lithium levels should be measured 12 hours after the last dose. However, above certain levels (1.5 mmol/l) lithium becomes toxic and unless this is managed effectively fatal (>4 mmol/l) consequences may occur. (See Chapter 4, p. 141 for lithium monitoring; toxicity in relation to plasma levels and management).**

PRESENTATION

Psychiatric wards/clinics, in casualty or other medical/surgical wards.

CAUSATION

- As a result of overdose
- Inadvertent prescribing/intake
- Renal failure, dehydration, vomiting, diarrhoea
- Due to drugs that increase lithium levels:
  — thiazide diuretics
  — indomethacin and NSAIDs
  — metronidazole
  — erythromycin, tetracycline.

The symptoms of toxicity are dose dependent and include:

- Nausea and vomiting
- Thirst, diarrhoea, dehydration
- Ataxia, drowsiness, confusion, severe (coarse) tremor
- Dysarthria, nystagmus, spasticity and hyperreflexia seizures
- Coma leading to death (>4.0 mmol/).

MANAGEMENT

- Stop lithium,
- Involve medical colleagues
- Give i.v. saline and osmotic diuretics
- Transfer to ICU may be required in severe cases.

SEROTONIN SYNDROME

Combining monoamine oxidase inhibitors (MAOIs) with serotonin augmenters (e.g. buspirone, SSRIs, trazodone or tricyclics) may lead to serotonin syndrome, the clinical features of which include:

- Ataxia, altered mental state
- Delirium, restlessness
- Fever, rigors
- Hyperreflexia
- Fits, myclonus
- Tremor.

It is best avoided by discontinuing MAOIs for at least 2 weeks before starting another antidepressant.

PRESENTATION

This iatrogenic condition may result from the inadvertent prescription of an antidepressant in addition to the MAOIs, without a previous 2 week washout. Patients may present in A&E with the features of the syndrome, or be seen as a newly admitted patient to the psychiatric ward.

HYPERTENSIVE CRISIS DUE TO MAOIs

This is a rare but potentially fatal condition which usually results from mixing a MAOI with food with a high tyramine content, or a pressor medication (see Chapter 4).

Features include:

- A sudden significant rise in blood pressure
- Nausea and vomiting
- Pounding occipital headache
- Stiff neck
- Sweating.

PRESENTATIONS

Common settings include psychiatric wards and A&E.

MANAGEMENT

- Treat immediately.

- Give α-adrenergic blocker such as phentolamine 5 mg intravenously and repeat as necessary, *or* phenoxybenzamine 100 mg in an intravenous drip over an hour.
- Alternative treatment includes asking the patient to bite a 10 mg capsule of nifedipine and swallow the contents with water. Repeat as necessary.
- Consult and involve medical colleagues in the management.

ANTIDOPAMINERGICS: ACUTE SIDE EFFECTS

AKATHISIA

Described as an inability to stay still (restlessness). This is one of the relatively early side effects of typical antipsychotics and occurs in approximately 4% of patients. It may be subjective, where the patient usually complains of an uncomfortable inner feeling or urge to move, but it is often objectively seen as an inability of the patient to stay still, and is described as motor restlessness. It is often distressing and may lead to attempted self-harm; curiously, it is worst in the afternoons.

PRESENTATION

- Commonly in a psychiatric ward
- The patient may come to casualty having recently been prescribed a typical antipsychotic.

MANAGEMENT

- Extremely difficult to treat
- Anticholinergics (procyclidine) often do not help
- Reduce the dose of typical antipsychotic or switch to an atypical one, such as olanzapine, or other low-potency antipsychotic such as thioridazine.

The following treatments may be tried but are not always effective:

- Low-dose β-blockers such as propranolol 5–30 mg t.d.s.
- Low-dose diazepam 2–5 mg t.d.s.

ACUTE DYSTONIA

Dystonias can be described as a brief or prolonged muscle contractions which may lead to abnormal movements or postures. They include an oculogyric crisis, tongue protrusion, torticollis, trismus, laryngopharangeal dystonia, and various dystonic postures of the limbs and the trunk. Commonly they result from typical antipsychotics, and young men under 30 appear to be particularly susceptible.

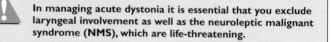

> **In managing acute dystonia it is essential that you exclude laryngeal involvement as well as the neuroleptic malignant syndrome (NMS), which are life-threatening.**

PRESENTATION

The most common presentation is likely to be a young man having his first dose of a high-potency typical neuroleptic on a psychiatric ward. The patient may also present in A&E or other wards. **Remember**, some non-psychiatric medications may also cause dystonia; these include:

- Antiemetics such as prochlorperazine (Stemetil)
- Antimalarials
- Levodopa
- Phenytoin (at toxic levels).

Conversion disorder and malingering are also diagnostic possibilities.

When dealing with the assessment ask about:

- The presence of breathing difficulties (suggesting laryngeal involvement)
- Tremor, fever (possibility of NMS)
- Vital signs (if practical)
- Identity of neuroleptics or other medications taken
- Details regarding rigidity (the part of the body where it began, sudden or gradual onset)
- Any other medical problem.

MANAGEMENT

Where dystonia leads to **breathing difficulties, abnormal vital signs** and **severe distress** it is essential that you attend immediately. If this is not possible, it may be prudent to advise on treatment prior to your arrival.
    Urgent treatment includes:

- Procyclidine 5–10 mg i.m.
- Benzotropine 2 mg.

In addition:

- Mild forms not involving laryngeal or pharyngeal muscles may be treated orally with procyclidine 5–10 mg or benzotropine 1–3 mg
- Avoid the causative drug in future
- Exclude NMS.

NEUROLEPTIC MALIGNANT SYNDROME (NMS)

This is a relatively rare (estimated incidence 0.5–2%) but particularly lethal condition, with a mortality rate that can rise to 20%. It is associated with high-potency antipsychotics (usually typical) and can occur within hours or months after the initial exposure. However, frequently this happens within the first few days of starting or increasing the dose: it is essential to consider it a medical emergency and attempt to exclude it.

The syndrome usually varies in its presentation and shows some overlap with other severe extrapyramidal syndromes, e.g. acute lethal catatonia. Its progression is, however, rapid, and approximately 40% of sufferers develop medical complications.

Essential features include:

- Fever, which may be mild
- Altered consciousness (such as in delirium)
- Autonomic instability, e.g. tachycardia, labile or unstable blood pressure, sweating, pallor and increase in respiratory rate
- Muscular rigidity not relieved by anticholinergics.

The following may also be present:

- Sialorrhoea
- Akinesia, bradykinesia
- Dyskinesia
- Dysphasia, dysarthria, dysphagia
- Other neurological features, such as ataxia, nystagmus and seizures.

Laboratory findings include:

- Grossly elevated creatinine phosphokinase (CPK): *this is the key finding*
  Note: repeated i.m. injections may also raise CPK levels
- Leucocytosis
- Increased potassium; low calcium, magnesium and iron
- Raised ESR
- Proteinuria; myoglobinuria
- EEG – excessive slow waves
- Lumbar puncture (LP) and MRI are usually negative, but may be needed to exclude other diagnostic possibilities.

RISK/PREDISPOSING FACTORS

- Young males (male:female ratio 2:1)
- Organic brain syndromes such as dementia, mental retardation, neurological disorders

- Physical exhaustion (e.g. agitated patient) and dehydration
- Affective disorders; MAOIs
- Patient new to antipsychotics
- High-potency/dose antipsychotics, e.g, high-dose haloperidol, high-potency phenothiazines and long-acting fluphenazines.

Note: Symptoms may develop over a 24–72-hour period and can last for 5–10 days after the last oral dose, and up to 30 days with depot injections.

CLARIFICATION OF THE REFERRAL

Both nursing and medical staff should be given information regarding this condition and why answers to the following questions are needed:

- Vital signs and their lability?
- An increase in temperature or the presence of fever?
- What were the current medications at onset, particularly neuroleptics?
- Onset of symptoms – sudden or gradual?
- Other medical and psychiatric disorders?
- Use of recent repetitive i.m. injections?

NMS is a medical emergency and prompt attendance is essential. Ask about the following:

- Vital signs, such as pulse, respiratory rate and blood pressure
- Temperature.

ASSESSMENT

- Medical/neurological – repeated checking of vital signs
- MSE (this varies)
- Laboratory investigations (see above and below).

The assessment should attempt to elicit the symptoms and signs described above and an attempt should be made to exclude other conditions.

Pay attention to the presence of:

- Autonomic instability
- Hypothermia
- Rigidity – leadpipe or cogwheel
- Mental state variation.

Note: Variation of NMS can occur with the presence of only one or two features.

Ask for **urine samples** for proteinuria and myoglobinuria. Send off blood for **urgent** creatinine phosphokinase (CPK), urea and electrolytes, and full blood count.

Management of NMS

- Have a high index of suspicion for this condition
- Stop neuroleptics
- Involve medical colleagues urgently
- Need to explain to nurses the seriousness of the condition and the need for accurate physical monitoring:
  — Temperature
  — BP, PR
  — Respiratory rate
  — Neurological observations every 15–30 min initially
- Cool and hydrate (may need i.v. hydration)
- Supportive treatment is required, depending on the degree of autonomic instability
- Transfer to ITU if clinical state worsens
  (for treatment of hypothermia, dehydration and cardiovascular support)
- Dialysis may be needed
- Drug prescribed (limited success)
  — Bromocriptine 7.5–60 mg daily
  — Dantrolene 0.8–2.5 mg/kg i.v. every 6 hours
  — Lorazepam i.v. (as second line treatment if above fails)
- ECT (in rare circumstances)
- History of NMS is not an absolute contraindication for the reintroduction of antipsychotics in the future. This should be done cautiously (with advice from senior colleagues) and it is better to use low-potency, different class of drugs or newer antipsychotics. This condition has a high recurrence rate.

For a comparison between iatrogenic syndromes in psychiatric practice see Table 6.4.

TABLE 6.4 Comparison of iatrogenic syndromes in psychiatric practice

	5-HT syndrome	Neuroleptic malignant syndrome	Central anticholinergic syndrome
Core symptoms	Variable temperature elevations (37.4–42.5°C)	Hyperthermia	Hyperthermia
	Mental state changes	Severe muscle rigidity (usually 'leadpipe')	Decreased sweating
	Hypomania	Diaphoresis	Hot, dry skin
	Restlessness	Delirium	Dilated, sluggish pupils
	Myoclonus	Muteness	Tachycardia
	Hyperreflexia	Incontinence	Constipation
	Diaphoresis	Rhabdomydysis	Urinary retention
	Shivering/teeth chattering	Mutism	Confusion
	Tremor	Autonomic instability (fluctuating blood pressure, pallor/flushing)	Impaired memory
	Diarrhoea		Delirium
	Incoordination	Most common temporal sequence: mental state	Hallucinations

TABLE 6.4 Comparison of iatrogenic syndromes in psychiatric practice *(contd)*

	5-HT syndrome	Neuroleptic malignant syndrome	Central anticholinergic syndrome
		change, rigidity, autonomic dysfunction, hypertermia	
Laboratory findings	No specific findings	Elevated CPK, WBC, LFTs, myoglobinuria	No specific findings

Adapted with permission from R. W. Pies, 1998. Handbook of Essential Psychopharmacology, American Psychiatric Press, Washington, D.C.

OTHER POSSIBLE MEDICAL PROBLEMS ON PSYCHIATRIC WARDS

- Cardiac arrest
- Chest pains
- Asthma attack
- Diabetic ketoacidosis
- Seizures
- Headaches
- Blood pressure changes
- Fever
- Unexplained physical symptoms.

While looking after psychiatric patients you may face some of the 'purely' medical problems listed above. The management is likely to vary with your particular experience/expertise and the availability of resources (investigative equipment, particular drugs, i.v. fluids and suitably qualified nurses). You will be expected to have at least some basic knowledge of investigations and management strategies.

It is essential that you think of and try to exclude life-threatening disorders, as well as consulting suitable experts at the earliest. It is always better to err on the side of caution.

Many psychiatric units run regular courses for cardiopulmonary resuscitation: you are strongly advised to attend these and continue to refresh your basic medical training.

CHAPTER 7

LEGAL ISSUES AND THE MENTAL HEALTH ACT

Nominated deputies 272

Definitions in the Mental
Health Act 1983 272

Civil sections 273

Assessment of patients 277

Forensic sections 278

Hospital orders (Section 37) 281

Mental Health Act
Commission 282

Mental Health Review
Tribunal 282

Other legal issues 284

Writing a psychiatric
report 287

Mental health legislation
in Scotland 293

Mental health legislation
in Northern Ireland 294

Mental health legislation
in Eire 295

Legislation in the USA, Canada,
Australia and New Zealand 296

In England and Wales the Mental Health Act (1983) encompasses both civil and forensic sections for dealing with individuals with mental disorder. It is important for the trainee psychiatrist to become familiar with certain sections of the Act that are relevant to clinical work.

It should be stated that at the time of writing plans are under way to introduce a new version of the Mental Health Act for England and Wales. Details are not yet available. It is believed that it would resemble the laws in Scotland and that the time of detention would be shortened, with judicial checks performed regularly and for each extension of detention.

NOMINATED DEPUTIES

Trainees can be appointed as nominated deputies by their consultants, who are the responsible medical officers (RMO) for their patients.

When two trainees swap their duties it should be shown on the hospital duty roster or noticeboard. Wards and switchboard also need to be informed, because in law the nominated deputy is the one officially named on the duty roster.

DEFINITIONS IN THE MENTAL HEALTH ACT 1983

Mental disorder is defined in the Mental Health Act as:

- Mental illness (itself undefined)
- Arrested or incomplete development of the mind
- Psychopathic disorder
- Any other disorder or disability of mind.

Detention under the Mental Health Act 1983 depends on the presence of mental disorders described in the Act and the need to detain the patient in hospital for their health and safety or for the protection of others. Dependence on alcohol or drugs, sexual deviation, promiscuity and immoral conduct are excluded as grounds for detention.

For a short-term section the presence of mental disorder is sufficient as a reason for detention.

For long-term sections the type of mental disorder must be distinguished from one of the following four categories:

- Mental illness
- Psychopathic disorder
- Mental impairment
- Severe mental impairment.

Mental impairment or **severe mental impairment** alone does not qualify for detention: it must be associated with seriously irresponsible conduct or abnormally aggressive behaviour.

Under the Mental Health Act mental impairment is defined as significant impairment of intellectual and social functioning, associated with aggressive and irresponsible conduct. In severe mental impairment the term significant is replaced by severe. No reference is made to IQ in the Mental Health Act, but this is usually 50–70 in mild mental impairment and below 50 in severe mental impairment.

Psychopathic disorder is also understood in behavioural terms. It is defined as 'a persistent disorder or disability of mind, whether or not including significant impairment of intelligence, which results in abnormally aggressive or seriously irresponsible conduct.'

This is a legal definition and can include all types of personality disorders, not just antisocial or psychopathic personality disorders.

In the Mental Health Act, for treatment orders, e.g. sections 3 and 37, the inclusion of the 'treatability' clause for psychopathic disorder and mental impairment is significant. In these cases the patient should only be detained if treatment is likely to alleviate or prevent a deterioration of the condition.

CIVIL SECTIONS (Table 7.1)

SECTION 5(2)

- Section 5(2) is an **emergency holding section** only. It does not give authority to treat, except in urgent situations.
- It is **only** for those who are **already admitted** to a psychiatric unit or ward.
- It is **not applicable** in the A&E or the outpatient department, or the day hospital.
- It is valid **up to 72 hours**.
- It is generally regarded as good practice for the consultant on call or the RMO to be consulted before applying the section.
- Appropriate psychiatric assessment should be carried out and patient's intentions must be assessed and recorded in detail before Section 5(2) is considered.
- Patients should not be threatened with being sectioned as this is considered coercive. Section 5(2) should only be applied on sound clinical grounds, ideally after consultation with the RMO.
- The patient will usually be in need of continued supervision as an inpatient. For them to leave the ward/unit is unlikely to be appropriate.

TABLE 7.1 Civil treatment orders under Mental Health Act 1983 (England and Wales)

Civil treatment order under Mental Health Act 1983	Grounds	Application by	Medical recommendations	Maximum duration	Eligibility for appeal to Mental Health Review Tribunal	Discharge
Section 5(2) Urgent detention of voluntary in-patient	Danger to self or to others		Doctor in charge of patient's care, or nominated deputy	72 hours		Discharge after 72 hours unless section applied
Section 5(4) Nurses holding power of voluntary in-patient	Mental disorder (danger to self or others)	Registered mental nurse or registered nurse for mental handicap	None	6 hours		Cases on approval of section 3
Section 2 Admission for assessment	Mental disorder	Nearest relative or approved social worker	Two doctors (one approved under Section 12)	28 days	Within 14 days	RMO Hospital managers Nearest relatives can be overridden by doctors if necessary
Section 3 Admission for treatment	Mental illness, psychopathic disorder, mental impairment, severe mental impairment	Nearest relative or approved social worker	Two doctors (one approved under Section 12)	6 months	Within first 6 months. If renewed, within second 6 months, then every year. Mandatory every 3 years.	As for Section 2 MHRT

(contd)

TABLE 7.1 Civil treatment orders under Mental Health Act 1983 (England and Wales) (contd)						
Civil treatment order under Mental Health Act 1983	Grounds	Application by	Medical recommendations	Maximum duration	Eligibility for appeal to Mental Health Review Tribunal	Discharge
	(If psychopathic disorder or mental impairment, treatment must be likely to alleviate or prevent deterioration)					
Section 4 Emergency admission for assessment	Mental disorder (urgent necessity)	Nearest relative or approved social worker	Any doctor	72 hours		After 72 hours unless Section 2 applied
Section 136 Admission by police	Mental disorder	Police officer	Allows patient in public place to be removed to 'place of safety'	72 hours		Cases after applied on non application of other section max 72 hours
Section 135	Mental disorder	Magistrates	Allows power of entry to home and removal of patient to place of safety	72 hours		

SECTION 5(4)

- This is the **nurse holding power**.
- It is used when a doctor/RMO or nominated deputy is not available and the patient, who should remain as an inpatient for his health and safety or the protection of others, is trying to leave hospital.
- This section can only last up to **6 hours**.
- In urgent situations the common law may be used to detain the patient in his or her best interests, if the use of Section 5(4) is not possible.

SECTION 2

ADMISSION FOR ASSESSMENT

- Recommendation is by two doctors, one of whom is Section 12(2) approved, usually a psychiatrist who has obtained at least the MRCPsych.
- Application is made by an approved social worker, but the nearest relative may also apply. Only in exceptional circumstances should the nearest relative be asked to make the application. It is normal practice for an approved social worker (ASW) to make the application.
- The psychiatric condition must be a mental disorder.
- Detention is up to 28 days. Termination of this section is through the patient's discharge or conversion to Section 3.
- The patient can appeal to the Mental Health Review Tribunal within 14 days.

Trainee psychiatrists cannot make recommendations under Section 2 unless they are Section 12(2) approved, but may do so if the second doctor is Section 12(2) approved. It is good practice that junior trainees do not do Section 2 recommendations, but for a consultant or senior trainee (SR/SpRs) to do so. This section is applied for assessment of the patient's mental state as an inpatient for up to 28 days.

It is not a treatment order. Treatment is given only when necessary or with the patient's consent.

- The diagnosis may not be clear.
- Admission is necessary for assessment of the patient's mental state, in their best interests, and for the safety of others.
- The section is usually applied when either the patient is not known to the service, or there is a significant change in their previous condition. In practice many patients are known to the service.

SECTION 3

ADMISSION FOR TREATMENT

- Medical recommendations are given by two doctors, one of whom is Section 12(2) approved.

- Application is made by the approved social worker (ASW), or the nearest relative.
- It is necessary in this case that the nearest relative is consulted, if possible.
- The psychiatric condition under which the person is detained is mental illness or severe mental impairment, psychopathic disorder or mental impairment.
- Detention is up to 6 months, renewable for a further 6 months, then at yearly intervals. It is terminated when the patient is discharged or remains in the hospital informally. An appeal to the Mental Health Review Tribunal (MHRT) can be made either by the patient or his nearest relative, or through the automatic appeals procedure via hospital managers. This becomes mandatory if 3 years elapse under Section 3.
- This is a section normally recommended by a consultant/RMO or involved SR/SpR who is Section 12(2) approved. A Section 12(2)-approved GP may also initiate Section 3.
- For both Section 2 and Section 3 two medical recommendations must be given to the ASW who makes the application. Once the application is made the section is considered to be in force.
- The patient is usually known to the service and inpatient treatment is considered necessary in their best interests.
- The patient may have been on Section 2 and an assessment completed, with the recommendation that the patient should be treated under Section 3.

SECTION 4

- This is applied for **emergency admission**.
- It can be recommended by any doctor.
- Application is made by an approved social worker or the nearest relative.
- The type of mental disorder that necessitates this emergency admission does not need to be specified.
- Its duration is 72 hours.
- It is terminated by the patient's discharge from the section or conversion to Section 2 or 3.
- There are technically no appeal procedures, but the patient may appeal to managers or have recourse to the courts.
- If two doctors are not immediately available or there is a significant delay in obtaining a second medical recommendation, and the patient's condition warrants immediate admission.

ASSESSMENT OF PATIENTS

The following should be taken into consideration when assessing a patient for a section of the MHA.

- The mental state of the individual
- A substantiated history
- Is the individual under the influence of alcohol or other substances?
- The social circumstances of the individual
- Whether the patient is in danger of harming himself or/and others?
- Whether the patient is causing serious management problems in the community, to his relatives and carers?
- Is the patient deteriorating, and what is the impact of such a deterioration on family/community?
- Is it in the patient's interest to be detained?
- What impact will detention have on the future of the individual?

Complete a detailed mental state assessment and apply the section in consultation with the consultant (RMO).

FORENSIC SECTIONS

These are other relevant sections in which compulsory admission is recommended for offenders under Part 3 of the Mental Health Act (see Table 7.2).

SECTION 35

This is a remand for report, where the Magistrates Court or the Crown Court orders admission of the patient for **up to 12 weeks**.

SECTION 36

Remand for treatment which is **up to 12 weeks**; it can only be made by a Crown Court.

SECTION 37 (see p. 281)

Hospital or **guardianship order** which is **up to 6 months**, renewable for another 6 months and thereafter yearly, which can be made by Magistrates or Crown Court for individuals convicted of an imprisonable offence, or under Section 37(3) if charged with such an offence.

SECTION 38

An **interim hospital order** which is valid **up to 12 weeks**, renewable at 28-day intervals for a maximum of 6 months. Magistrates or Crown Courts can make this order.

TABLE 7.2 Forensic treatment orders for mentally abnormal offenders

	Grounds	Made by	Medical recommendations	Maximum duration	Eligibility for appeal to Mental Health Review Tribunal
Section 35 Remand to hospital for report	Mental disorder	Magistrates or Crown Court	Any doctor	28 days. Renewable at 28-days intervals. Maximum 12 weeks	
Section 36 Remand to hospital for treatment	Mental illness, severe mental impairment (not if charged with murder)	Crown Court	Two doctors: one approved under Section 12	28 days. Renewable at 28-days intervals. Maximum 12 weeks	
Section 37 Hospital and guardianship orders	Mental disorder. (If psychopathic disorder or mental impairment must be likely to alleviate or prevent deterioration.) Accused of, or convicted for, an imprisonable offence	Magistrates or Crown Court	Two doctors, one approved under Section 12	6 months. Renewable for further 6 months and then annually	During second 6 months. Then every year. Mandatory every 3 years.
Section 38 Interim hospital order	Mental disorder. For trial of treatment	Magistrates or Crown Court	Two doctors, one approved under Section 12	12 weeks. Renewable at 28-day intervals. Maximum 6 months	None
Section 41 Restriction order	Added to Section 37. To protect public from serious harm	Crown Court	Oral evidence from one doctor	Usually without limit of time. Effect: leave, transfer, or discharge only with consent of Home Secretary	As Section 37

(contd)

TABLE 7.2 Forensic treatment orders for mentally abnormal offenders (contd)

	Grounds	Made by	Medical recommendations	Maximum duration	Eligibility for appeal to Mental Health Review Tribunal
Section 47 Transfer of a sentenced prisoner to hospital	Mental disorder	Home Secretary	Two doctors, one approved under Section 12	Until earliest date of release from sentence	Once in the first 6 months. Then once in the next 6 months. Thereafter, once a year.
Section 48 Urgent transfer to hospital of remand prisoner	Mental disorder	Home Secretary	Two doctors, one approved under Section 12	Until date of trial	Once in the first 6 months. Then once in the next 6 months. Thereafter, once a year.
Section 49 Restriction direction	Added to Section 47 or Section 48	Home Secretary	—	Until end of Section 47 or 48. Effect: leave, transfer or discharge only with consent of Home Secretary	As for Section 47 and 48, to which applied

SECTION 41 (RESTRICTION ORDER)

A restriction on discharge to protect the public from serious harm, added to a Section 37 order. It is a restriction usually **without limit of time**, but may be made for a defined period. It is made by the Crown Court only and requires oral evidence from a psychiatrist in court.

SECTION 49

This is a restriction on discharge which **lapses on the earliest date of release from prison** for a patient who was transferred from prison and admitted to hospital for assessment under Section 47. The Home Secretary makes this order.

SECTION 25/SUPERVISED DISCHARGE ORDER

This is a new addition to the Mental Health (Patients in the Community) Act 1995, and is similar to the guardianship order, Section 7. It does not give the power to impose treatment in the community, e.g. take medication, only to attend for psychiatric treatment. It requires two medical recommendations. The patient should already be on Sections 3, 37, 47 and 48, to be eligible for Section 25. It gives the RMO the power of formal supervision through a key worker in the community, usually a CPN or social worker. The agreement of all agencies involved in the patient's care to make resources available is necessary for Section 25 to be administered effectively. This section is not commonly used, as it has long and tedious paperwork requirements. It does not allow for treatment to be given without consent, and Section 3 must be applied if treatment becomes essential. It is usually dealt with by a consultant and trainees are not usually involved.

HOSPITAL ORDERS (SECTION 37)

These are made by courts for a person with a mental disorder who has committed an imprisonable offence. They are similar to admission and treatment under Section 3, but the individual is not eligible for a Mental Health Review Tribunal in the first 6 months.

The courts must be satisfied by evidence from a doctor or from the hospital managers that a bed is available for the patient.

The RMO/consultant may send the patient on leave of absence or discharge him whenever he sees fit, irrespective of the length of sentence that the court might have imposed in the place of a hospital order. However, Home Office authorization is required if the patient is also made subject to

S41 restrictions, which allow for discharge with conditions of treatment, psychiatric and social worker supervision and specification of place of residence.

SECTION 117

This section of the Act deals with aftercare for those who have been detained under the long-term treatment sections, i.e. Section 3. The Local Authority is required to provide such care to support the patient in the community. GPs and all other professionals involved should always be invited to attend Section 117 meetings, as well as the relatives and the patient.

There is an automatic provision in the section for review, and this should continue as long as there is a need for psychiatric help.

You are quite likely to be asked to attend these meetings for your patients, and it may be your responsibility to ensure that the proceedings are recorded in the case notes.

MENTAL HEALTH ACT COMMISSION

This is an independent body that monitors the application of the Mental Health Act in all cases. It has over 100 part-time members, including lay people, lawyers, doctors, nurses and social workers.

All psychiatric facilities which exercise the Act in the treatment, assessment and detention of patients are visited twice annually, and special hospitals are visited monthly.

The Commission calls upon psychiatrists to act on its behalf when second opinions are required under the Act. It scrutinizes sections and detention documents, and acts to protect the legal rights of detained patients, helping them deal with their complaints. It also produces the Code of Practice of the Mental Health Act.

The visits of the Commission may include formal meetings with staff or informal, patient-oriented visits. It has no clinical jurisdiction.

MENTAL HEALTH REVIEW TRIBUNAL (MHRT)

This is an independent judicial body that has rights of discharge or making other recommendations about detained patients. Its main purpose is to determine the continued need for detention.

Tribunals can **reclassify the type of mental disorder** under which the patient is detained, **make recommendations** about conditions of leave, and **recommend transfer** to another hospital.

The patient has the **right to legal aid**, to commission independent reports and to be represented by a lawyer.

It is the right of each detained patient to have a hearing from the Mental Health Review Tribunal according to rules and regulations. It is up to the managers to arrange the tribunal in accordance with the Mental Health Act.

The tribunal has the power to:

- Discharge patients from the section or, in the case of S41, conditionally discharge
- Defer discharge to enable appropriate arrangements to be made
- Continue the section
- Reclassify the type of mental disorder.

The tribunal consists of the President, a lawyer and, in the case of restricted patients, a QC or a judge; a psychiatrist; and a lay person.

Other people who should attend:

- The RMO (or nominated deputy)
- Social worker
- Relatives or nurses, or other interested parties, may also be allowed to attend the tribunal.

The consultant writes the report and is usually present at the hearing. Junior trainees may also perform these duties, after consultation with senior colleagues and guidance. The psychiatric report must be detailed and appropriate to the occasion. Its main question is, why is it necessary to continue to detain the patient, and to oppose their being treated informally or in the community?

If you have to write a report, bear the following in mind:

- The patient's full history
- Their current mental state
- Reasons for the original detention (avoid jargon)
- Keep the report simple and to the point
- Give clinical reasons why it is recommended that the detention continues.
- Explain why discharge will jeopardize treatment and mental health. This is the main question that the tribunal will discuss.

You may have to appear before the tribunal yourself, and if so defend your report by focusing on the clinical reasons that led to detention and which still require it.

- Only write what you are prepared to defend.
- Only document what you have been formally told by nursing staff, and check that reported entries match your information and are contained in the nursing report.
- Discuss the matter with the social worker and nursing colleagues, and see their reports.

Tribunals do not exist to make you feel awkward: their job is to protect the patient by seeing that the law is followed and legal procedures are carried out. Some may appear adversarial but you should not take comments personally.

- As a professional you may not be cross-examined by patient's legal representative but may be asked to clarify certain points.
- Only the tribunal can ask you questions. Normally, your diagnosis will not be discussed, but again, eleborative questions may be asked.
- You cannot be asked to comment on facts, episodes or research that you have not heard, seen, or had the opportunity to consider, but your opinion may be asked after ample time for preparation.
- Tribunals may not ask you to alter treatment, but may ask questions about your management.

OTHER LEGAL ISSUES

CONSENT TO TREATMENT (Table 7.3)

Consent is 'the voluntary and continuing permission for the patient to receive a particular treatment based on an adequate knowledge of the purpose, the likely effects and risks of that treatment, including the likelihood of its success and any alternatives to it'. The doctor must therefore assess the patient's competence to consent, as well as disclosing sufficient information about the suggested treatment.

Competence is a legal concept exercised through the clinical judgement of the doctor.

The House of Lords has reaffirmed the doctor's duty in common law to provide treatment for an incompetent patient so long as such treatment is in the best interests of the patient.

BEST INTERESTS OF THE PATIENT

If a doctor's practice is in line with the accepted practice of his colleagues and peers, it would generally be considered appropriate and in the best interests of the patient. However, there are cases where the courts have taken a differing view from that of the medical profession.

Disclosure of information by the doctor to the patient about the nature of the treatment, its likely effects and consequences is essential. Such disclosure has been determined by the House of Lords to be one aspect of a 'reasonable level of care'. The doctor is not considered negligent if he discloses information in accordance with standards accepted by a body of skilled and experienced medical people.

TABLE 7.3 Consent to treatment under Mental Health Act 1983. Consent should be both informed and voluntary (implies mental illness, e.g. dementia, does not affect judgement)		
Type of treatment	**Informal**	**Detained**
Urgent	No consent	No consent
Section 57 Irreversible, hazardous or non-established treatments, e.g. psychosurgery (e.g. leukotomy), hormone implants (for sex offenders), surgical operations (e.g. castration)	Consent and second opinion	Consent and second opinion
Section 58 Psychiatric drugs, ECT	Consent	Consent or second opinion

1. For first 3 months of treatment a detained patient's consent is not required for Section 58 medicines, but is for ECT.
2. Patients can withdraw voluntary consent at any time.

For detained patients consent must be obtained under Section 58. For consenting patients the consultant/RMO is required to complete a certificate of consent, which contains a statement that the patient is capable of understanding the nature, the purpose and the likely effects of medication given. **Treatment given for the first 3 months to a detained patient does not require a Section 58 form, or for Section 58 to be applicable**.

For patients detained under section 62 urgent treatment may be given without consent, in good faith, under the duty of care. This means that in an acute emergency modified electroconvulsive therapy **(ECT)** may also be given under S62. This treatment may be given as part of life-saving measures.

In common law, when there is immediate danger to the health or safety of the patient or others, the treatment given must be reasonable and in proportion to the danger.

TESTAMENTARY CAPACITY

This deals with a person's **ability to make a will** and his capacity to understand the nature and effect of the task. Doctors may be called to assess the testamentary capacity of patients who have who have mental disorders or psychiatric history. There are three essential components:

- Does the patient understand the nature and implications of making a will?
- Does he have some appreciation of the extent of his estate?
- Does he appreciate which people may reasonably expect to be beneficiaries (although he may choose to exclude them)?

Individuals with mental disorders can and do make valid wills when there is no evidence that their mental disorder directly impinges on their capacity to do so.

CONFIDENTIALITY OF MEDICAL INFORMATION

All communications between doctors and patients should be confidential. Medical notes are confidential documents, except in certain circumstances when people's lives and safety may be under threat, or when reports are written for the court.

In such cases disclosure is legally defensible.

Patients have a right of access to their case notes, but a doctor may refuse access to all or certain parts of medical records where disclosure may not be in the best interest of the patient or others.

OTHER DUTIES

While on call a psychiatric trainee may be contacted by the police, a police surgeon, or by the GP with a request of an assessment, at the police station, of an individual who is accused of committing a crime or picked up as in need of care (S136). In such circumstances it is important before committing yourself to anything to find out what your hospital's policy is for dealing with such situations.

Usually it is the consultant on call or the specialist registrar (SpR)/senior registrar (SR) who carries out the assessment in the police cells. Normally, experienced police sergeants, aware of these protocols, inform the police surgeon and the approved social worker (ASW). ASWs coordinate such assessments by contacting the consultant (RMO)/SR/SpR on call.

Junior trainees should not be expected to assess cases that require more experienced and senior attendance. If in doubt, contact the on call consultant/ SR/SpR, who will normally respond.

MEDICAL DEFENCE COVER

It is important that you join a **private medical defence body**, such as the Medical Defence Union, Medical Protection Society etc. Sensitive cases may require giving of evidence and may involve the trainee in legal proceedings which are not always covered by Crown indemnity, e.g. prison assessments. It is believed that doctors involved in enquiries are better represented by their medical defence bodies than by Trust solicitors. If you are in doubt about any of the legal aspects of sections, or demands made by managers, staff or even colleagues, it is prudent to consult your defence union.

COURT DIVERSION SCHEMES

Many health authorities now have court diversion schemes designed to divert mentally disordered people out of the criminal justice system. They work in different ways, and there may be a professional available daily or weekly sitting in the courts. Referrals are taken from magistrates or lawyers, and sometimes from the police. Cases are also identified from those awaiting court appearance.

THE COMMON LAW

This allows professionals to treat patients urgently, in their best interests, especially when the patient is either incompetent or refusing consent. For very invasive but non-life threatening situations, such as planned operations, it is better to seek legal advice, e.g. thorough Trust solicitors. In an emergency always act to save the patient's life, whatever the circumstances, e.g. following an overdose when the patient refuses medical treatment.

Normally treatment of patients is protected by common law: it is presumed that when the patient comes voluntarily to the doctor and when the doctor examines the patient, consent is implied; otherwise it would be an assault. When giving ECT to a patient who is not detained, consent should be and usually is acquired in writing. If the patient changes his or her mind the treatment cannot be given.

> ⚠️ **Patients must never be threatened with detention under the Mental Health Act, to encourage informal admission or consent to treatment. This constitutes coercion and is unlawful.**

WRITING A PSYCHIATRIC REPORT

A patient under your care may be involved in legal proceedings, whether of a criminal nature or not, and you may be asked to write a psychiatric report. The request for the report may come from number of parties, including:

- a court of law
- solicitors acting for that individual or the prosecution services
- probation services
- social services
- employers

Prior to writing a report

- Seek advice and guidance from your senior colleagues (e.g. your consultant) before agreeing to provide the report.
- Specific questions may be asked. Read and address these carefully.
- Communicate with the person who has asked for the report, for clarification of medical, legal and other issues in question.
- Payment of your fees for the report should be clarified in advance, since this is usually not part of your duties and you are not indemnified against any cases ensuing from your legal report. However, it may be indemnified by your consultant's protection policy if it has been prepared under the guidance and supervision of your consultant.
- Do not write reports if you are not protected by a medical defence body.
- Seek written permission from the patient for disclosing your opinion to the involved parties, e.g. the courts.
- Always assess the patient and carry out a comprehensive examination before writing the report.
- Give the opinion about the diagnosis. Try to avoid jargon and if using medical or technical terms provide meanings, which could be understood by a lay person.
- Discuss treatment and services available.
- Discuss prognosis.

If you feel that you are unable to or do not have sufficient experience in order to write the report, then ask the referrer to write to a more appropriate person.

A FRAMEWORK FOR A PSYCHIATRIC REPORT PREPARED AT THE REQUEST OF A SOLICITOR

PSYCHIATRIC REPORT ON: DATE:

Date of Birth

Home Address

Prison Number

I have prepared this report at the request of (name of solicitors).
For the preparation of the report I conducted an interview with (Patient's name) at (location) on (date).

Prior to interviewing (Patient's name), I had access to a number of documents provided by (solicitors) which were as follows:

1. Defendant's proof of evidence.
2. Advance disclosures.
3. Interview transcripts.
4. Recent discharge summary from (name of psychiatric hospital).

I understand that (Patient's name) is charged with the offence of (name of offence) and is currently on remand at (location).
He has entered a Guilty/not Guilty plea.

At the interview I informed (Patient's name) and he understood that I would be preparing a report for the Court, and that any discussion we had would not be confidential.

At the time of the interview (Patient's name) was not receiving any medication and informed me that no alcohol or illicit substances had been taken.

(The patient) appeared to comprehend the purpose and nature of our interview and took part willingly.

BACKGROUND

Describe defendant's background.

FAMILY HISTORY

Give relevant details of parents and siblings and the relationships.

FAMILY PSYCHIATRIC HISTORY

Family history of either psychiatric disorder or criminal behaviour if any.

PERSONAL HISTORY

Describe birth, developmental history, early and late childhood. Describe any significant events (death, divorce of parents, abuse, etc.) and their impact.

Educational and occupational record.

PSYCHOSEXUAL HISTORY

Give an account of the development of significant relationships, and any known sexual problems.

→

Consider particularly whether the accused shows a capacity to develop long-term relationships.

PREVIOUS FORENSIC HISTORY

List and describe record of previous convictions. Comment on the development of criminal behaviour, response to previous probation orders, previous hospitalizations under the Mental Health Act following conviction.

Describe if there is any indication of the development of a particular type of offence, and whether there is any indication of previous dangerous behaviour.

Describe particularly any offences involving the use of violence, weapons, or sexual offences.

Describe premorbid personality

PREVIOUS PSYCHIATRIC HISTORY

Account for previous admissions to hospital, whether informal, under Civil Sections, or following criminal conviction. If known, comment on response to treatment, and compliance with treatment following discharge.

HISTORY OF ALCOHOL CONSUMPTION AND ILLICIT SUBSTANCE USAGE

Account of use of alcohol and or use of illicit drugs and any evidence of dependency.

Describe if there have been periods of abstinence, dependency and whether any treatment had been successful.

Use of alcohol/illicit drugs and its relationship with criminal behaviour.

MEDICAL HISTORY

Account of any medical history, emphasizing particularly any history of head injury, epilepsy.

DRUG HISTORY

Account of all prescribed drugs and their use.

SOCIAL HISTORY

Account of occupation, financial status, dwellings and use of social resources.

→

ACCOUNT OF INDEX OFFENCE

It may be omitted if the defendant is pleading not guilty. If the defendant is pleading guilty or has been convicted, the defendant's account of the circumstances of the offence should be given.

Comment on any areas of dispute between the defendant's account, the allegations, and the witness statements. Comment on any evidence of mental disorder and likely mental state (if at all possible) at the time of the alleged offence.

PROGRESS SINCE ARREST

Describe defendant's progress whilst in custody. Comment on evidence of mental disorder, further evidence of violent behaviour, and whether the defendant has been willing or not to accept treatment on a voluntary basis whilst in custody.

Comment also on the results of any special investigations, which may have a bearing on the diagnosis.

MENTAL STATE ON (DATE)

Describe the defendant's mental state when assessed.

Explain any technical terms which are readily understandable to colleagues but may not be clearly understood by the court. Avoid obscure technical terms.

CONCLUSION, OPINION AND RECOMMENDATIONS

Set this out as a series of numbered paragraphs.

Comment on the defendant's fitness to plead and fitness to stand trial.

Comment on the presence of mental disorder within the meaning of the Mental Health Act, specifying the form of disorder (mental illness, mental impairment, severe mental impairment, or psychopathic disorder).

Give psychiatric diagnosis.

Briefly elaborate on the symptomatology of the particular psychiatric disorder the defendant is suffering from, e.g. the defendant suffers from a paranoid schizophrenic illness characterized by the development of persecutory delusions (he believe that others are conspiring to harm him), command type auditory hallucinations (he hears voices which give him instructions).

State if this is a mental disorder for which admission to hospital is or is not appropriate under the terms of the Mental Health Act.

Discuss which hospital is prepared to offer admission and a Hospital Order.

Comment on the likely prognosis.

Conclude the report with a statement of your professional status (SHO/SpR/Lecturer/Medical Research Fellow/Consultant, etc.), and whether or not you are approved under Section 12 of the Mental Health Act.

Sign the report over your typed name, which should be followed by your professional qualifications.

Copies of the report should be sent, with the agreement of the instructing agent, to all relevant parties, which should include normally the Clerk to the Court, the defence Solicitors, the relevant Probation Service, the Prison Medical Service, and the accepting Consultant.

WHAT TO DO WHEN YOU ARE ASKED TO APPEAR BEFORE THE COURT

- Make adequate preparations.
- Seek guidance from experienced colleagues.
- Try to attend court proceedings as an observer well before your own case.
- Take your report and medical records with you and refer to them when necessary.
- Do not contradict your report.
- Remain focused the on psychiatric assessment.
- Do not attempt to make up answers.
- Always address the judge or the jury, never the lawyer asking the question.
- Only narrate facts.
- Numbering the paragraphs in your report assists referral to its contents in court.
- Avoid giving an opinion on any issue outside psychiatry that you know.
- If asked to give an opinion on research or a report that you have not seen or do not know about, ask for time to consider it in order to allow you to respond to it properly at a later stage.
- If a mistake is highlighted in your report ask the judge to allow you to address it, emphasizing that the bulk and purpose of your report was correct.
- If legal representatives challenge your whole report or discredit it by identifying small mistakes or omissions, ask the judge to allow you to respond. Respond by identifying minor points as oversights or mistakes and assert that the psychiatric evidence overall was correct and your opinion stands.

Always prepare theoretically before appearance in court.

MENTAL HEALTH LEGISLATION IN SCOTLAND

The definitions of mental disorder are similar, although there is no formal category of psychopathic disorder. It appears that short-term application of the sections is easier, and that it is the sheriff who decides on long-term sections.

In England and Wales Section 4 is seldom used, but its equivalent in Scotland, Section 24, is commonly used. For comparative sections in Scotland: (see Box and Table 7.4).

MHA Scotland (1984)	MHA England & Wales (1983)		
Section 24 One recommendation by a doctor and the patient's relative or a social worker. No appeal. May be extended to 28 days after second recommendation (S26). Appeal to sheriff.	**Section 4**	**Emergency admission**	**72 hours**
Section 26 Two recommendations. Application by social. worker or nearest relative. Appeal to sheriff.	**Section 2**	**28-day, short-term involuntary admission**	
Section 18 Two recommendations. Approval of sheriff. Reviewed at 28 days, then in the last 6 months for rescinding or renewal. Patient has right to appeal. Nearest relative can authorize discharge. Discharge by consultant.	**Section 3**	**Detention for treatment 6 months**	
Section 118 Removal to a place of safety. Information to responsible person or nearest relative by police.	**Section 136**	**Up to 72 hours**	

TABLE 7.4   Equivalent sections of Scottish and English Mental Health Acts

Treatment order		
Treatment Order	Mental Health (Scotland) 1984	Mental Health (England & Wales) Act 1983
Emergency admission	Section 24	Section 4
Short-term detention	Section 26	Section 2
Admission for treatment	Section 18	Section 3
Nurses holding power of a voluntary inpatient	Section 25(2) for 2 h	Section 5(4) (for 6 hours)
Guardianship	Section 37	Section 37
Committal to hospital pending trial	Sections 25 & 330 of the 1975 Act	Section 36
Remand for enquiry into mental condition	Sections 180 & 381 of the 1975 Act	Section 35
Removal to hospital of persons in prison awaiting trial or sentence	Section 70	Section 48
Interim hospital order	Sections 174a & 375a of the 1975 Act amended by the Mental Health (Amendment) (Scotland) Act 1983	Section 38
Hospital order	Sections 175 & 376 of the 1975 Act	Section 37
Restriction order	Sections 178 & 379 of the 1975 Act	Section 41
Transfer of prisoner under sentence to hospital	Section 71	Section 47

The Scottish Mental Welfare Commission does the work of the English Mental Health Act Commission and the Mental Health Review Tribunals. Those who are in the criminal justice system are dealt with by the Mental Health (Scotland) Act 1984 and the Criminal Procedure (Scotland) Act 1975.

MENTAL HEALTH LEGISLATION IN NORTHERN IRELAND

Mental illness and medical treatment are defined in the Mental Health Act (Northern Ireland) Order 1986.

Mental illness is an abnormality in emotions, perception, thinking and judgement that requires, in the interest of the person and others, care and medical treatment. This is defined as nursing and other care under medical supervision.

Detention applied by registered nurses lasts up to 48 hours; applied by a junior doctor up to 72 hours; and applied by psychiatrists can be for 6 months.

Mental handicap, severe mental handicap and mental impairment are defined; it is also stated that no person should be treated as suffering from mental disorder if he or she is suffering only from personality disorder, promiscuity or other immoral conduct, sexual deviancy, or abuse of alcohol and drugs.

Some features of the order include:

- Compulsory admission for assessment for up to 14 days before being admitted for treatment (Part II of the order).
- Temporary holding powers (6 hours by RMN and 48 hours by a doctor) are similar to those in the English and Scottish Acts.
- Patients may be detained for up to 6 months (renewable for a further 6 months and then annually, subject to independent approval) should they be diagnosed as suffering from mental illness or severe mental impairment and at high risk of serious physical harm to self or others.
- Provisions for consent to treatment and guardianship are similar to those in the English Act.
- Provisions similar to those in the English Act also exist for individuals involved in criminal proceedings.
- The Mental Health Commission, in addition to covering those detained and suffering with a mental disorder, also deals with voluntary patients, people on guardianship and those in residential accommodation.

Other aspects, e.g. consent, medication renewal, etc., are similar to the Mental Health Act 1983 of England and Wales.

MENTAL HEALTH LEGISLATION IN EIRE

THE MENTAL TREATMENT ACT 1945

Civil mental health matters are dealt with by the above Act. Compulsory detention for treatment takes two forms:

- **Temporary certification (under S184–189)** The mentally ill (including addict) person is adjudged to require hospital treatment and is unfit to be treated as a voluntary patient. Temporary certification requires an application from the nearest relative (or social worker, if the relative is unavailable or unwilling) and two medical recommendations, one of which is the receiving consultant. It may last up to 6 months initially and can be renewed.

- **Detention of a person of unsound mind (under S162–163)** This is rarely used nowadays. It is applied when 'there is a reason to believe that a person is of unsound mind, is a proper person to be taken charge of and detained under care and treatment, and is likely to recover within 6 months from the date of such examination'. It requires an application from a relative, one other person with knowledge of the patient, and two medical recommendations, one of which is the receiving consultant.

A detained patient can appeal to the Minister of Health (who is empowered to have the Inspector of Mental Hospitals investigate the circumstances of the case), or can initiate legal proceedings seeking their release. The statutory review of the organization and running of the mental hospital is undertaken by the Inspector of Mental Hospitals, who reports to the Minister of Health.

THE CRIMINAL JUSTICE SYSTEM IN IRELAND

Currently Irish law does not have provisions to divert someone away from the criminal justice system once arrested and charged, including those who are considered mentally ill or disordered at the time of arrest.

SECTION 165 OF THE CURRENTLY APPLICABLE IRISH MENTAL HEALTH LEGISLATION (MENTAL TREATMENT ACT 1945)

This allows a policeman to remove a person 'believed to be of unsound mind' from a public place to a police station, where this is believed necessary for the safety of the public or the mentally ill person. This may lead to an urgent psychiatric assessment.

There are no legislative provisions to allow the transfer of an individual on remand to a district psychiatric hospital for assessment or treatment. The only option available following remand in custody is for the accused to be transferred to the Central Mental Hospital, Dundrum (the only specifically forensic psychiatric institution in the country).

LEGISLATION IN USA, CANADA, AUSTRALIA AND NEW ZEALAND

USA

There are different laws in different states in the USA. The practice of detention under such legislation is called 'certifying'. The current emphasis is whether or not the patient is a danger to him or herself and others. As in the UK patient confidentiality can be compromised and a patient detained if he or she is dangerous. A psychiatrist applies the regulations by certifying the patient and subsequent extensions are subject to legal review. There are panels and boards that review cases under detention.

CANADA

In Canada legislation is similar to that in the USA. Provinces have different criteria and policies for detaining people under the mental health regulations. Patients are certified and there are review boards that oversee the detentions. These are constituted by the provincial government.

AUSTRALIA AND NEW ZEALAND

Here the law is similar to the UK regulations but is updated according to provincial requirements. The provincial Mental Health Acts of 1986 and 1990 are the basis of such practices.

APPENDICES

Descriptive
psychopathology   300

Classification in psychiatric
practice: ICD-10 and
DSM-IV   311

DESCRIPTIVE PSYCHOPATHOLOGY

ABNORMAL BEHAVIOUR

This can be subdivided into:

- Underactivity
- Overactivity
- Bizarre behaviour.

UNDERACTIVITY

A decrease in activity compared to what is considered normal and the usual activity of the patient, determined by a detailed past history, consists of:

- **Retardation**, which may be due to depressive illness. The patient becomes slow in active movements and in all other faculties.
- **Obsessional slowness**, caused by doubts about a particular action, which is made difficult to carry out by obsessional vacillations and abnormal indecisiveness.
- **Stupor**, an extreme of retardation normally defined in neurological illness as responsiveness only to loud sounds, pain and occasional monosyllabic sounds. It consists of lack of movement and diminished responsiveness. In psychiatry it may occur in depressive disorders, catatonia, hysteria and mania, which may be accompanied by periods of excitement.

OVERACTIVITY

- **Manic overactivity** is characterized by incessant physical movement owing to excessive energy experienced by the patient.
- **Depressive agitation** is seen when depressive disorder leads to undirected psychomotor restlessness.
- **Anxious overactivity** is due to subjective feelings of anxiety, leading to purposeless excessive activity, accompanied by other features of anxiety.
- **Hyperkinesis** is usually found in children and is usually accompanied by overactivity, impulsivity and excitability.
- **Obsessional overactivity** may take various forms. It may not appear as overt overactivity, but may be excessive with regard to specific behaviours, e.g. excessive checking, drinking, gambling. cleaning, counting etc.

BIZARRE MOVEMENTS AND POSTURES

- **Mannerisms and stereotypy** are present in many psychiatric disorders. They appear to be similar in presentation, but the difference is that mannerisms are repetitive, involuntary, purposive, goal-directed actions, whereas stereotypies are repetitive, fixed, non-goal directed and apparently purposeless.

- **Echopraxia** is imitative automatic repetition of movements, carried out by the patient despite requests by the psychiatrist/assessor to cease them.
- **Ambitendency** is characterized by repetitive, incomplete, voluntary movements while trying to carry out an action.
- **Catatonic phenomena** consist of waxy flexibility, posturing, tremor, phantom phenomena, negativism, automatic obedience and catatonic frenzy.
  — **Waxy flexibility** is characterized by waxlike moulding of the posture: the patient is unable to resist the 'moulding' by the examiner and maintains the made postures, despite wishing not to do so.
  — **Posturing** is described as the maintenance of abnormal, inappropriate postures for long periods, such as hours or days, without apparent control over bodily movements.
  — **Tremor** in catatonia is reflected as shaking of the hands and other parts of the body.
  — **Phantom phenomena** are the adoption of postures, as if something were supporting the body. The patient may keep the head above the bed, as if supported by a pillow but without a pillow, for long periods. They may similarly adopt postures with the legs or the trunk, as if supported by some object.
  — **Negativism** is inappropriate, purposeless resistance against attempts to be moved, either verbally or physically.
  — **Automatic obedience** is the opposite of negativism, where the patient follows a verbal or physical command in a tentative, involuntary manner.
  — **Catatonic frenzy** is undirected, incessant, purposeless physical activity, which may appear as running in circles, turning round and round, or shaking the body while uttering bizarre sounds of excitement. Sometimes inappropriate aggressive actions may also occur.
- **Compulsive behaviours** may sometimes appear bizarre. They may include dressing or undressing rituals; rituals before any movements, e.g. writing, going to work, walking on lines or squares, touching walls at precise intervals; or any action associated with bizarre, compulsive rituals.
- **Tics** are repetitive, irregular, jerky movements involving one or a collection of muscles. They are very common and may appear as facial or limb movements. One particular syndrome, called Gilles de la Tourette, is characterized by involuntary motor or verbal tics, with obscenities, in some. **Schnauzkraumpf** means making bizarre faces, and is a psychotic feature.
- **Parkinsonism** may be seen in patients taking neuroleptics; its features include:
  — Cogwheel rigidity
  — A festinant gait
  — Postural abnormalities
  — A resting tremor.

SPEECH DISORDERS

Disorders of the **rate of speech** refer to a fast, slow, irregular or interrupted rhythm, or the complete absence of speech. **Irregular** speech may be due to stammering or interruption of the flow of thoughts. The irregularity caused by stammering may be due to the repetition of sounds and words.

- **Dysarthria** is difficulty in articulation.
- **Mutism** is the virtual absence or loss of speech.
- **Dysprosody** is the absence of the normal melody of speech, the ups and downs, and the emphasis on words found in normal speech. **Monotonous** speech lacks normal melody.

These disorders must be considered in relation to the premorbid history of the patient and cannot be determined entirely on the first examination, unless clearly abnormal.

- **Pressure of speech** describes an increase in the rate and quantity of speech.
- **Disorders of quantity** describe excess or poverty of speech.
  - **Excessive speech** or **logorrhoea** consists of increased, rambling and unnecessary use of words when significantly fewer words could be used.
  - **Poverty of speech**, in contrast, consists of abnormally less use of words that could be appropriate for any given situation. Answers may consist of monosyllables or sounds.

Disorders of the **form of speech** or thought consist of perseverative speech, neologisms, word salad, tangentiality, thought block, loosening of associations, talking past the point **(vorbeireden, vorbeigehen)**, circumstantiality, flight of ideas and desultory thinking.

- **Perseverative speech** describes irrelevant and repetitive speech which continues beyond the point.
- **Palilalia** is repetition of a word, with increasing frequency.
- **Echolalia** is automatic imitation and repetition of sentences or portions of another person's speech.
- **Logoclonia** is imitative repetition of the last syllable or sound uttered by another person.
- **Neologisms** are the creation of new, objectively meaningless words, and may occur in schizophrenia.
- **Word salad** is an inappropriate and incomprehensible mixture of words and phrases which are meaningless.
- **Loosening of associations** includes tangentiality, knight's move thinking and derailment. These are descriptions of loss in the normal flow of speech and thoughts.
  - Thoughts reflected in speech may move suddenly from one direction to another and go off at a tangent, not clearly but oddly related, i.e. **tangentiality**.

    — Thoughts and speech may suddenly change direction to an unrelated one, as in the **knight's move** of chess.

    — **Derailment** occurs when a thought moves on to a less important, less relevant, subsidiary thought.

- **Fusion of thought**, reflected in speech, is the interweaving of contrasting and different ideas.
- **Drivelling** occurs when odd, disordered components are presented as one complex thought.
- **Omissions and substitutions** occur when an integral part of a thought is inappropriately removed and an important part is replaced by an unimportant part, in either speech or thought.
- **Circumstantiality** is the excessive and copious description of trivial detail, but ultimately focusing on the target of thought.
- **Talking past the point (vorbeireden)** is when it appears that the patient is about to reach the point of conversation being talked about, but never actually does so. It is clear that the patient understands the question, but talks past the answer. The other variant of this phenomenon is **vorbeigehen**, when a patient understands the question but gives the wrong answer.
- **Flight of ideas** is reflected by fast speech and ideas moving from topic to topic, connected by rhyming words, punning or clang associations, chance relationships and distractions by environmental stimuli.
- **Thought block** is an abrupt gap in the flow of thoughts, evidenced by silence; the thought is never recalled and the train of previous thoughts is lost.
- **Alexithymia** is considered by some as an emotional disorder, and is characterized by an inability to express inner emotions owing to a subjective lack of awareness of such thoughts.

DISORDERS OF EMOTION

DISORDERS OF AFFECT

Affect is observable behaviour, which change over time in response to changing emotional states, and is the expression of a subjectively experienced emotional state. The following types are described:

- **Inappropriate** or **incongruous**, i.e. not appropriate for the situation and its associated speech or thoughts
- **Labile**, i.e. variable and inappropriate, fluctuating between extremes
- **Blunted:** reduced responsiveness to external stimuli
- **Flat:** there is an absence of expression and response to environmental stimuli.

MOOD DISORDERS

- **'Mood'** refers to a pervasive and sustained emotion which significantly colours one's perception of the world.

- **Diurnal variation** of mood refers to a mood state which is worse in the morning and improves as the day progresses. Mood can also be described as **congruous** (appropriate to situations and feelings, e.g. depression) or **incongruous** (inappropriate to feelings and situations, e.g. schizophrenia).
- **Apathy** is an inability to experience pleasure or other emotions, and is characterized by indifference and detachment.
- **Tension** describes an increase in psychomotor activity which is experienced as unpleasant.
- **Agitation** is inner tension with an increase in purposeless motor activity.
- **Elation** is a state of heightened happiness and wellbeing.
- **Euphoria** is a state of abnormally contented pleasure and indifference.
- **Dysphoria** is unpleasant mood.
- **Dysthymia** is disturbed mood, i.e. low and unhappy.
- **Euthymia** is one's normal and usual mood.
- **Cyclothymia** is changing mood from unhappy to sad.
- **Depression** describes a pervasive and seriously low mood, which may be mild, moderate or severe, causing serious dysfunction in normal life.
- **Irritability** is reduced self-control over anger and negative impulses, and may result in the expression of anger towards others.
- **Anxiety** is a feeling of apprehension or fear due to external or internal stimuli. It may be related to real fear owing to actual danger, and recognized as such. When it is pathological it is due to internal factors not clearly understood, causing dysfunction in life.

DISORDERS OF THE CONTENT OF THOUGHT

These can be subdivided into disorders of **type** and of **intensity**:

- Disorders of **type** consist of **psychotic** and **anxiety-related (neurotic) content**.
- Disorders of **intensity** determine the **severity and degree of morbidity**, whether mild, moderate or severely psychotic or neurotic. These are two criteria against which thought content should be described.

Disorders of **intensity** consist of overvalued ideas and delusions:

- **Overvalued ideas** are intense, unreasonable, alien to the patient's subculture, yet strongly held, with intense emotional investment, but with the acknowledged doubt that they may not be true. The patient tends to live his or her life around the overvalued idea, but it is not as strongly held as a delusion. The difference between them is one of intensity.
- A **delusion** is a falsely developed belief as regards reality, which is firmly held, incorrigible, impervious to reason and contrary to the patient's religious, cultural and educational context. Delusions can be of any type, content or quality, and may have hypochondriacal, compulsive or phobic components. They may be:

— **Primary** or **secondary:** a fully formed delusion occurs without any relation to preceding events. It may be preceded by a **delusional mood (wahnstimmung)**, in which there is a sense of foreboding or bewildering apprehension. Once the delusion surfaces, sometimes associated with delusional perception, the delusional mood disappears. A similar mood state has also been seen prior to the onset of severe neurotic disorders.

- **Mood congruent** or **incongruent:** if the delusion is depressive and so is the mood, then it is a mood-congruent delusion, i.e. the delusion is appropriately related to the mood. When this is not the case it is called mood incongruent.

- The most commonly mentioned delusions are **paranoid** or **delusions of suspicion**. Some other examples are:
    — **Grandiose**, i.e. when the patient believes that he/she is great
    — **Heredity**, when they believe they belong to royalty
    — **Controlling**, i.e. when they believe they have and control supernatural powers, genies, spirits
    — **Spiritual**, **satanic** or **religious**: the patient believes he or she has spiritual or satanic or religious powers, or some form of religious position
    — **Status**, **power:** they may believe they are a powerful entity, or have great status
    — **Infestation:** the patient believes he or she is infested with germs, insects or aliens
    — **Disease:** the patient believes they suffer from a serious disease
    — **Death** or **nihilistic:** believing that he or she is dead, or that parts of the body are dead
    — **Somatic** or bodily functions: believes that body parts are not working properly, or are altered
    — **Being loved** (de Clérambault syndrome): the patient believes that someone, usually of a higher social and financial position, maybe a celebrity, is in love with them without fully realizing it. Letters and contacts are believed to have been received. Any unrelated gesture, even on TV or in the newspapers, from the victim, may be considered as proof of love. Stalking and persistent attempts to contact occur
    — **Recognition:** there are two syndromes, **Capgras** *(illusion de sosies)* and **Fregoli**. Capgras syndrome is when a patient believes that a persecutor or someone else has replaced a person closely known to the patient. Fregoli syndrome describes when the patient believes that the persecutor can change faces: strangers may be recognized as changed persecutors
    — **Change in identity:** it is believed that the patient has a different identity, was swapped at birth, or was someone else
    — **Change in shape:** believes that their body changes shape, or parts of the body have changed

— **Poverty:** patient believes that he or she is poverty stricken, which is not the reality

— **Passivity:** believes they are being controlled by outside powers, waves, etc. May also believe that their thoughts are known by others **(thought broadcasting)**, through radio, TV or newspapers. **Thought insertion:** believes that others are putting thoughts into their mind. **Made actions:** when actions are controlled by others. **Made feelings:** when others control and create feelings in the patient's mind. **Thought withdrawal:** when thoughts are removed from the patient's mind. **Made impulses:** when impulses are believed to be under the control of others

— **Reference:** believes that others are talking about or conspiring against the patient

— **Guilt:** believes he or she is guilty of a crime, when in reality they are not

— **Self-reproach:** blames self for some occurrence which is not true

— **Jealousy** or **Othello syndrome:** believes in the infidelity of a spouse, and may become violent

— **Delusional perception:** an abnormal, delusional meaning is attributed to a familiar event, without a logical reason

— **Anxiety-related (neurotic) abnormal thought content** consists of phobias, obsessions, impulses and urges.

A **phobia** is an irrational, out of proportion, intense fear of any situation, leading to avoidance.

There are many types of phobias, named after the situation in which they occur:

● **Agoraphobia** (fear of open places)
● **Claustrophobia** (fear of confined spaces)
● **Acrophobia** (fear of heights)
● **Social phobia** (fear of public or social situations etc.)
● **Specific animal, object or situational phobias** e.g. spiders, snakes, rats, dogs, other animals or insects, dead or alive, as well as fear of strangers.

Hypochondriasis is defined as an unrealistic interpretation of bodily symptoms, resulting in an unfounded fear and preoccupation with serious illness. There is no avoidance, but intense attempts to check and investigate whether a disease is present or not. Reassurance works, albeit temporarily.

Obsessions are recurrent thoughts, owned and considered irrational by the patient; resistance to these thoughts may or may not be present. Common obsessional themes concern contamination, illness, checking, aggression, sex etc. Obsessions are usually accompanied by **compulsions** or **rituals**, which result from an intense wish to act on the obsession. Resistance results in anxiety, which may be relieved temporarily when the action is performed, only to recur later.

DISORDERS OF PERCEPTION

Perceptual disorders are divided into distortions or **illusions**, and **hallucinations**.

Illusions are distortions of actual perceptions, i.e. distorted or altered sensory perceptions with sensory input. Sensory distortions may be:

- **Visual**, i.e. visual perceptions are altered, for example shadows in the fire may become images of people, demons, etc. Light in a room may appear to be an apparition. The colour of the environment may appear changed: if it appears yellow it is called xanthopsia. Similarly, red, black and other colours are given their respective Latin names.
- **Auditory:** auditory perception is altered, e.g. the patient may hear his or her name being called when no-one has actually called. They may hear murmuring, or people talking between themselves, when in a noisy hostile neighbourhood.

With **sensory illusions** there may be a change in perception of bodily sensations, e.g. noises may appear louder or quieter than they actually are. This is known as **hyperacusis** and **hypoacusis**, respectively. **Hyperaesthesia** and **hypoaesthesia** refer to increased or decreased sensations of pain or touch.

Hallucinations are perceptions without any external stimuli, which are perceived as real and objective. In other words, hallucinations are **sensory perceptions without sensory input**. They are perceived to be in external space, real and unchangeable, and may occur in various modalities:

- **Auditory:** patient 'hears' voices talking in the second or third person.
- **Pseudoauditory:** hears voices inside the head. These may have no pathological significance. They occur in subjective space and lack the perception of reality.
- **Hypnagogic:** these occur at the time of falling asleep. They are not pathological. May frequently occur in grief reactions.
- **Hypnapompic:** these occur while one is waking and have the same significance as the former.
- **Visual:** patient sees images, people, objects or other phenomena in objective space. Usually occur in organic brain disease.
- **Autoscopy:** patient sees a mirror image, being able to step outside his body.
- **Extracampine:** awareness of the presence of someone (persecutor) who is outside their field of vision.
- **Reflex:** a sensation in one field leads to hallucinations in another, e.g. seeing cars may lead to hearing voices.
- **Tactile:** sensations of insects crawling or other superficial bodily hallucinations.
- **Deep visceral:** pain and other sensations are felt in the viscera. One may actually experience manipulation of the intestines or ovaries.

- **Olfactory:** smells of various types may be experienced; a burning smell is associated with localization disorder of the temporal lobe.
- **Gustatory:** tastes are experienced in the mouth.
- **Kinaesthetic:** the body experiences being moved, with speed, or from place to place.
- **Lilliputian:** a complex visual experience of small people performing complex actions.
- **Functional:** hallucinations occur only when another perception is experienced. Hearing water flow may lead to voices in the ears.
- **Hallucinosis:** usually frightening hallucinations, in clear consciousness, related to alcoholism.

Depersonalization and **derealization** are changes in perception of self and the environment. With **depersonalization** there is a perception that one is not real, or is changed. There are perceptions about being fragmented, disunited as a person, or that the self may be merging with the environment.

Derealization is a perception that the environment is not real or has changed, or that one feels detached from it. These are uncomfortable sensations which distress the patient.

There can also be an alteration of perception regarding the size of objects in the environment:

- **Micropsia:** when items appear smaller than they actually are.
- **Macropsia:** when they appear bigger than normal.
- **Phantom limb:** a limb is felt when it has been amputated. It is believed that this is caused by sensations in the neuronal pathways leading to the sensory cortex.
- **Reduplication:** patient feels that part of or the whole body has been duplicated.
- **Hemisomatognosis:** a limb which is intact may be perceived as having been removed.
- **Somatic distortion:** a limb may be experienced as growing bigger or smaller, or distorted.

DISORDERS OF COGNITION

DISORDERS OF CONSCIOUSNESS

Clouding of consciousness can be classified as:

- **Drowsiness:** falls asleep but awoken by mild stimuli; speaks coherently, but only for a short time
- **Torpor:** a state of drowsiness and ready sleepiness
- **Delirium:** disorientation and fearful restlessness, with hallucinations
- **Oneroid state:** a dreamlike state when not asleep
- **Twilight state:** a prolonged dreamlike state with disturbed consciousness and perceptual experiences

- **Fugue state:** a state of wandering without loss of consciousness, but there is no recall after the event.

From the normally awake state there are degrees of levels of consciousness in which a person may be sleepy, excessively drowsy, and then the following:

- **Stupor:** may be awoken by pain and loud sounds; gives incomprehensible and short answers; minimal spontaneous activity.
- **Coma:** semicoma is a state where there is no response or spontaneous motor activity but painful stimuli are responded to by withdrawal. **Deep coma** is when there are no responses to any degree of stimulus, and no spontaneous activity.
- **Disorientation** is described in time, place, person and situation.
- **Disorders of attention** or **inattention** is an inability or refusal to attend to a task.
- **Distractibility** is when the attention is drawn to other, trivial stimuli in the environment.
- **Selective inattention** is when unpleasant stimuli are not attended to but others are paid due attention.

DISORDERS OF MEMORY

Memory is the ability to recall past events. **Amnesia** is an inability to recall past events. Amnesia for the time prior to the event is called **retrograde,** and for the time after the event is called **anterograde**. **Hyperamnesia** is when the ability to recall or retain information is exaggerated.

Paramnesiae are distortions of recall or memory. They consist of:

- *Déjà vu*: an unfamiliar situation is recognized
- *Jamais vu*: a familiar situation is not recognized
- *Déjà etendu*: an unfamiliar sound is recognized
- Unconscious, **retrospective falsification:** false details are added to a real memory
- **Confabulation:** gaps in memory are unconsciously filled with false details.

DISORDERS OF INTELLIGENCE AND MENTAL FUNCTIONING

A patient's status can be assessed by cognitive function and other measures, to determine their level of intellectual functioning. Intelligence can be assessed by IQ tests, general knowledge, arithmetic, basic awareness of common knowledge and skills.

- **Amentia** (learning disability or LD): there is incomplete or arrested development of the brain, leading to impaired functioning ability and capacity. A statistical method of classification is used to describe people suffering from these disorders.

- **IQ** (intelligence quotient) is determined and compared with the predetermined norm.
  — IQ less than 20 is profound LD
  — less than 35 is severe LD
  — less than 50 is moderate LD
  — less than 70 (or 69) is mild LD
  — Between 70 and 100 is borderline, and above 100 normal.
- **Dementia** describes progressive global, organic deterioration in mental function and ability, without altered consciousness.
- **Pseudodementia:** cognitive abilities may not function normally, and may deteriorate as part of a psychiatric syndrome without organic degeneration. This is not actual, organic dementia, and can be treated.

NEUROLOGICAL SYMPTOMS AND SIGNS RELEVANT TO PSYCHIATRY

AGNOSIAS

These are the inability to recognize and interpret sensory information. There should be no disorder of sensory pathways, disorders of consciousness, unfamiliarity or mental deterioration.

- **Prosapagnosia:** inability to recognize one's own body, face, or parts of the body
- **Agraphagnosia:** inability to recognize numbers or letters traced on the palm with the eyes closed
- **Anosognosia:** lack of recognition of illness, sometimes of the diseased part of the body
- **Astereognosia:** inability to recognize common objects by palpation
- **Finger agnosia:** inability to recognize one's own or other person's fingers
- **Autotopagnosia:** inability to point out and name various parts of the body
- **Coenestopathia:** perception of a part of the body as distorted
- **Visual agnosia:** familiar objects, seen but not recognized, can be recognized by touch or hearing.

APHASIAS

Disturbances in comprehension and the meaning of words.

- **Visual asymbolia:** words can be written but not read
- **Nominal aphasia:** objects cannot be named
- **Syntactical aphasia:** words cannot be properly arranged, according to linguistic syntax

- **Word deafness:** words are not comprehended, but there is no problem with hearing
- **Agnosic alexia:** words are seen but cannot be read
- **Expressive (motor) non-fluent (Broca's) aphasia:** comprehension but disturbance in expression of words
- **Receptive** (Wernicke's): expression of words but no comprehension

Both **receptive** and **expressive** aphasias may be present. Jargon aphasia refers to incomprehensible, neologistic speech.

Apraxias are motor equivalents of aphasias. In the absence of paresis, sensory or motor loss there is an inability to perform volitional acts. Apraxias include:

- **Constructional** (visuospatial agnosia): inability to construct an object, draw or copy
- **Ideational:** inability to perform a sequential series of movements
- **Dressing:** inability to dress one self
- **Ideomotor:** inability to carry out progressively difficult tasks.

CLASSIFICATIONS IN PSYCHIATRIC PRACTICE: ICD-10 AND DSM-IV

Both ICD-10 and DSM-IV are well established classification systems. ICD-10 is favoured in the UK, Europe and most other countries, whereas DSM-IV is used mainly in North America and is favoured by psychiatric researchers.

As a trainee in the UK you are more than likely to deal with ICD-10, but a detailed knowledge is not usually required. Most psychiatric units/wards have their own copy; you are likely to refer to it when confirming diagnostic categories and preparing discharge summaries (Parts I and II). Tables A1 and A2 outline these classifications.

SUMMARY OF PSYCHIATRIC CLASSIFICATION: ICD-10

Organic, including symptomatic, mental disorders

F00	Dementia in Alzheimer's disease
F01	Vascular dementia
F02	Dementia in other diseases classified elsewhere
F03	Unspecified dementia
F04	Organic amnesic syndrome, not induced by alcohol and other psychoactive substances
F05	Delirium, not induced by alcohol and other psychoactive substances
F06	Other mental disorders due to brain damage and dysfunction and to physical disease
F07	Personality and behavioural disorders due to brain disease, damage and dysfunction

F09   Unspecified organic or symptomatic mental disorder

Mental and behavioural disorders due to psychoactive substance use

F10   Mental and behavioural disorders due to use of alcohol

F11   Mental and behavioural disorders due to use of opioids

F12   Mental and behavioural disorders due to use of cannabinoids

F13   Mental and behavioural disorders due to use of sedatives or hypnotics

F14   Mental and behavioural disorders due to use of cocaine

F15   Mental and behavioural disorders due to use of other stimulants, including caffeine

F16   Mental and behavioural disorders due to use of hallucinogens

F17   Mental and behavioural disorders due to use of tobacco

F18   Mental and behavioural disorders due to use of volatile solvents

F19   Mental and behavioural disorders due to multiple drug use and use of other psychoactive substances

Schizophrenia, schizotypal and delusional disorders

F20   Schizophrenia

F21   Schizotypal disorder

F22   Persistent delusional disorders

F23   Acute and transient psychotic disorders

F24   Induced delusional disorder

F25   Schizoaffective disorders

F28   Other nonorganic psychotic disorders

F29   Unspecified nonorganic psychosis

Mood (affective) disorders

F30   Manic episode

F31   Bipolar affective disorder

F32   Depressive episode

F33   Recurrent depressive disorder

F34   Persistent mood (affective) disorders

F35   Other mood (affective) disorders

F39   Unspecified mood (affective) disorder

Neurotic, stress-related and somatoform disorders

F40   Phobic anxiety disorders

F41   Other anxiety disorders

F42   Obsessive–compulsive disorder

F43   Reaction to severe stress, and adjustment disorders

F44   Dissociative (conversion) disorders

F45   Somatoform disorders

F48   Other neurotic disorders

Behavioural syndromes associated with physiological disturbances and physical factors

F50   Eating disorders

F51   Non-organic sleep disorders

F52   Sexual dysfunction not caused by organic disorder or disease

F53   Mental and behavioural disorders associated with the puerperium, not elsewhere classified

F54   Psychological and behavioural factors associated with disorders or diseases classified elsewhere

F55   Abuse of non-dependence-producing subtances

F59 Unspecified behavioural syndromes associated with physiological disturbances and physical factors

Disorders of adult personality and behaviour

F60 Specific personality disorders
F61 Mixed and other personality disorders
F62 Enduring personality changes not attributable to brain damage and disease
F63 Habit and impulse disorders
F64 Gender identity disorders
F65 Disorders of sexual preference
F66 Psychological and behavioural disorders associated with sexual development and orientation
F68 Other disorders of adult personality and behaviour
F69 Unspecified disorder of adult personality and behaviour

Mental retardation

F70 Mild mental retardation
F71 Moderate mental retardation
F72 Severe mental retardation
F73 Profound mental retardation
F78 Other mental retardation
F79 Unspecified mental retardation

Disorders of psychological development

F80 Specific developmental disorders of speech and language
F81 Specific developmental disorders of scholastic skills
F82 Specific developmental disorders of motor function
F83 Mixed specific developmental disorders
F84 Pervasive developmental disorders
F88 Other disorders of psychological development
F89 Unspecified disorder of psychological development

Behavioural and emotional disorders with onset usually occurring in childhood and adolescence

F90 Hyperkinetic disorders
F91 Conduct disorders
F92 Mixed disorders of conduct and emotions
F93 Emotional disorders with onset specific to childhood
F94 Disorers of social functioning with onset specific to childhood and adolescence
F95 Tic disorders
F98 Other behavioural and emotional disorders with onset usually occuring in childhood and adolescence

Unspecified mental disorders

F99 Mental disorder not otherwise specified

SUMMARY OF PSYCHIATRIC CLASSIFICATION: DSM-IV

This is a multiaxial classification with the following five axes:

Axis I   Clinical disorders
          Other conditions that may be a focus of clinical attention
Axis II   Personality disorders
          Mental retardation
Axis III General medical conditions
Axis IV   Psychosocial and environmental problems

Axis V Global assessment of functioning

In the following summary, NOS stands for 'not otherwise specified'.

Axis I: Clinical disorders; other conditions that may be a focus of clinical attention

Disorers usually first diagnosed in infancy, childhood or adolescene (excluding mental retardation, which is diagnosed on Axis II)

Learning disorder

Motor skills disorder

Communication disorders

Pervasive developmental disorders

● Autistic disorder
● Rett's disorder
● Childhood disintegrative disorder
● Asperger's disorder
● NOS

Attention-deficit and disruptive behaviour disorders

Feeding and eating disorders of infancy and early childhood

Tic disorders

Elimination disorders

● Encopresis
● Enuresis

Other disorders of infancy, childhood, or adolescence

Delirium, dementia, and amnestic and other cognitive disorders

Delirium

Dementia

Amnestic disorders

Other cognitive disorders

Mental disorders due to a general medical condition
Substance-related disorders

Alcohol-related disorders

Amphetamine (or amphetamine-like)-related disorders

Caffeine-related disorders

Cannabis-related disorders

Cocaine-related disorders

Hallucinogen-related disorders

Inhalant-related disorders

Nicotine-related disorders

Opioid-related disorders

Phencyclidine (or phencyclidine-like)-related disorders

Sedative-, hypnotic-, or anxiolytic-related disorders

Polysubstance-related disorders

Other (or unknown) substance-related disorders

Schizophrenia and other psychotic disorders

Schizophrenia

Schizophreniform disorder

Schizoaffective disorder

Delusional disorder

Brief psychotic disorder

Shared psychotic disorder

Psychotic disorder due to a general medical condition

Substance-induced psychotic disorder

Psychotic disorder NOS

Mood disorders

Depressive disorders

Bipolar disorders

Anxiety disorders

Panic disorder without agoraphobia

Panic disorder with agoraphobia

Agoraphobia without history of panic disorder

Specific phobia

Social phobia

Obsessive–compulsive disorder

Post-traumatic stress disorder

Acute stress disorder

Generalized anxiety disorder

Anxiety disorder due to a general medical condition
Substance-induced anxiety disorder
NOS

Somatoform disorders
Somatization disorder
Undifferentiated somatoform disorder
Conversion disorder
Pain disorder
Hypochondriasis
Body dysmorphic disorder
NOS

Factitious disorders

Dissociative disorders
Dissociative amnesia
Dissociative fugue
Dissociative identity disorder
Depersonalization disorder
NOS

Sexual and gender identity disorders
Sexual dysfunctions
- Sexual desire disorders
- Sexual arousal disorders
- Orgasmic disorders
- Sexual pain disorders
- Sexual dysfunction due to a general medical condition

Paraphilias
- Exhibitionism
- Fetishism
- Frotteurism
- Paedophilia
- Sexual masochism
- Sexual sadism
- Transvestic fetishism
- Voyeurism
- NOS

Gender identity disorders

Eating disorders
Anorexia nervosa
Bulimia nervosa
NOS

Sleep disorders
Primary sleep disorders

- Dyssomnias
- Parasomnias

Sleep disorders related to another medical disorder
Other sleep disorders

Impulse-control disorders not elsewhere classified

Adjustment disorders

Other conditions that may be a focus of clinical attention

Axis II: Personality disorders; mental retardation

Personality disorders
Paranoid personality disorder
Schizoid personality disorder
Schizotypal personality disorder
Antisocial personality disorder
Borderline personality disorder
Histrionic personality disorder
Narcissistic personality disorder
Avoidant personality disorder
Dependent personality disorder
Obsessive–compulsive personality disorder
NOS

Mental retardation
Mild mental retardation
Moderate mental retardation
Severe mental retardation
Profound mental reterdation
Mental retardation, severity unspecified

Axis III: General medical conditions

Infectious and parasitic diseases

Neoplasmas

Endocrine, nutritional and metabolic diseases and immunity disorders

Diseases of the blood and blood-forming organs

Diseases of the nervous system and sense organs

Diseases of the circulatory system

Diseases of the respiratory system

Diseases of the digestive system

Diseases of the genitourinary system

Complications of pregnancy, childbirth and the puerperium

Diseases of the skin and subcutaneous tissue

Diseases of the musculoskeletal system and connective tissue

Congenital anomalies

Certain conditions originating in the perinatal period

Symptoms, signs and ill-defined conditions

Injury and poisoning

Axis IV: Psychosocial and environmental problems

Problems with primary support group

Problems related to the social environment

Educational problems

Occupational problems

Housing problems

Economic problems

Problems with access to health-care services

Problems related to interaction with the legal system/crime

Other psychosocial and environmental problems

Axis V: Global assessment of functioning

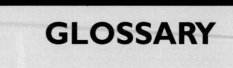

GLOSSARY

Acute intoxication: a transient condition resulting from the administration of a psychoactive substance, causing changes in physiological, psychological or behavioural functions and responses.

Affect: observable behaviours expressing subjectively experienced feeling state (emotion) and which varies over time in response to changing emotional states.

Agitation: excessive motor activity with a feeling of inner tension.

Agoraphobia: literally, a fear of the marketplace. A high anxiety level and multiple phobic symptoms occur. It may include a fear of crowds, open and closed spaces and travelling by public transport.

Alexithymia: inability to describe or feel one's emotions.

Ambitendency: a series of tentative, incomplete movements carried out during voluntary action.

Ambivalence: simultaneous presence of opposing impulses/thoughts towards the same thing.

Amnesia: the inability to recall past experiences/events.

Anxiety: feeling of apprehension or tension caused by anticipating an external or internal danger.

Apathy: detachment or indifference and a loss of emotional tone and the ability to feel pleasure.

Attention: ability to focus on an activity.

Automatism: an act over which the individual has no control, e.g. sleepwalking.

Autoscopy (phantom mirror image): an hallucination in which one sees and recognizes oneself.

Autotopagnosia: the inability to name, recognize or point on command to parts of the body.

Bereavement: an event encompassing loss, particularly of a negative nature, from loss of a relative by death to unemployment or divorce.

Blunted affect: a reduction in or absence of emotional expression.

Capgras syndrome: the patient believes that a familiar person has been replaced by a double.

Clanging: speech in which words are chosen because of their sounds rather than their meanings including rhyming and punning.

Clouding of consciousness: the patient is drowsy and does not react completely to stimuli. There is disturbance of attention, concentration, memory, orientation and thinking.

Coma: if the coma is deep, there is no response to deep pain or any spontaneous movement. Tendon, pupillary and corneal reflexes are usually absent.

Compulsions or compulsive rituals: repetitive, stereotyped, seemingly purposeful behaviour that is the motor component of obsessional thoughts. Examples include checking and cleaning rituals.

Concentration: the ability to sustain attention.

Concrete thinking: a lack of abstract thinking, normal in childhood, and occurring in adults with organic brain disease (e.g. frontal lobe disorders) and schizophrenia.

Confabulation: gaps in memory are unconsciously filled with false memories.

Cotard's syndrome: a nihilistic delusional disorder in which, for example, the patient believes their money, friends or body parts do not exist.

Countertransference: the therapist's emotions and attitudes to the patient.

Couvade syndrome: an hysterical disorder in which a prospective father develops symptoms characteristic of pregnancy.

Culture-bound syndromes: specific psychiatric disorders occurring in certain cultures/countries.

Defence mechanisms: mental mechanisms that protect consciousness from the affects, ideas and desires of the unconscious.

Déjà-vu: an illusion of recognition of a situation.

Delirium: a disorder of consciousness in which the patient is bewildered, disorientated and restless. There may be associated fear and hallucinations.

Delusion: a false belief firmly sustained contrary to the evidence and is out of keeping with the individual's sociocultural and educational norm.

Dementia: a global organic impairment of intellectual functioning without impairment of consciousness.

Denial: a defence mechanism in which the subject acts as if consciously unaware of a wish or reality.

Dependence syndrome: use of psychoactive substances takes higher priority than other behaviours and there is a desire, often strong and overpowering, to take the substance(s) on a continuous or periodic basis, usually leading to harm.

Depersonalization: a feeling that one is altered or not real in some way.

Depression: a low or depressed mood that may be accompanied by anhedonia, in which the ability to enjoy regular and pleasurable activities is lost.

Derealization: a feeling that the surroundings do not seem real.

Disease: the pathological abnormality occurring in an organism as a result of some specific noxious insult(s).

Disorders (loosening) of association (formal thought disorder): a disorder language seen in schizophrenia, e.g. knight's-move thinking and word salad.

Displacement: a defence mechanism in which thoughts and feelings about one person or object are transferred on to another.

Dissociative disorder: a disorder in which there is a disturbance in the normal integration of awareness of identity, consciousness, memory and control of bodily movements.

Distractability: the attention is frequently drawn to irrelevant external stimuli.

DSM-IV: the *Diagnostic and statistical manual of mental disorders*, 4th edition. Published by the American Psychiatric Association, Washington DC, 1994.

Dysphoria: an unpleasant mood.

Dysthymia (depressive neurosis): a chronic depression of mood, which does not fulfil the criteria for recurrent depressive disorder.

Ecstasy: a feeling of intense pleasure.

Ego: part of the mental apparatus that is present at the interface of the perceptual and internal demand systems. It controls voluntary thoughts and actions and, at an unconscious level, defence mechanisms.

Eidetic image: a vivid and detailed reproduction of a previous perception, e.g. a photographic memory.

Elevated mood: a mood more cheerful than normal. It is not necessarily pathological.

Erotomania (de Clerambault's syndrome): the delusional belief that another person is deeply in love with one. It usually occurs in women, with the object often being a man of much higher social status.

Euphoric mood: an exaggerated feeling of wellbeing. It is pathological.

Expansive mood: feelings are expressed without restraint, and one's self-importance may be overrated.

Flat affect: almost no emotional expression is seen and the patient typically has an immobile face and monotonous voice.

Formication: a somatic hallucination in which insects are felt to be crawling under one's skin.

Free association: articulation, without censorship, of all thoughts that come to one's mind.

Free-floating anxiety: pervasive and unfocused anxiety.

Fregoli syndrome: the patient believes that a familiar person, who is often believed to be the patient's persecutor, has taken on different appearances.

Freudian slips (parapraxes): unconscious thoughts slipping through.

Fugue: a state of wandering from usual surroundings and loss of memory.

Generalized anxiety disorder: a neurotic disorder characterized by unrealistic or excessive anxiety and worry which is generalized and persistent and not restricted to particular environmental circumstances, that is, it is free-floating.

Grief: psychological and emotional processes, expressed both internally and externally, that accompany bereavement.

Hallucination: a false sensory perception in the absence of a real external stimulus. It is perceived as being located in objective space and as having the same realistic qualities as normal perceptions. It is not subject to conscious manipulation and only indicates a psychotic disturbance when there is also impaired reality testing.

Hallucinosis: hallucinations (usually auditory) occurring in clear consciousness, e.g. in alcoholism.

Health: defined by the World Health Organization as being a state of complete physical, mental and social wellbeing.

Hyperacusis: an increased sensitivity to sounds.

Hyperaesthesia: a sensory distortion in which sensations appear increased.

Hypnagogic hallucination: hallucination occurring while falling asleep, described as normal.

Hypnopompic hallucination: hallucination occurring while waking from sleep, described as normal.

Hypoaesthesia: sensory distortion in which sensations appear decreased.

Hypochondriasis: preoccupation not based on real organic pathology, with a fear of having a serious physical illness.

ICD-10: the tenth revision of the International classification of diseases published by the World Health Organization, Geneva, 1992.

Id: an unconscious part of the mental apparatus which is partly made up of inherited instincts and partly by acquired, but repressed, components.

Illusion: a false perception of a real external stimulus.

Inappropriate affect: an affect that is inappropriate to the circumstances, for example appearing cheerful immediately following the death of a loved one.

Induced psychosis (folie à deux): a delusional disorder is shared by two (or more) individuals who are closely related emotionally. One has a genuine psychotic disorder and their delusional system is induced in the other, who may be dependent or less intelligent.

Introjection and identification: defence mechanisms by which the attitudes and behaviour of another are transposed into oneself, helping one cope with separation from that person.

Isolation: a defence mechanism in which certain thoughts are isolated from others.

Jamais vu: the illusion of failure to recognize a familiar situation.

Jargon aphasia: incoherent, meaningless, neologistic speech.

Knight's-move thinking: odd, tangential associations between ideas, leading to disruptions in the smooth continuity of speech.

Labile affect: the affect repeatedly and rapidly shifts, for example from anger to sadness.

Learning disability (mental retardation): classified by DSM-IV and ICD-10 as an IQ of less than or equal to 70.

Logoclonia: the last syllable of the last word is repeated.

Logorrhoea (volubility): fluent and rambling speech using many words.

Macropsia: objects appear larger or nearer than they really are.

Mannerisms: repeated involuntary movements that appear to be goal directed.

Mens rea: a guilty state of mind at the time of a criminal offence.

Mental apparatus: the id, ego and superego in psychodynamic theory.

Mild mental retardation: IQ of 50–70.

Moderate mental retardation: IQ of 35–49.

Mood: a pervasive and sustained emotion that colours the person's perception of the world.

Mood-congruent delusion: content of the delusion is appropriate to the patient's mood (e.g. in depression).

Mood-incongruent delusion: content of the delusion is not appropriate to the patient's mood (e.g. in schizophrenia).

Mutism: total loss of speech.

Negativism: a motiveless resistance to commands and attempts to be moved.

Neologism: a word newly made up, or an everyday word used in a special way.

Neurosis or neurotic disorder: a psychiatric disorder in which the patient has insight into the illness, can distinguish between subjective experiences and reality, and does not construct a false environment based on misconceptions.

Nihilistic delusion: the delusional belief that others, oneself, or the world do not exist or are about to cease to exist.

Obsessions: repetitive senseless thoughts, recognized by the patient, as being irrational which, at least initially, are unsuccessfully resisted.

Overvalued idea: an unreasonable and sustained intense preoccupation maintained with less than delusional intensity (e.g. fear of fatness in anorexic)

Pallilalia: a word is repeated with increasing frequency.

Panic attacks: acute episodic intense anxiety attacks with or without physiological symptoms.

Parasuicide (deliberate self-harm): act deliberately undertaken by a patient who mimics the act of suicide, but which does not result in a fatal outcome.

Passivity phenomenon: the delusional belief that an external agency is controlling aspects of the self which are normally entirely under one's own control (e.g. made feelings, made impulses, made actions, somatic passivity).

Perseveration (of speech and movement): mental operations carried on beyond the point at which they are appropriate.

Personality disorders: deeply ingrained and enduring behaviour patterns resulting in inflexible responses to a broad range of personal and social situations.

Phantom limb: following the amputation of a limb there is a continued awareness of its presence.

Phobia: a persistent irrational fear of an activity, object or situation, leading to avoidance. The fear is out of proportion to the real danger and cannot be reasoned away.

Phobic anxiety: avoidance of the focus of anxiety.

Physical dependence: an adaptive state in which intense physical disturbance occurs when the administration of a psychoactive substance is suspended. The substance is taken to avoid the physical symptoms of the withdrawal state.

Poverty of speech: very reduced speech, sometimes with monosyllabic answers to questions.

Premenstrual syndrome (PMS): includes emotional, physical and behavioural symptoms occurring regularly during the second half of each menstrual cycle. These subside during menstruation and are completely absent between menstruation and ovulation.

Pressure of speech: increased quantity and rate of speech, which is difficult to interrupt.

Primary delusion: a delusion arising fully formed without any discernible connection with previous events. It may be preceded by a delusional mood in which there is an awareness of something unusual and threatening occurring.

Profound mental retardation: IQ of less than 20.

Projection: a defence mechanism in which repressed thoughts and wishes are attributed to other people or objects.

Projective identification: a defence mechanism in which another person is both seen as possessing and constrained to take on repressed aspects of oneself.

Pseudodementia: similar clinically to dementia, but has a non-organic cause, e.g. depression.

Pseudohallucination: a form of imagery arising in the subjective inner space of the mind and lacking the substantiality of normal perceptions. It is not subject to conscious manipulation.

Psychiatry (psychological medicine): the branch of medicine dealing with mental disorder and its treatment.

Psychoactive substance: a substance that can lead to relatively rapid effects in the central nervous system, including a change in the level of consciousness or the state of mind. Examples include alcohol, illicit drugs (e.g. cocaine, heroin and LSD) and licit drugs (e.g. nicotine and caffeine).

Psychological dependence: a psychoactive substance produces a feeling of satisfaction and a psychological drive that requires periodic or continuous administration of the substance to produce pleasure or to avoid the psychological discomfort of its absence.

Psychology: the science investigating behaviour, experience and the phenomena of mental and emotional life.

Psychomotor agitation: overactivity and restlessness (e.g. in agitated depression).

Psychosis: the patient is out of touch with reality, does not have insight, has the whole of his or her personality distorted by illness, and constructs a false environment out of subjective experiences. Delusions and/or hallucinations may occur.

Rationalization: a defence mechanism in which an attempt is made to explain in a logically consistent or ethically acceptable way affects, ideas and wishes whose true motive is not consciously perceived.

Reaction formation: a defence mechanism in which an attitude diametrically opposed to an oppressed wish is held.

Reduplication phenomenon: part or all of the body is felt to be duplicated.

Regression: defence mechanism in which there is a return to an earlier stage of development.

Repression: a defence mechanism in which there is a pushing away of unacceptable ideas and wishes which remain in the unconscious.

Retrospective falsification: false details are added to the recollection of an otherwise real memory.

Schneiderian first-rank symptoms: provided there is no organic cerebral pathology the presence of any of Schneider's first-rank symptoms is indicative of, though not pathognomonic of, schizophrenia.

Sections: orders under the Mental Health Act 1983 (England and Wales), allowing the detention of patients.

Severe mental retardation: IQ of 20–34

Sick-role behaviour: activity by individuals who consider themselves as ill.

Simple phobia: fear of discrete objects (e.g. snakes) or situations.

Social phobia: fear of personal interactions in a public setting (e.g. public speaking).

Somatic passivity: the delusional belief that one is a passive recipient of bodily sensations from an external agency.

Somnambulism: sleepwalking.

Stammering: the flow of speech is broken by pauses and the repetition of parts of words.

Stereotypy: a repeated regular fixed pattern of movement or speech that is not goal directed.

Sublimation: a defence mechanism allowing unacceptable thoughts or impulses are satisfied by means of socially acceptable activities.

Superego: partly conscious and partly unconscious, derivative of the ego that exercises self-judgement and holds ethical and moralistic values.

Systematized delusion: a group of delusions united by a single theme or a delusion, with multiple elaboration.

Tactile (haptic) hallucinations: superficial somatic hallucinations.

Testamentary capacity: the capacity to make a legally valid will.

Thought blocking: a sudden interruption in the train of thought occurs, leaving a 'blank', after which what was being said cannot be recalled.

Thought broadcasting: the delusional belief that one's thoughts are being 'read' by others, as if they were being broadcast (e.g. on radio).

Thought insertion: the delusional belief that thoughts are being put into one's mind by an external agency.

Thought withdrawal: the delusional belief that thoughts are being removed from one's mind by an external agency.

Tics: repeated irregular movements involving a particular muscle group.

Tolerance: effects of psychoactive substances diminish with repeated use, so that increasing doses are needed to achieve the same effects.

Transference: the unconscious process in which emotions and attitudes experienced in childhood are transferred to the therapist.

Undoing: a defence mechanism in which previous thoughts or actions are made not to have occurred.

Visceral hallucinations: somatic hallucinations of deep sensations.

Withdrawal state: physical and psychological symptoms which occur following absolute or relative withdrawal of a psychoactive substance after its repeated use.

USEFUL ADDRESSES

Alcoholics Anonymous
PO Box 1
Stonebow House
Stonebow
York YO1 2NJ
Tel: (01904) 644026

British Medical Association
Tavistock Square
London WC1H 9JP
Tel: (0207) 387 4499

CSM (for reporting adverse drug reaction)
Freepost
London SW8 5BR
Tel: (0207) 627 3291

Department of Health
Alexander Fleming House
Elephant and Castle
London SE1 6BY
Tel: (0207) 210 5983

Royal College of Psychiatrists
17 Belgrave Square
London SW1X 8PG
Tel: (0207) 235 2351

GENERAL ADDRESSES

African Carribean Mental Health
Association (ACMHA)
35–37 Electric Avenue
Brixton
London SW9 8JP
Tel: (0207) 737 3603

Age Concern Greater London
54 Knatchbull Road
London SE5 9QU
Tel: (0207) 274 6723

Age Concern Northern Ireland
3 Lower Crescent
Belfast BT7 1NR
Tel: (01232) 245729

Age Concern Scotland
54A Fountainbridge
Edinburgh EH3 9PT
Tel: (0131) 228 5656

Age Concern Wales
1 Cathedral Road

Cardiff CF1 9SD
Tel: (02920) 371566

Alzheimer's Disease Society
Gordon House
10 Greencoat Place
London SW1P 1PH
Tel: (0207) 306 0606

Asian Family Counselling Services
74 The Avenue
London W13 8LB
Tel: (0208) 997 5749

British Association for Counselling
1 Regent Place
Rugby CV21 2PJ
Tel: (01788) 550899

British Association of Occupational
Therapists
6 Marshalsea Road
London SE1 1HL
Tel: (0207) 357 6480

British Association of Psychotherapists
37 Mapesbury Road
London NW2 4HJ
Tel: (0208) 452 9823

British Geriatrics Society (BGS)
1 St Andrews Place
Regent's Park
London NW1 4LB
Tel: (0207) 935 4004

British Red Cross
9 Grosvenor Crescent
London SW1X 7EJ
Tel: (0207) 235 5454

Chartered Society of Physiotherapy
14 Bedford Row
London WC1R 4ED
Tel: (0207) 242 1941

Community Service Volunteers
237 Pentonville Road
King's Cross
London N1 9NG
Tel: (0207) 278 6001

Counsel and Care for the Elderly
Twyman House

16 Bonny Street
London NW1 9PG
Tel: (0207) 485 1550

Court of Protection
Stewart House
24 Kingsway
London WC2B 6HD
Tel: (0207) 269 7000

Cruse: Bereavement Care
126 Sheen Road
Richmond TW9 1UR
Tel: (0208) 940 4818

Disability Alliance
Universal House
Wentworth Street
London E1 7SA
Tel: (0207) 247 8776

Help the Aged
St James' Walk
London EC1R 0BE
Tel: (0207) 253 0253

Jewish Care
221 Golders Green Road
London NW11 9DZ
Tel: (0208) 458 3282

King's Fund Centre
126 Albert Street
London NW1 7NF
Tel: (0207) 267 6111

Manic Depression Fellowship
8–10 High Street
Kingston-upon-Thames KT1 1EY
Tel: (0208) 974 6550

Mental Health Foundation
37 Mortimer Street
London W1N 8JU
Tel: (0207) 580 0145

MIND—National Association for Mental
Health
22 Harley Street
London W1N 2ED
Tel: (0207) 637 0741

Nafsiyat Intercultural Therapy Centre
278 Seven Sisters Road

Finsbury Park
London N4 2HY
Tel: (0207) 263 4130

National Association of Citizens Advice
Bureaux
115 Pentonville Road
London N1 9LZ
Tel: (0207) 833 2181

National Council for Voluntary
Organizations (NCVO)
20 Bedford Square
London WC1B 3HU
Tel: (0207) 636 4066

National Schizophrenia Fellowship
(NSF)
28 Castle Street
Kingston-upon-Thames KT1 1SS
Tel: (0208) 547 3937

Parkinson's Disease Society
36 Portland Place
London W1N 3DG
Tel: (0207) 383 3513

Refugee Council
3 Bondway
London SW8 1SJ
Tel: (0207) 820 3000

Relate—National Marriage Guidance
Council
Herbert Gray College
Little Church Street
Rugby CV21 3AP
Tel: (01788) 537241

Royal National Institute for the Blind
224 Great Portland Street
London W1N 4XX
Tel: (0207) 388 1266

St John Ambulance
1 Grosvenor Crescent
London SW1X 7EE
Tel: (0207) 235 5231

Terrence Higgins Trust
52/54 Gray's Inn Road
London WC1X 8JU
Tel: (0207) 242 1010
(12 noon to 7 pm daily)

GOVERNMENT OFFICES

Central Office of Information
Hercules Road
London SE1 7DU
Tel: (0207) 928 2345

Commission for Racial Equality
Elliot House
10–12 Allington Street
London SW1E 5EH
Tel: (0207) 828 7022

Crown Prosecution Service
50 Ludgate Hill
London EC4M 7EX
Tel: (0207) 273 3000

Equal Opportunities Commission
Overseas House
Quay Street
Manchester M3 3HN
Tel: (0161) 833 9244

Health and Safety Executive
(General Enquiries)
Broad Lane
Sheffield S3 7HQ
Tel: (01142) 892000

Health, Department of
Richmond House
79 Whitehall
London SW1A 2NS
Tel: (0207) 210 4850

Home Office
50 Queen Anne's Gate
London SW1H 9AT
Tel: (0207) 273 3000

National Audit Office
157–197 Buckingham Palace Road
London SW1W 9SP
Tel: (0207) 798 7000

Office of Population Censuses &
Surveys/General Register Office
St Catherine's House
10 Kingsway
London WC2B 6JP
Tel: (0207) 242 0262

Social Security, Department of
Richmond House
79 Whitehall
London SW1A 2NS
Tel: (0207) 210 5983

REGIONAL TRIBUNAL OFFICES

Mental Health Review Tribunals
Hepburn House
Marsham Street
London SW1P 4HW
Tel: (0207) 211325/211356

Mental Health Review Tribunals
3rd Floor
Cressington House
249 St Mary's Road
Garston
Liverpool L19 0NF
Tel: (0151) 494 0095

Mental Health Review Tribunals
Spur A, Block 5
Government Buildings
Chalfont Drive
Western Boulevard
Nottingham NG8 3RZ
Tel: (0115) 94222/3

Mental Health Review Tribunals
2nd Floor
New Crown Buildings
Cathays Park
Cardiff CF1 3NQ
Tel: (02920) 825798

OTHER

United Kingdom Advocacy Network
(UKAN)
Premier House
14 Cross Burgess Street
Sheffield S1 2HG
Tel: (0114) 275 3131

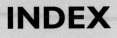

INDEX

Absorption, 119
Abstract thinking, 49
Acamprosate, 130
Acupuncture, 199
Adjustment disorder, 76–77
Adolescence, 40
Aetiological factors, 58–59
Affect/mood, 46
Aggression assessment scale, 230
Aggressive patient, *see* Violent/
    homicidal patient
Agitated patient, 217
Agoraphobia, 248
    management, 133–134
Akathisia, 265
Akinetic mutism, 240
Alcohol consumption/abuse
    associated psychiatric disorders/
        comorbidity, 92, 121–130, 165
    CAGE questionnaire, 37, 62
    dementia/cognitive impairment, 123
    hallucinations, 123, 236
    history taking, 37, 41
    physical examination, 56
    violent behaviour, 228
Alcohol dependence syndrome, 122–123
    criteria, 37
    psychotherapy, 211–212
Alcohol intoxication, 252–253
Alcohol withdrawal, 126–128
    major (delerium tremens), 127–128
    minor (abstinence), 126–127
    planned (detoxification), 128–130, 212
    seizures, 128
Alcoholics Anonymous 12 Steps, 212
Alprazolam, 132
    withdrawal management, 138
Alzheimer's disease, 56
Amitriptyline, 137
Amnesic patient, 217
Amoxipine, 164
Amphetamines, 254–255, 262
Anankastic (obsessive–compulsive)
        personality disorder, 96
    assessment, 98
    management, 169
Angel dust (phencyclidine), 257
Angry mood, 228
Anorexia nervosa, 72–74
    appearance, 45

management, 130–131
    overvalued ideas, 48
Antabuse (disulfiram), 130
Anticholinergics
    central anticholinergic syndrome, 269–270
    elderly patients, 114
Anticonvulsants
    aggressive behaviour, 231
    bipolar affective disorder, 145–148
    elderly patients, 114
    liver disease, 118
    pretreatment/maintenance laboratory
        investigations, 148
Antidepressants, 155
    adjustment disorder, 76
    alcohol-related anxiety/depression, 124
    anorexia nervosa, 131
    bulimia nervosa, 131
    depression, 152–165
    duration of therapy, 154
    elderly patients, 115
    generalized anxiety disorder, 132
    liver disease, 117
    mixed anxiety/depressive disorder
        (anxiety–depression), 134
    panic disorder, 132
    personality disorder, 167, 168, 169
    phobias, 133–134
    post-traumatic stress disorder, 136–137
    schizophrenia, 179
    selection criteria, 153–154
    switching drugs, 109–110
Antihistamines, 248
Antiparkinsonian drugs, 189–191
    side effects, 189
Antipsychotics
    anorexia nervosa, 131
    anxiety, 248
    atypical/novel, 180
    depot injections, 187, 188
    dosage, 181–182, 188, 189
    dosage equivalents, 112
    elderly patients, 114
    emergency intramuscular
        administration, 188
    hallucinating patient, 238
    indications, 180
    liver disease, 118
    oral/parenteral dose equivalents, 112
    personality disorders, 167, 168

Antipsychotics (contd)
    paranoid, 166
    pretreatment tests, 182
    rapid tranquillization of manic
        patient, 230, 234
    schizophrenia, 175–176, 177–179, 180–182
    side effects, 183–185
        acute emergencies, 217, 265–266
        management, 185
    switching drugs, 111–113
    treatment monitoring, 182
    withdrawal, 109
Antisocial personality disorder,
        see Dissocial personality disorder
Anxiety disorders, 76–83
    adjustment disorder, 76–77
    alcohol-related, 124
    appearance, 45
    assessment, 244
    drug-related, 244, 245
    emergencies, 243–248
    history taking, 34, 36
    hyperventilation, 77, 247
    management, 131–138, 246–248
    medical causes, 245
    personality disorder comorbidity, 92
    signs/symptoms, 243
    speech/talk, 46
Anxiety rating scales, 63
Anxiolytics, 246
    aggressive behaviour, 232
    liver disease, 118
    overdose, 253–254
    personality disorder, 168, 169
    switching drugs, 110, 111
Anxious (avoidant) personality disorder, 96
    assessment, 99
    management, 169
Appearance, 44–45
Approved social workers (ASW), 22, 286
Art therapist, 24–25
Assertiveness skills, 11
Assessment, 32–70
    A&E department, 216
    clinical psychologist's role, 25
    history taking, 32–43
    investigations, 59–62
    management plan, 59
    Mental Health Act, 277–278
    mental state examination, 43–44

Mini Mental State Examination, 51–53
    new outpatient referrals, 17
    physical examination, 54–58
    summary/record of findings, 58
Assessment room, 33
Attention assessment, 49
Atypical (masked) depression, 91
Auditory hallucinations, 48, 172, 237–238
Australian mental health legislation, 297
Aversive therapy, 207

Barbiturates overdose, 254
Beck Depression Inventory, 63, 151
Behaviour abnormalities, 300–301
    bipolar affective disorder, 86
    mental state examination, 44–45
Behaviour therapy, 26, 206–208
    alcohol-related addiction/
        dependence disorders, 212
    obsessive–compulsive disorder, 135
    phobias, 133
Benzodiazepines
    acute manic episodes, 139
    adjustment disorder, 76
    aggressive behaviour, 232
    alcohol withdrawal, 127, 128, 129
    dosage equivalents, 111
    elderly patients, 114
    emergency use, 246, 247
    generalized anxiety disorder, 132
    mixed anxiety/depressive disorder
        (anxiety–depression), 134
    obsessive–compulsive disorder, 135, 136
    overdose, 253–254
    panic disorder, 132
    phobias, 133, 134
    post-traumatic stress disorder, 137
    rapid tranquillization of manic/
        violent patient, 229, 234
    schizophrenia, 178
Benzodiazepines dependence/
        abuse, 137–138
    withdrawal management, 138
    withdrawal symptoms, 138
Benzotropine, 266
Bereavement
    history taking, 39, 40
    mute/unresponsive patient, 241
Beta-blockers

Beta-blockers (contd)
  aggressive behaviour, 232
  anxiety, 248
  anxious (avoidant) personality
    disorder, 169
  social phobia, 133
Biochemical values, 61–62
Biological (somatic/vegetative)
    symptoms, 88
Bipolar affective disorder (manic
    depressive psychosis), 83–86, 173
  electroconvulsive therapy (ECT), 145
  history taking, 39
  ICD-10 diagnostic categories, 83–84
  initial stabilization, 139, 140
  management, 139–141
  mental state examination, 86
  mood stabilizers, 140, 141
    carbamazepine, 145–147
    clonazepam, 149–150
    lithium, 141–145
    sodium valproate (valproic acid),
      147–150
  psychosocial therapies, 140
Birth history, 39
Bleuler's four As, 102
Blood tests, 59
Borderline personality disorder, 95, 173
  assessment, 98
  chronically suicidal patients, 225–226
  hallucinations, 236
  history taking, 38
  management, 167–168
  physical examination, 56
  violent/homicidal behaviour, 229
Brief Psychiatric Rating Scale, 62
Brief reactive psychosis, 174
Briquet's syndrome, 92
Bulbar palsy, 57
Bulimia nervosa, 74–75
  appearance, 45
  management, 130–131
Buspirone
  antidepressants augmentation, 153
  anxiety, 124, 248
  obsessive–compulsive disorder, 135
  post-traumatic stress disorder 137

CAGE questionnaire, 37, 62

Canadian mental health legislation, 297
Cannabis (marijuana), 256
Carbamazepine
  aggressive behaviour, 231
  bipolar affective disorder, 145–147
  drug interactions, 146
  mania, 235
  post-traumatic stress disorder, 137
  side effects, 146
  switching to valproate, 111
Care programme approach (CPA),
    29–30, 175
Case notes, 10
Catatonic schizophrenia, 100, 241, 242
Central anticholinergic syndrome, 269
Chaperon, 33, 34, 54
Childhood history, 39–40
Children, pharmacotherapy, 116
Chlordiazepoxide, alcohol withdrawal,
    126, 127, 129
Chlorpromazine
  hallucinating patient, 238
  rapid tranquillization of manic patient,
    234
Citalopram, 156
  alcohol-related depression, 124
  elderly patients, 115
Clarification in history taking, 34, 35
Classical conditioning, 206
Clerking patients, 12–13
Clinical duties, 8–10
  emergency psychiatric clinics, 18
  multidisciplinary team members, 18–19
Clomipramine
  anankastic personality disorder, 169
  anorexia nervosa, 131
  bulimia nervosa, 131
  obsessive–compulsive disorder, 135
Clonazepam, 149, 150
  aggressive behaviour, 231
  mania, 235
Clonidine, 262
  Wernicke–Korsakoff syndrome, 125
Closed questions, 34
Clozapine
  contraindication in liver disease, 118
  patient monitoring service, 186
  schizophrenia, 178, 186
  side effects, 186
  treatment-resistant psychosis, 111

Cocaine, 172, 254–255
  withdrawal, 262
Cognitive (cognitive behavioural) therapy,
    26, 205–206
  alcohol-related addiction/
      dependence disorders, 212
  post-traumatic stress disorder, 137
  schizophrenia, 175
Cognitive distortions, 206
Cognitive impairment, 308–309
  alcohol-related, 123
  rating scales, 63
  violent/homicidal behaviour, 228
Cognitive state assessment, 48–51
  abstract thinking, 49
  attention/concentration, 49
  bipolar affective disorder, 86
  general knowledge, 50
  insight, 51
  intelligence, 51
  memory, 49
  orientation, 48
Command hallucinations, 217, 228, 239
Common law, 287
Communication
  colleagues, 10–11
  daily informaion exchange, 12
  emergencies, 215
  history taking skills, 34, 35
Comorbidity, 8, 58
  personality disorders, 92, 165
Competence, 284
Complaints of patient, 36
Compliance, 107
Compulsions, 81
Compulsory admissions, 223
Compulsory treatment
  acute mania, 235
  Mental Health Act, 230, 235
  violent/homicidal behaviour, 230
Concentration assessment, 49
Concrete thinking, 49
Confidentiality, 286
Congenital rubella, 57
Consent, 243, 276, 284–285
  common law, 287
  disclosure of information to patient, 284
  electroconvulsive therapy, 193, 287
Counselling, 203–204
  schizophrenia, 175

Countertransference, 209
Court appearances, 292
Court diversion schemes, 287
Cranial nerves assessment, 56–58
Criminal Procedure (Scotland) Act (1975),
    294
Cultural camouflage, 67
Cultural issues, see Transcultural
    psychiatry
Culture-bound syndromes, 69–70
Cushinoid appearance, 45
Cyproterone, 232

Day hospital, 15
  patient follow-up, 24
  professionals, 15
  services, 15
  ward rounds, 14
Defence mechanisms, 209
Delerium, 239–240
  affect/mood, 46
  electroconvulsive therapy, 192
Delerium tremens, 127–128, 259
Deliberate self-harm, 220
  risk assessment/management, 219–220
  supervision register placement, 30
  see also Suicidal patient
Delusional perception, 171
Delusions, 48, 171, 173, 174, 217, 218
  clarification of beliefs, 171
  management, 174
  primary/secondary, 48
Dementia
  alcohol-related, 123
  appearance, 45
  personality disorder comorbidity, 165
  speech/talk, 45, 46
Dependence disorders, 211–212
Dependent personality disorder,
    97, 99, 169
Depression, 87–91, 150–165
  alcohol-related, 123
  appearance, 45
  atypical syndromes, 90–91
  clarification of symptoms, 150–151
  delusions, 48
  drug treatment, 152–165
  drug-induced, 152
  electroconvulsive therapy, 192

Depression (contd)
  history taking, 36, 40, 41
  ICD-10 categories, 87, 150–151
  light therapy, 198
  medical causes, 151–152
  personality disorder comorbidity, 92
  psychosocial issues, 152
  psychosocial treatment, 152
  psychotic, 173
  rating scales, 63
  somatic (vegetative/biological)
    symptoms, 88
  speech/talk, 45, 46
  treatment-resistant, 165
Depressive episode, 88–90
Depressive stupor, 89
Descriptive psychopathology, 300–310
Detoxification (alcohol withdrawal), 128–130
Developmental history, 39
Dhat syndrome, 69
Diabetes, 58
Diagnosis, 58–59
Diagnostic categories, 7, 8
Diazepam
  alcohol withdrawal, 127, 128
  benzodiazepines withdrawal
    management, 138
  equivalent benzodiazepine doses, 138
  generalized anxiety disorder, 132
Differential diagnosis, 58–59
Digoxin, 108
Directive psychotherapy, 203
Discharge planning, 28–29
Discharge summary
  part I, 63, 64–65
  part II, 64, 66–67
Disordered behaviour, 172
Dissocial (antisocial) personality disorder, 94
  assessment, 98
  history taking, 40, 41
  management, 167
  violent/homicidal behaviour, 229
Dissociative states, 241, 242
Distribution, 119
Disulfiram (Antabuse), 130
Djinn syndrome, 69
Documentation policy, 12
Dopamine agonists
  acute side effects management, 265–266
  schizophrenia, 178

Double learning theory, 206
Dream interpretation, 209
Droperidol, 234
Drug abuse, see Substance abuse
Drug history, 37
Drug interactions, 113
Drug-induced anxiety states, 244, 245
Drug-induced depression, 152
Drug-induced psychosis, 172
Drug-related emergencies, 249–259
DSM-IV classification, 314–317
  personality disorders, 91–92
Dual diagnosis, 8, 58
Dysthymia, 90
Dystonia, acute, 242, 265–266

Echolalia, 46
Ecstasy, 254–255
Educational record, 40
Eire mental health legislation, 295–296
Elderly patients
  alcohol withdrawal, 127
  drug treatment, 114–115
  personality disorder, 166
  social history taking, 42
Electroconvulsive therapy (ECT), 191–197
  bipolar affective disorder, 145
  consent/legal issues, 193, 287
  drug interactions, 194
  indications/contraindications, 192
  investigations, 194
  preparations, 193
  procedure, 195–197
  schizophrenia, 178
  side effects, 193
  suicidal patient, 223
Emergencies, 12, 214–270
  admission procedure, 217
  alternatives to admission, 217
  assessment in A&E, 216
  behavioural, 220–249
  common law consent, 287
  drug/alcohol-related, 249–259
  history-taking, 217–218
  legal aspects, 216, 273, 277, 287
  management, 214–215, 218
  preliminary diagnosis, 218
  risk assessment/management, 219–220
Emergency admission, 217, 277

Emergency holding powers, 273
Emergency psychiatric clinics, 17–18
Emotion disorders, 303–306
Emotional incontinence, 46
Emotionally unstable personality
      disorder, 95
Environment of assessment room, 33
Espanto syndrome, 70
EU trainees, 5–6
Excretion, 119–120
Experiential psychotherapies, 208
Exploratory psychotherapies, 208
Extrapyramidal side effects
   antiparkinsonian drug treatment, 189
   elderly patients, 114
   switching antipsychotic drugs, 111, 113
Eye movement desensitization and
      reprocessing, 137

Facial expression, 45
   cranial nerve lesions, 57
Factitious disorder, 248–249
Family events, 38
Family history, 38–39
Family therapy, 202, 212
Family tree, 38
Flamboyant clothes, 45
Flight of ideas, 46, 233
Flooding/implosion, 207
Flumazenil, 253
Fluoxetine, 156
   anorexia nervosa, 131
   bulimia nervosa, 131
   elderly patients, 115
   liver disease, 117
   obsessive–compulsive disorder, 135
   panic disorder, 132
   personality disorders, 169, 170
   post-traumatic stress disorder, 137
   withdrawal, 108
Fluvoxamine, 156
   elderly patients, 115
Forensic history, 41
Forensic treatment orders, 279–280
Form of speech, 46
Free association, 209
Frontal lobe impairment
   affect/mood, 46
   concrete thinking, 49

Gabapentin, 114
Gas syndrome, 69
Gene therapy, 200
General Health Questionnaire, 62
General knowledge assessment, 50
General practice (vocational) trainees, 5
Generalized anxiety disorder (GAD), 77–78
   management, 132
Geriatric Depression Scale, 63
Glutethemide overdose, 254
Grandiose delusions, 171
Group psychotherapy, 202, 210, 212
Guardianship order, 278

Haematological values, 60
Hallucinations, 48, 171–172
   assessment, 237
   emergencies, 217, 218, 235–239
   management, 238–239
Hallucinogens overdose, 255–257
Haloperidol
   agitation/paranoid delusion, 240
   alcohol-related paranoia/pathological
      jealousy, 126
   hallucinating patient, 238
   paranoid personality disorder, 166
   rapid tranquillization of manic/
      violent patient, 230, 234
   schizophrenia, 181
   substance withdrawal, 260, 262
Hamilton Rating Scale for Anxiety, 63
Hamilton Rating Scale for Depression,
      3, 151
Hebephrenic schizophrenia, 100
Hepatotoxic drugs, 117
Herbal treatments, 199
High expressed emotion, 173, 175
History of presenting complaint, 36
History taking, 32–43
   assessment room preparation, 33
   background information, 32–33
   emergencies, 217–218
   format, 35–43
   informant history (supplemental
      information), 42–43
   interview, 34–35
   note taking, 34
   personal history, 39–42
   safety, 33

History taking *(contd)*
  sexually disinhibited patient, 34
  social history, 42
  transcultural psychiatry, 67–68
Histrionic personality disorder, 95–96
  assessment, 98
  comorbidity, 92
  management, 168
HIV infection, 58
Holistic treatment approach, 204–205
Homicidal patient, *see* Violent/
      homicidal patient
Homicidal thoughts, 47
Hospital orders, 278, 281–282
Huntington's chorea, 200
Huqa/Hubbly Bubbly, 38
Hyperacusis, 48
Hypericum perforatum (St John's Wort), 199
Hyperventilation, 77, 247
Hypomania, 83–84

Iatrogenic syndromes, 269
ICD-10 classification, 311, 312–314
  depression, 150–151
  personality disorders, 91–92
  schizophrenia, 99–101
Idiosyncratic drug interactions, 113
Illusions, 48, 236
Imipramine
  dependent personality disorder, 170
  nocturnal incontinence, 154
  panic disorder, 132
Impulsive personality disorder, 95
Inappropriate affect, 46
Individual psychotherapy, 202
Informant history (supplemental
      information), 42–43
Inhalants intoxication, 258
Insight assessment, 50
Intelligence assessment, 50
Intelligence disorders, 309–310
Interim hospital order, 278
Interpreter, 68
Interpretive psychotherapy, 208, 209
Interview, 34–35
Intoxication, 46, 249–252
  assessment, 251–252
  management, 252
Investigations

A&E setting, 216
  primary physical, 59, 60, 61–62
  secondary physical, 59–61
Isocarboxazid, 159, 160

Key worker, 30
Khat, 38
Koro syndrome, 69

L-thyroxine, 153
Labile affect, 46
Lactating women, pharmacotherapy,
      115–116
Latah syndrome, 69
Learning disability, 39
Leave arrangements
  detained patients, 14, 20
  trainees, 11
Legal aspects, 272–297
  Canadian legislation, 297
  Eire legislation, 295–296
  electroconvulsive therapy, 193
  emergencies, 216
  mania, 235
  New Zealand legislation, 297
  Northern Ireland legislation, 294–295
  Scottish legislation, 293–294
  USA legislation, 296–297
  violent/homicidal patient, 230
  see also Mental Health Act (1983)
Light therapy (phototherapy), 198–199
Lithium, 141–145
  aggressive behaviour, 231
  antidepressants augmentation, 153
  bipolar affective disorder, 139, 140
  drug interactions, 141–143
  duration of therapy, 144
  elderly patients, 114
  levels in milk, 116
  mania, 235
  nephrotoxicity, 117
  obsessive–compulsive disorder, 135
  pretreatment/maintenance laboratory
      investigations, 143
  side effects, 142, 143
  switching drugs, 111
  therapeutic monitoring, 108, 142, 262–263
  toxicity, 262–263

Liver disease, 117–118
Lofepramine, 154
  elderly patients, 115
Logoclonia, 46
Long-term memory assessment, 49
Lorazepam
  aggressive behaviour, 232
  agitation/paranoid delusion, 240
  alcohol withdrawal, 126, 127
  emergency use, 247
  hallucinogens overdose, 257
  marijuana (cannabis) intoxication, 256
  rapid tranquillization of manic/
    violent patient, 229, 234
  substance withdrawal, 260, 262
  withdrawal management, 138
Lysergic acid diethylamide (LSD), 256

Magnesium sulphate, 127
Major ward rounds, 13
Malingering, 241
Management (mini) ward rounds, 14
Management plan, 59
Mania, 232–235
  acute episode, 139, 140
  affect, 46
  appearance, 45
  assessment, 232–233
  differential diagnosis, 233
  disorders mimicking, 85
  electroconvulsive therapy, 192
  history taking, 36, 38
  legal aspects, 235
  management, 233–235
  presentation, 232
  rating scales, 63
  speech/talk, 45, 46
  violent/homicidal behaviour, 229
  with/without psychotic symptoms, 84
Manic depressive psychosis see Bipolar
    affective disorder
Manic-State Rating Scale, 63
Marijuana (cannabis), 256
Masked (atypical) depression, 91
Medical defence cover, 286
Medical problems, 270
Meditation, 199
Memory assessment, 49
Memory disorders, 309

Mental functioning disorders, 309–310
Mental Health Act (1983), 272
  admission for assessment, 276
  admission for treatment, 276
  assessment of patient, 277–278
  civil sections, 273–277
  civil treatment orders, 274–275
  compulsory treatment, 230, 235
  consent to ECT, 193
  definitions, 272–273
  emergencies management, 215
  emergency admission, 277
  emergency holding powers, 273
  forensic sections, 278–281
  hospital order, 278, 281–282
  interim hospital order, 278
  involuntary admissions, 223
  nurse holding powers, 22, 276
  nurses' roles, 22
  remand for report, 278
  remand for treatment, 278
  restriction order, 281
  section 136, 216
  supervised discharge order, 281
Mental Health Act Commission, 282
Mental Health Act (Northern Ireland)
    Order (1986), 294
Mental Health Review Tribunal, 282–284
Mental Health (Scotland) Act (1984), 294
Mental state examination, 44–51
  abnormal experiences/perceptions, 48
  affect/mood, 46
  appearance/behaviour, 44–45
  cognitive state, 48–51
  history taking, 35
  psychiatric assessment, 43–44
  speech/talk, 45–46
  substance withdrawal, 260
  summary, 50
  thought, 46–48
  violent/homicidal patient, 228
Mental Treatment Act (1945), 295, 296
Meprobamate overdose, 254
Metabolism, 119–120
Methadone, 262
Mini Mental State Examination (MMSE),
    51–53, 63
Mini ward rounds, 14
Mirtazapine, 159
  elderly patients, 115

Mixed affective episode, 90
Mixed anxiety/depressive disorder
    (anxiety–depression), 134
Moclobemide, 163–164
    bulimia nervosa, 131
Modelling, 207
Monoamine oxidase inhibitors (MAOIs),
    159–164
    bulimia nervosa, 131
    dietary advice, 161–163
    elderly patients, 115
    food/drug interactions, 161
    hypertensive crisis, 264–265
    irreversible, 159–163
    phobias, 134
    post-traumatic stress disorder, 137
    reversible, 163–164
    side effects, 160–161
    switching drugs, 109, 110, 160
    withdrawal, 109
Mongomery–Asperger Depression Rating
    Scale, 63, 151
Mood assessment
    bipolar affective disorder, 86
    depression, 87
Mood stabilizers, 141–150
    aggressive behaviour, 231
    bipolar affective disorder, 139, 140, 141
    comparative side effects, 149–150
    dosages, 141
    elderly patients, 114
    mania, 235
    personality disorders, 167
    pretreatment/maintenance laboratory
        investigations, 148
    switching drugs, 111
Morbid jealousy, 229
Movement abnormalities, 45
Multidisciplinary team, 5, 7, 13, 18–20
    art therapist, 24–25
    clinical psychologist, 25–26, 27–28
    day hospital, 15
    emergency clinics, 17–18
    medical staff, 18
    meetings, 19
    non-medical staff, 19
    occupational therapist, 23–24, 27
    psychiatric nursing staff, 20–22, 26–27
    rehabilitation activities, 175
    social workers, 22, 27

    trainees' roles, 19, 26–28
Multiple sclerosis, 58
Munchausen's syndrome, 241, 248–249
Mute/unresponsive patient,
        217, 218, 240–243
    assessment, 241
    management, 241–243

Naloxone, 258
Narcissistic personality disorder, 95, 96
Nefazadone, 164
Nephrotoxic drugs, 117
Neuroimaging, 60
Neuroleptic malignant syndrome,
        113, 242, 266, 267–268, 269
    electroconvulsive therapy, 192
    management, 269
Neuroleptics, see Antipsychotics
Neurological signs/symptoms, 310–311
Neurotransmitters, 119
    drug actions, 120, 121
New Zealand mental health legislation, 297
Nifidipine, 265
Night rounds, 14
Nominated deputies, 272
Noradrenergic and specific serotoninergic
        antidepressants (NaSSA), 158–159
    elderly patients, 115
Northern Ireland mental health
        legislation, 294–295
Nortriptyline, 108
Nursing staff, 20–22, 26–27
    emergency clinics, 17, 18
    emergency holding power, 22, 273
    handovers, 12, 26
    roles, 21–22
    service structure, 21

Obsessions, 47, 81
Obsessive–compulsive disorder, 81–83, 248
    history taking, 34, 44
    management, 135
    personality disorder comorbidity, 92
Obsessive–compulsive personality disorder,
    see Anankastic personality disorder
Occupational record, 40
Occupational therapist, 23–24, 27, 175
Oestrogen therapy, 232

Olanazapine, 166
Olfactory hallucinations, 172
Open-ended questions, 34, 40, 41, 151
Operant conditioning, 206
Opioids
    overdose, 258–259
    withdrawal, 261–262
Organic brain impairment
    hallucinations, 236
    mute/unresponsive patient, 240
    violent/homicidal behaviour, 229
Organizational skills, 10–11
Orientation assessment, 48
Outpatient clinics, 16
    new referrals, 17
Over-the-counter medication, 37
Overseas doctors training scheme
    (ODTS), 6
Overseas trainees, 5–6
Overvalued ideas, 48

Panic disorder, 78–79, 248
    management, 132
Paranoia
    alcohol-related, 125–126
    violent/homicidal behaviour, 228
Paranoid delusions, 171
Paranoid personality disorder, 93
    management, 166
Paranoid schizophrenia, 99
Parapraxes, 209
Parkinsonism
    appearance, 45
    electroconvulsive therapy, 192
Paroxetine, 156
    anorexia nervosa, 131
    elderly patients, 115
    mixed anxiety/depressive disorder
        (anxiety-depression), 134
    obsessive–compulsive disorder, 135
    panic disorder, 132, 248
    personality disorders, 169, 170
    phobias, 134
    post-traumatic stress disorder, 137
    withdrawal, 108
Part I clinical summary, 63, 64–65
Part II clinical summary, 64, 66–67
Passivity of thoughts, 47, 171
Past medical history, 36

Past psychiatric history, 36
Pathological jealousy
    alcohol-related, 125–126
    violent/homicidal behaviour, 228
Patient advocate, 28
Patient data in history taking, 35
Perception disorders, 307–308
Perceptual distortions, 236
Performance anxiety, 133
Perpetuating factors, 58, 59
Persecutory delusions, 171
Personal history, 39–42
    adolescence, 40
    birth/development, 39
    childhood, 39–40
    education, 40
    forensic history, 41
    occupational record, 40
    premorbid personality, 42
    psychosexual history, 40–41
Personality Assessment Schedule, 63
Personality disorders, 91–99
    assessment, 97–98
    classification systems, 91–92
    comorbidity, 165
    management, 165–170
    psychosocial treatments, 166
    rating scales, 63
Personality traits, 91
Pharmacodynamics, 118–119
Pharmacokinetics, 119–120
Pharmacology, 118
Pharmacotherapy, 106–200
    children, 116
    discharge planning, 29
    drug interactions, 113
    elderly patients, 114–115
    liver disease, 117–118
    mode of action, 107
    pregnant/lactating women, 115–116
    renal impairment, 117
    review, 107–108
    switching drugs, 109–110
    withdrawal, 108–109
Phencyclidine (PCP; angel dust), 257
Phenelzine, 159, 160
    bulimia nervosa, 131
    phobias, 133
    post-traumatic stress disorder, 137
Phenobarbitone

Phenobarbitone *(contd)*
  elderly patients, 114
  overdose, 254
Phenothiazines, 118
Phentolamine, 265
Phenytoin
  aggressive behaviour, 232
  therapeutic monitoring, 108
Phobias, 47
  management, 133–134
Phototherapy (light therapy), 198–199
Physical examination, 54–58
  cranial nerves assessment, 56–58
  emergencies, 216, 218
  implications of findings, 54–55
Police
  detentions under section 136,
    227, 232, 286
  emergencies management, 216
Polio, 57
Post-traumatic stress disorder, 79–81
  management, 136–137
Posture, 45
Precipitating factors, 58, 59
Predisposing factors, 58, 59
Pregnant women, pharmacotherapy
    115–116
Premorbid personality, 42
Preoccupations/worries, 47
Prescribing, 106
Present State Examination, 62
Primary delusions, 171
Primidone, 232
Prioritizing, 11
Procyclidine, 242, 265
  elderly patients, 114
Propranolol
  aggressive behaviour, 232
  social phobia, 133
Pseudobulbar pathology, 46
Pseudohallucinations, 236
Psychiatric report, 287–292
Psychiatric services, 15–16
Psychoanalysis, 210
Psychodynamic psychotherapy, 209
Psychological tests, 60–61
Psychological treatments, 202–212
  alcohol-related addiction/
    dependence disorders, 211–212
Psychologist, 25–26, 27–28

assessment skills, 25
  treatment programmes, 26
Psychopathic disorder, 273
Psychosexual history taking, 34, 40–41
Psychosis
  acute emergencies, 217
  clarification of symptoms, 170–171
  hallucinations, 236
  management, 170–173
  medical aetiology, 172
  psychiatric diagnostic categories,
    172–173
  psychomotor retardation, 241, 242
  psychosocial/cultural issues, 173
  treatment, 173
  violent/homicidal behaviour, 229
Psychosocial issues, psychotic symptoms
    assessment, 173
Psychosocial treatments
  acute transient psychotic disorder/
    brief reactive psychosis, 174
  anxiety, 247
  borderline personality disorder, 167–168
  delusional disorders, 174
  depression, 152
  holistic approach, 204–205
  NHS services, 211
  patient selection, 202–203, 211
  personality disorders,
    166, 167–168, 169, 170
  schizophrenia, 175
Psychostimulant overdose, 254–255
Psychosurgery, 197–198
Psychotherapy, *see* Psychosocial treatments
Psychotic depression, 173
Puerperal depression/psychosis, 192

Quality of speech, 46
Questions in history taking, 34

Rapid tranquillization
  manic patient, 234–235
  violent patient, 229–230
Rapidly cycling bipolar affective disorder,
    147, 235
Rapport, 45
Rate of speech, 45
Rating Scale for Mania, 63

Rating scales, 62–63
Rational emotive therapy, 205
Reason for Living Inventory, 63
Receptors, drug actions, 120, 121
Records
    clerking patients, 12, 13
    emergencies, 215
    violent/homicidal behaviour, 230–231
    see also Psychiatric report
Recurrent brief depressive disorder, 90
Referral
    background information gathering,
        32–33
    source, 35
Refractory epilepsy, 192
Rehabilitation in schizophrenia, 175
Rehearsal, 137
Remand for report, 278
Remand for treatment, 278
Renal impairment, 117
Repetitive transcranial magnetic
        stimulation, 199–200
Residual schizophrenia, 100
Responsible medical officer, 4
Restraint, 234
Restricted affect, 46
Restriction order, 281
Reversible inhibitors of monoamine
        oxidase A (RIMAs), 163–164
Risk assessment/management, 30, 219–220
Risperidone
    liver disease, 118
    paranoid personality disorder, 166

Safety
    history taking environment, 33
    violent/homicidal patient
        assessment, 227
Scale for the Assessment of Negative
        Symptoms, 63
Scale for the Assessment of Positive
        Symptoms, 63
Schedule for Affective Disorders and
        Schizophrenia, 62
Schizoaffective disorder, 173
Schizoid personality disorder, 93–94
    assessment, 98
    management, 167
Schizophrenia, 99–103, 170

affect, 46
appearance, 45
auditory hallucinations, 48
Bleuler's four As, 102
catatonic, 241, 242
delusions, 48
drug treatment, 175–176, 177–179,
        180–182
electroconvulsive therapy, 178, 191
hallucinations, 236
history taking, 34, 35, 36, 38, 39, 40, 41
ICD-10 diagnostic categories, 99–100
management, 174–191
prognostic factors, 102–103
psychosocial interventions, 175
psychotic symptoms, 170, 171, 172, 173
rating scales, 63
schneiderian first-rank symptoms,
        47, 101
speech/talk, 45, 46
thought disorders, 47
treatment resistance, 176, 178
Schizotypal disorder, 94, 173
Schneiderian first-rank symptoms, 47, 48
    bipolar affective disorder, 84
    manic patients, 233
    schizophrenia, 101, 171, 172
Scottish mental health legislation, 293–294
Scottish Mental Welfare Commission, 294
Seasonal affective disorder (SAD)/
        seasonal mood disorder, 91
    light therapy, 198
Seclusion policy, 12
Security arrangements, 12
Seizures
    alcohol withdrawal, 128
    antipsychotics-induced, 123
Selective serotonin reuptake inhibitors
        (SSRIs), 156–157
    aggressive behaviour, 232
    alcohol-related depression, 124
    anankastic personality disorder, 169
    anorexia nervosa, 131
    bulimia nervosa, 131
    drug interactions, 157
    generalized anxiety disorder, 132
    mixed anxiety/depressive disorder
        (anxiety–depression), 134
    obsessive–compulsive disorder,
        82, 83, 135

Selective serotonin reuptake inhibitors (SSRIs) *(contd)*
panic disorder, 132, 248
phobias, 134
post-traumatic stress disorder, 137
side effects, 158
switching drugs, 109, 110, 160
withdrawal, 108–109
Selegiline, 178
Self-awareness disorders, 48
Self-neglect, 30, 45
Self-referrals, 17, 18, 25
Sensory deceptions, 48
Sensory distortions, 48, 236
Serotonin syndrome, 264, 269
Serotonin-noradrenergic reuptake inhibitors (SNRIs), 158
elderly patients, 115
Sertraline, 156
elderly patients, 115
Services, psychiatric, 15–16
Sexual abuse, 39, 41
Sexually disinhibited patient, 34
Shinkeishitsu syndrome, 70
Short-term memory assessment, 49
Simple phobia, 133
Simple schizophrenia, 100
Sleep deprivation treatment, 199
Smokers, 38, 56
Social history, 42
Social phobia, 133
Social workers, 17, 18, 22, 27, 175
Sodium valproate, 147–150
aggressive behaviour, 231
drug interactions, 147–148
elderly patients, 114
mania, 235
side effects, 148–150
switching to carbamazepine, 111
Somatic delusions, 171
Somatic (vegetative/biological) symptoms, 88
Somatization, 92
Specialist training, 3
Specialization in psychiatry, 2
Speech assessment
bipolar affective disorder (manic depressive psychosis), 86
mania, 233
mental state examination, 45–46

Speech disorders, 301–303
psychosis, 172
Stroke, 57
Structured Interview for DSM-III-R Personality Disorders, 63
Subspecialties, 3
Substance abuse
appearance, 45
hallucinations, 236
history taking, 38, 41
personality disorder comorbidity, 92, 165
physical examination, 56
violent/homicidal behaviour, 228
Substance withdrawal, 259–262
Suicidal intent evaluation, 63, 222
Suicidal Intent Scale, 63
Suicidal patient, 217, 218, 220–226
admission criteria, 223–224, 226
cocaine/amphetamine withdrawal, 262
common presentations, 221
interview, 224–225
management, 223
repeated attempts, 225–226
risk factors, 221–222
supervision, 225
Suicidal thoughts, 47
Suicide
epidemiology, 220, 221
family history recording, 39
procedures following, 226
Sulpiride, 111
Supervised discharge order, 281
Supervision register, 30, 175
Supervision of training, 4, 7
Supportive psychotherapy, 203, 208, 212
schizophrenia, 175
Susto, 70
Suxamethonium sensitivity, 113
Syphilis, 58
Systematic desensitization, 207

Tactile hallucinations, 172
Talking down, 234
Temazepam withdrawal management, 138
Testamentary capacity, 285, 286
Tetracyclic antidepressants, 154
Therapeutic alliance, 209
Therapeutic communities, 211
Therapeutic monitoring, 108

Therapeutic monitoring *(contd)*
anticonvulsants, 148
lithium, 144
Therapeutic window, 108
Thiamine therapy, 125, 127, 129, 253
Thioridazine
anxiety, 248
paranoid personality disorder, 166
Thought assessment
bipolar affective disorder
(manic depressive psychosis), 86
mental state examination, 46–48
Thought broadcasting, 47
Thought disorder
history taking, 34, 44
psychosis, 172
Thought echo, 47
Thought insertion, 47
Thought withdrawal, 47
Thyrotoxicosis, 45, 55, 56
Time management, 10
Token economy, 207
Tradazone, 164
Training, 2
basic, 2
higher, 3
supervision, 4, 7
Training posts, 7–8
clinical duties, 8–10
Transcranial magnetic stimulation, 199–200
Transcultural psychiatry, 67–70
culture-bound syndromes, 69–70
history taking, 67–68
psychotic symptoms assessment, 173
Transference, 209
Transient psychotic disorder, acute, 174
Tranylcypromine, 159, 160
Trauma story, 137
Tricyclic antidepressants, 154
anorexia nervosa, 131
bulimia nervosa, 131
contraindications, 155
depression, 154–156
elderly patients, 115
generalized anxiety disorder, 132
liver disease, 117
obsessive–compulsive disorder, 135
post-traumatic stress disorder, 137

side effects, 156
switching drugs, 109, 110, 160
withdrawal, 109
Trigeminal neuralgia, 57

Unipolar depression, 87–88, 90
Unresponsive patient, 240–243
Urine tests, 59
USA mental health legislation, 296–297

Vegetative (somatic/biological)
symptoms, 88
Vigabatrin, 114
Violent/homicidal patient,
30, 217, 218, 226–232
assessment, 227–228
behavioural management, 229
diagnosis, 228–229
documentation, 230–231
drug treatment, 226, 229–230, 231–232
history taking environment, 33
legal aspects, 230
mental state examination, 44
presentations, 227
risk assessment/management, 219–220
risk factors, 226, 227
signs of impending violence, 227, 228
Visual hallucinations, 172, 238

Ward rounds, 13–14
Ward work, 11–12
Weight loss, 45
Wernicke–Korsakoff syndrome, 124–125
Wernicke's encephalopathy, 57, 129
Windigo syndrome, 70
Withdrawal states
psychotropic drugs, 108–109
violent/homicidal behaviour, 228
Working through, 209

Yoga, 199

Zuclopenthixol acetate, 230, 235